OTHER PMIC TITLES OF INTEREST

MW00658162

CODING AND REIMBURSEMENT

Coding Guides by Medical Specialty
Collections Made Easy!
CPT Plus!
DRG Plus!
E/M Coding Made Easy!
HCPCS Coders Choice®
Health Insurance Directory
HIPAA Compliance Manual
ICD-9-CM, Coders Choice®
ICD-9-CM Coding for Physicians Offices
ICD-9-CM Coding Made Easy!
ICD-9-CM Home Health Edition
Medical Procedure Coding Made Easy!
Medicare Compliance for Physicians
Medical Fees in the United States
Medicare Rules & Regulations
Reimbursement Manual for the Medical Office
The Coder's Handbook
Working with Insurance and Managed Care Plans

PRACTICE MANAGEMENT

Accounts Receivable Management for the Medical Practice
Achieving Profitability with a Medical Office System
Encyclopedia of Practice and Financial Management
Managed Care Organizations
Managing Medical Office Personnel
Marketing Healthcare
Marketing Strategies for Physicians
Medical Marketing Handbook
Medical Practice Forms
Medical Practice Handbook
Medical Staff Privileges
Negotiating Managed Care Contracts
Patient Satisfaction
Performance Standards for the Laboratory
Professional and Practice Development
Starting in Medical Practice

**PMIC Titles are Available From Your Local Medical Book Store,
Online at PmicOnline.com or by Phone at 1-800-633-7467**

OTHER PMIC TITLES OF INTEREST

FINANCIAL MANAGEMENT

A Physician's Guide to Financial Independence
Business Ventures for Physicians
Encyclopedia of Practice and Financial Management
Financial Valuation of Your Practice
Personal Money Management for Physicians
Personal Pension Plan Strategies for Physicians
Securing Your Assets
Selling or Buying a Medical Practice

RISK MANAGEMENT

Malpractice Depositions
Malpractice: Managing Your Defense
Medical Risk Management
Preparing for Your Deposition
Preventing Emergency Malpractice
Testifying in Court

DICTIONARIES AND OTHER REFERENCE

Drugs of Abuse
Health and Medicine on the Internet
Medical Acronyms, Abbreviations and Eponyms
Medical Phrase Index
Medical Word Building
Medico Mnemonica
Medico-Legal Glossary
Spanish/English Handbook for Medical Professionals

MEDICAL REFERENCE AND CLINICAL

Advance Medical Directives
Clinical Research Opportunities
Manual of IV Therapy
Medical Procedures for Referral
Patient Care Emergency Handbook
Patient Care Flowchart Manual
Pulmonary Medicine: Problems in Primary Care
Patient Care Procedures for Your Practice
Questions and Answers on AIDS

**PMIC Titles are Available From Your Local Medical Book Store,
Online at PmicOnline.com or by Phone at 1-800-633-7467**

Introduction To The

ICD•10

Coding System

A Comprehensive Guide to ICD•10•CM and ICD•10•PCS For Health Care Professionals

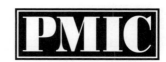

ISBN: 978-1-57066-532-5

Practice Management Information Corporation (PMIC)
4727 Wilshire Boulevard
Los Angeles, California 90010
http://www.pmiconline.com

Printed in the United States of America

FOREWORD

On September 30, 2013 you will file your health insurance claims using ICD-9-CM diagnosis codes. On the very next day, October 1, 2013, you must file your health insurance claims using ICD-10-CM codes.

Unlike the annual revisions of an existing code set, for example ICD-9 2012 replacing ICD-9 2011 on October 1, 2011, this is not a revision, but a complete replacement of an entire code set. The ICD-10 code set is different from the ICD-9 code set in format and the number of possible digits, and also has many more codes to choose from. The draft ICD-10-CM code set includes 69,370 codes excluding the potential for placeholders and 7th digits. The draft ICD-10-PCS code set includes 72,083 codes. That's a total of 141,453 (even more with 7th digits and placeholders) codes in the ICD-10 system compared to 22,202 codes in the ICD-9 coding system.

The transition will require business and systems changes throughout the health care industry. Everyone who is covered by the Health Insurance Portability and Accountability Act (HIPAA) must make the transition, not just those who submit Medicare or Medicaid claims.

DISCLAIMER

This publication is designed to offer basic information regarding the ICD-10 coding system. The information presented is based upon extensive review of existing literature and the experience and interpretations of the author. Though all of the information has been carefully researched and checked for accuracy and completeness, neither the authors nor the publisher accepts any responsibility or liability with regard to errors, omissions, misuse or misinterpretation.

CONTENTS

ICD-10-PCS PROCEDURES IN THE MEDICAL AND SURGICAL SECTION 277

ICD-10-PCS PROCEDURES IN THE MEDICAL AND SURGICAL-RELATED SECTIONS 309

PROCEDURES IN THE ANCILLARY SECTIONS 326

TERMINOLOGY

Acute Conditions – The medical conditions characterized by sudden onset, severe change, and/or short duration.

Additional Diagnosis – The secondary diagnosis code used, if available, to provide a more complete picture of the primary diagnosis..

Alteration -- Modifying the anatomic structure of a body part without affecting the function of the body part

Applied mapping – Distillation of a reference mapping to conform to the needs of a particular application (e.g., data quality, research).

Approach (5th character) – Defines the technique used to reach the site of the procedure.

Backward mapping – mapping that proceeds from a newer code set to an older code set, for example from ICD-10-CM to ICD-9-CM.

Bilateral – For bilateral sites, the final character of the codes in the ICD-10-CM indicates laterality. An unspecified side code is also provided should the side not be identified in the medical record. If no bilateral code is provided and the condition is bilateral, assign separate codes for both the left and right side.

Body Part or Region (4th character) – Defines the specific anatomical site where the procedure is performed.

Body System (2nd character) – Defines the general physiological system on which the procedure is performed or anatomical region where the procedure is performed.

Bypass -- Altering the route of passage of the contents of a tubular body part.

Category – The three-digit diagnosis code classifications that broadly define each condition (e.g., 250 for diabetes mellitus).

Centers for Disease Control and Prevention (CDC) – A federal health data organization that helps maintain several code sets included in the HIPAA standards, including the ICD-9-CM codes. A division of the Department of Health and Human Services responsible for monitoring, researching and developing public health policies for the prevention of disease, injury and disability and the promotion of healthy behaviors. The National Center for Health Statistics is the part of the CDC that maintains health related statistics including the coordination with World Health Organization (WHO) on use of International Classification of Diseases (ICD) in North America.

Centers for Medicare & Medicaid Services (CMS) – The federal agency that runs the Medicare program. In addition, CMS works with the States to run the Medicaid program. CMS works to make sure that the beneficiaries in these programs are able to get high quality healthcare.

Change -- Taking out or off a device from a body part and putting back an identical or similar device in or on the same body part without cutting or puncturing the skin or a mucous membrane

Character – One of the seven components that comprise an ICD-10-PCS procedure code.

Chronic Conditions – Medical conditions characterized by long duration, frequent recurrence over a long period of time, and/or slow progression over time.

Cluster – in a combination entry, one instance where a code is chosen from each of the choice lists in the target system entry, that when combined satisfies the equivalent meaning of the corresponding code in the source system

Combination Codes – A single code used to classify any of the following: two diagnoses; a diagnosis with an associated secondary process (manifestation); or a diagnosis with an associated complication.

Control -- Stopping, or attempting to stop, postprocedural bleeding.

Conventions of ICD-10 – The general rules for use of the classification independent of guidelines. These conventions are incorporated within the Index and Tabular of the ICD-10-CM as instructional notes.

Creation -- Making a new genital structure that does not take over the function of a body part.

Crosswalk/mapping – A new test is determined to be similar to an existing test, multiple existing test codes, or a portion of an existing test code. The new test code is then assigned to the related existing local fee schedule amounts and resulting national limitation amount. In some instances, a test may only equate to a portion of a test, and, in those instances, payment at an appropriate percentage of the payment for the existing test is assigned.

Current Procedural Terminology (CPT) Codes – This is the procedural coding system that is currently used in America primarily to report physician professional services. Frequently called "CPT", the Current Procedural Terminology, is a code set, developed in 1966 and maintained by the American Medical Association (AMA), used to describe what healthcare professional services were provided or utilized by healthcare professionals. CPT codes are also known as "Level I" codes. Additional codes to describe use of healthcare facilities and services provided by healthcare professionals are known as "Level II" or "Healthcare Common Procedure Coding System" (HCPCS). Level II codes were developed are maintained by CMS.

Destruction -- Physical eradication of all or a portion of a body part by the direct use of energy, force or a destructive agent.

Detachment -- Cutting off all or a portion of the upper or lower extremities.

Dilation -- Expanding an orifice or the lumen of a tubular body part.

Division -- Cutting into a body part without draining fluids and/or gases from the body part in order to separate or transect a body part.

Drainage -- Taking or letting out fluids and/or gases from a body part.

Excision -- Cutting out or off, without replacement, a portion of a body part.

External (approach) -- Procedures performed directly on the skin or mucous membrane and procedures performed indirectly by the application of external force through the skin or mucous membrane.

Extirpation -- Taking or cutting out solid matter from a body part.

Extraction -- Pulling or stripping out or off all or a portion of a body part by the use of force.

Federal Register – The "Federal Register" is the official daily publication for rules, proposed rules and notices of federal agencies and organizations, as well as Executive Orders and other Presidential documents.

Forward mapping – mapping that proceeds from an older code set to a newer code set, for example from ICD-9-CM Volume 3 to ICD-10-PCS.

Fragmentation -- Breaking solid matter in a body part into pieces.

Fusion -- Joining together portions of an articular body part rendering the articular body part immobile.

GEMs - This reference mapping attempts to include all valid relationships between the codes in the ICD-9-CM diagnosis classification and the ICD-10-CM diagnosis classification.

General Equivalence Map (GEM) – reference mapping that attempts to include all valid relationships between the codes in the ICD-9- CM diagnosis classification and the ICD-10-CM diagnosis classification

Health Insurance Portability & Accountability Act (HIPAA) – A law passed in 1996 which is also sometimes called the "Kassebaum-Kennedy" law. This law expands healthcare coverage for patients who have lost or changed jobs, or have pre-existing conditions. HIPAA does not replace the states' roles as primary regulators of insurance. The HIPAA legislation has the following broad goals, to provide: 1) a way to uniquely identify providers, employers and health plans, 2) a uniform level of protection of health information, known as the "Security Rule," 3) a uniform level of protection of the privacy of health data associated with patients, known as the "Privacy Rule" and 4) a simpler healthcare electronic transaction process by describing standards by which all healthcare administrative entities would use, which is known as the "Transactions and Code Sets Rule".

Healthcare Common Procedure Coding System (HCPCS) – A medical code set that identifies healthcare procedures, equipment, and supplies for claim submission purposes. It has been selected for use in the HIPAA transactions. HCPCS Level I contains numeric CPT codes which are maintained by the AMA. HCPCS Level II contains alphanumeric codes used to identify various items and services that are not included in the CPT medical code set. These are maintained by Health Care Financing Administration (HCFA), Blue Cross and Blue Shield Association (BCBSA), and the Health Insurance Association of America (HIAA). HCPCS Level III contains alphanumeric codes that are assigned by Medicaid state agencies to identify additional items and services not included in levels I or II. These are usually called "local codes", and must have "W", "X", "Y", or "Z" in the first position. HCPCS Procedure Modifier Codes can be used with all three levels, with the WA - ZY range used for locally assigned procedure modifiers.

HIPAA 4010 – The original healthcare transactions version of HIPAA (officially known as Version 004010 of the ASC X12 transaction implementation guides) named as part of HIPAA's Electronic Transaction Standards regulation. Version 4010 was required to be used by HIPAA covered healthcare entities by Oct. 16, 2003.

HIPAA 5010 – Required by Jan. 1, 2012 to be the new version of the HIPAA healthcare transactions. Officially known as Version 005010 of the ASC X12 transaction Technical Report Type 3. This new version was required as a result of Department of Health and Human Services (HHS) final rules published on Jan. 6, 2009.

ICD-10 – The mortality and morbidity classification coding system implemented by WHO in 1993 to replace ICD-9.

ICD-10-CM – The updated version of the clinical modification coding set defined by the National Center for Health Statistics that will replace ICD-9-CM on Oct. 1, 2013.

ICD-10-PCS – The updated procedural coding system defined by CMS that will replace Volume 3 of ICD-9-CM for hospital inpatient services.

ICD-9 – The mortality and morbidity classification coding system that is currently used throughout most of the world, including the United States. The ICD-9 classification of death and disease is based a series of classifications systems first adopted in 1893.

ICD-9-CM – The "clinical modification" to the ICD-9 code set that is currently used in America to report medical diagnoses. The "Clinical Modification" refers to the base WHO defined ICD-9 code set that has been defined for use in United State by the National Center for Health Statistics (NCHS) division of the Centers for Disease Control (CDC).

ICD-9-PCS – The procedural coding system currently used in America primarily for hospital inpatient services. It is contained in Volume 3 of ICD-9-CM.

Index (to diseases) – The ICD-10-CM is divided into the Alphabetic Index, an alphabetical list of terms and their corresponding code, and the Tabular List, a chronological list of codes divided into chapters based on body system or condition. The Alphabetic Index consists of the following parts: the Index of Diseases and Injury, the Index of External Causes of Injury, the Table of Neoplasms and the Table of Drugs and Chemicals.

Insertion -- Putting in a nonbiological device that monitors, assists, performs or prevents a physiological function but does not physically take the place of a body part.

Inspection -- Visually and/or manually exploring a body part.

International Classification of Diseases (ICD) – A medical code set maintained by the World Health Organization (WHO). The primary purpose of this code set is to classify both causes of death or mortality and diseases or morbidity. A U.S. extension, known as ICD-CM, "Clinical Modification," is maintained by the NCHS within the CDC to more precisely define ICD use in the U.S.

Manifestation Codes – Certain conditions have both an underlying etiology and multiple body system manifestations due to the underlying etiology. For such conditions, the ICD-10-CM has a coding convention that requires the underlying condition be sequenced first followed by the manifestation. Wherever such a combination exists, there is a "use additional code" note at the etiology code, and a "code first" note at the manifestation code. These instructional notes indicate the proper sequencing order of the codes, etiology followed by manifestation.

Map -- Locating the route of passage of electrical impulses and/or locating functional areas in a body part.

Medical Necessity – Services or supplies that: are proper and needed for the diagnosis or treatment of a medical condition; are provided for the diagnosis, direct care, and treatment of a medical condition; meet the standards of good medical practice in the local area; and are not mainly for the convenience of the patient or doctor.

Morbidity – Term refers to the disease rate or number of cases of a particular disease in a given age range, gender, occupation, or other relevant population based grouping.

Mortality –Term refers to the death rate reflected by the population in a given region, age range, or other relevant statistical grouping

National Center for Health Statistics (NCHS) – A federal organization within the CDC that collects, analyzes, and distributes healthcare statistics. The NCHS helps maintain the ICD-CM codes.

No Map Flag – attribute in a GEM that when turned on indicates that a code in the source system is not linked to any code in the target system .

Occlusion -- Completely closing an orifice or the lumen of a tubular body part.

Open (approach) -- Cutting through the skin or mucous membrane and any other body layers necessary to expose the site of the procedure.

Percutaneous (approach) -- Entry, by puncture or minor incision, of instrumentation through the skin or mucous membrane and any other body layers necessary to reach the site of the procedure.

Percutaneous Endoscopic (approach) -- Entry, by puncture or minor incision, of instrumentation through the skin or mucous membrane and any other body layers necessary to reach and visualize the site of the procedure.

Principle Diagnosis – First-listed/primary diagnosis code. The code sequenced first on a medical record defines the primary reason for the encounter as determined at the end of the encounter.
Procedure – The complete specification of the ICD-10-PCS seven characters.

Reattachment -- Putting back in or on all or a portion of a separated body part to its normal location or other suitable location.

Release -- Freeing a body part from an abnormal physical constraint by cutting or by use of force.

Removal -- Taking out or off a device from a body part.

Repair -- Restoring, to the extent possible, a body part to its normal anatomic structure and function.

Replacement -- Putting in or on biological or synthetic material that physically takes the place and/or function of all or a portion of a body part.

Reposition -- Moving to its normal location, or other suitable location, all or a portion of a body part.

Resection -- Cutting out or off, without replacement, all of a body part.

Restriction -- Partially closing an orifice or the lumen of a tubular body part.

Reverse lookup – using a GEM by looking up a target system code to see all the codes in the source system that translate to it.

Revision -- Correcting, to the extent possible, a portion of a malfunctioning device or the position of a displaced device.

Root Operation/Type (3rd character) – Defines the objective of the procedure.

Section (1st character) – Defines the general type of procedure.

Sequelae – A late effect is the residual effect (condition produced) after the acute phase of an illness or injury has terminated. There is no time limit on when a late effect code can be used. The residual may be apparent early, such as in cerebral infarction, or it may occur months or years later, such as that due to a previous injury.

Signs/Symptoms – Codes that describe symptoms and signs, as opposed to diagnoses, are acceptable for reporting purposes when a related definitive diagnosis has not been established (confirmed) by the provider.

Source system -- code set of origin in the mapping; the set being mapped 'from'

Supplement -- Putting in or on biological or synthetic material that physically reinforces and/or augments the function of a portion of a body part

Tabular List – It is essential to use both the Alphabetic Index and Tabular List when locating and assigning a code. The Alphabetic Index does not always provide the full code. Selection of the full code, including laterality and any applicable 7th character can only be done in the Tabular List. A dash (-) at the end of an Alphabetic Index entry indicates that additional characters are required. Even if a dash is not included at the Alphabetic Index entry, it is necessary to refer to the Tabular List to verify that no 7th character is required.

Target system – destination code set in the mapping; the set being mapped 'to'.

Transfer -- Moving, without taking out, all or a portion of a body part to another location to take over the function of all or a portion of a body part.

Transplantation -- Putting in or on all or a portion of a living body part taken from another individual or animal to physically take the place and/or function of all or a portion of a similar body part.

Uniform Hospital Discharge Data Set (UHDDS) – The UHDDS definitions are used by hospitals to report inpatient data elements in a standardized manner. These data elements and their definitions can be found in the July 31, 1985, Federal Register (Vol. 50, No, 147), pp. 31038-40.

Value – Individual units defined for each character of ICD-10-PCS and represented by a number or letter.

Via Natural or Artificial Opening (approach) -- Entry of instrumentation through a natural or artificial external opening to reach the site of the procedure.

Via Natural or Artificial Opening Endoscopic (approach) -- Entry of instrumentation through a natural or artificial external opening to reach and visualize the site of the procedure.

Via Natural or Artificial Opening With Percutaneous Endoscopic Assistance (approach) -- Entry of instrumentation through a natural or artificial external opening and entry, by puncture or minor incision, of instrumentation through the skin or mucous membrane and any other body layers necessary to aid in the performance of the procedure.

Volume I – The detailed, tabular list of diagnosis codes in the ICD-9-CM manual.

Volume II – The alphabetical index to diseases in the ICD-9-CM diagnosis coding manual.

Volume III – The ICD-9/ICD-10 list of procedure codes, used in inpatient settings.

World Health Organization (WHO) – An organization that maintains the International Classification of Diseases (ICD) medical code set.

INTRODUCTION

On October 1, 2013, the most significant change in medical coding requirements since the 1992 replacement of CPT visit codes with E & M codes will take place. On that date ICD-10 replaces ICD-9 as the mandated diagnosis coding system in the United States. All health insurance claims processed on or after October 1, 2013 must include ICD-10 codes. This change will have a tremendous impact on the health care industry.

- All health care providers must use ICD-10 instead of ICD-9 for new claims.
- All computer software that provides for storage of diagnosis codes must be revised to accommodate the additional digits of ICD-10 and maintain ICD-9 codes for previously filed claims.
- The conversion and implementation costs will be in the billions of dollars.

HISTORY OF THE INTERNATIONAL CLASSIFICATION OF DISEASES

For students of medical nomenclature and coding systems, the following history of the International Classification of Diseases excerpted from Wikipedia may be interesting.

HISTORICAL SYNOPSIS

In 1893, a French physician, Jacques Bertillon, introduced the *Bertillon Classification of Causes of Death* at a congress of the International Statistical Institute in Chicago. A number of countries and cities adopted Dr. Bertillon's system, which was based on the principle of distinguishing between general diseases and those localized to a particular organ or anatomical site, as used by the City of Paris for classifying deaths. Subsequent revisions represented a synthesis of English, German and Swiss classifications, expanding from the original 44 titles to 161 titles. In 1898, the American Public Health Association (APHA) recommended that the registrars of Canada, Mexico, and the United States also adopt it. The APHA also recommended revising the system every ten years to ensure the system remained current with medical practice advances. As a result, the first international conference to revise the International Classification of Causes of Death convened in 1900; with revisions occurring every ten years thereafter. At that time the classification system was contained in one book, which included an Alphabetic Index as well as a Tabular List. The book was small compared with current coding texts.

The revisions that followed contained minor changes, until the sixth revision of the classification system. With the sixth revision, the classification system expanded to two volumes. The sixth revision included morbidity and mortality conditions, and its title was modified to reflect the changes: *International Statistical Classification of Diseases, Injuries and Causes of Death (ICD).* Prior to the sixth revision, responsibility for ICD revisions fell to the Mixed Commission, a group composed of representatives from the International Statistical Institute and the Health Organization of the League of Nations. In 1948, the World Health Organization (WHO) assumed responsibility for preparing and publishing the revisions to the ICD every ten years. WHO sponsored the seventh and eighth revisions in 1957 and 1968, respectively. It later become clear that the established ten-year interval between revisions was too short.

The ICD is currently the most widely used statistical classification system for diseases in the world. International health statistics using this system are available at the WHO Statistical Information System (WHOSIS).

In addition, some countries—including Australia, Canada and the United States—have developed their own adaptations of ICD, with more procedure for classification of operative or diagnostic procedures.

HISTORY AND USAGE IN THE UNITED STATES

In the United States, the U.S. Public Health Service published *The International Classification of Diseases, Adapted for Indexing of Hospital Records and Operation Classification (ICDA)*, completed in 1962 and expanding the ICD-7 in a number of areas to more completely meet the indexing needs of hospitals. The U.S. Public Health Service later published the *Eighth Revision, International Classification of Diseases, Adapted for Use in the United States*, commonly referred to as ICDA-8, for official national morbidity and mortality statistics. This was followed by the *ICD, 9th Revision, Clinical Modification*, known as ICD-9-CM, published by the U.S. Department of Health and Human Services and used by hospitals and other healthcare facilities to better describe the clinical picture of the patient. The diagnosis component of ICD-9-CM is completely consistent with ICD-9 codes, and remains the data standard for reporting morbidity. National adaptations of the ICD-10 progressed to incorporate both clinical code (ICD-10-CM) and procedure code (ICD-10-PCS) with the revisions completed in 2003. In 2009, the U.S. Centers for Medicare and Medicaid Services announced that it would begin using ICD-10 on April 1, 2010, with full compliance by all involved parties by 2013.

BRIEF HISTORY OF ICD-10

ICD-10 was first published by the World Health Organization (WHO) in 1992. The National Center for Health Statistics (NCHS), the Federal agency responsible for use of the International Statistical Classification of Diseases and Related Health Problems, 10th revision (ICD-10) in the United States, has developed a clinical modification of the classification for morbidity purposes. The ICD-10 is used to code and classify mortality data from death certificates, having replaced ICD-9 for this purpose as of January 1, 1999. ICD-10-CM is planned as the replacement for ICD-9-CM, volumes 1 and 2. ICD-10-PCS is the replacement for ICD-9-CM volume 3, Procedures.

ICD-10-CM was developed following a thorough evaluation by a Technical Advisory Panel and extensive additional consultation with physician groups, clinical coders, and others to assure clinical accuracy and utility. Notable improvements in the content and format include: the addition of information relevant to ambulatory and managed care encounters; expanded injury codes; the creation of combination diagnosis/symptom codes to reduce the number of codes needed to fully describe a condition; the addition of a sixth character; incorporation of common 4th and 5th digit subclassifications; laterality; and greater specificity in code assignment. The new structure will allow further expansion than was possible with ICD-9-CM.

ICD-10 IS THE CHRONOLOGICAL SUCCESSOR TO ICD-9

The new classification system provides significant improvements through greater detailed information and the ability to expand in order to capture additional advancements in clinical medicine. ICD-10 consists of two different code sets:

- **ICD-10-CM** – The diagnosis classification system developed by the Centers for Disease Control and Prevention for use in all U.S. health care treatment settings. Diagnosis coding under this system uses 3–7 alpha and numeric digits and full code titles, but the format is very much the same as ICD-9-CM; and

- **ICD-10-PCS** – The procedure classification system developed by the Centers for Medicare & Medicaid Services (CMS) for use in the U.S. for inpatient hospital settings only. The new procedure coding system uses 7 alpha or numeric digits while the ICD-9-CM coding system uses 3 or 4 numeric digits.

The current system, International Classification of Diseases, 9th Edition, Clinical Modification (ICD-9-CM), does not provide the necessary detail for patients' medical conditions or the procedures and services performed on hospitalized patients. ICD-9-CM is 30 years old, has outdated and obsolete terminology, uses outdated codes that produce inaccurate and limited data, and is inconsistent with current medical practice. It cannot accurately describe the diagnoses and inpatient procedures of care delivered in the 21st century.

ICD-10 BASICS FOR MEDICAL PRACTICES

Begin preparing now for the ICD-10 transition to make sure you are ready by the October 1, 2013, compliance deadline. The following quick checklist will assist you with preliminary planning steps.

☑ **Identify your current systems and work processes that use ICD-9 codes.**

This could include your clinical documentation, encounter forms/superbills, practice management system, electronic health record system, contracts, and public health and quality reporting protocols. It is likely that wherever ICD-9 codes now appear, ICD-10 codes will take their place.

☑ **Talk with your practice management system vendor about accommodations for both Version 5010 and ICD-10 codes.**

Contact your vendor and ask what updates they are planning to your practice management system for both Version 5010 and ICD-10, and when they expect to have it ready to install. Check your contract to see if upgrades are included as part of your agreement. If you are in the process of making a practice management or related system purchase, ask if it is Version 5010 and ICD-10 ready.

☑ **Discuss implementation plans with all your clearinghouses, billing services, and payers to ensure a smooth transition.**

Be proactive, don't wait. Contact organizations you conduct business with such as your payers, clearinghouse, or billing service. Ask about their plans for the Version 5010 and ICD-10 compliance and when they will be ready to test their systems for both transitions.

☑ **Talk with your payers about how ICD-10 implementation might affect your contracts.**

Because ICD-10 codes are much more specific than ICD-9 codes, payers may modify terms of contracts, payment schedules, or reimbursement.

☑ **Identify potential changes to work flow and business processes.**

Consider changes to existing processes including clinical documentation, encounter forms, and quality and public health reporting.

☑ **Assess staff training needs.**

Identify the staff in your office who code, or have a need to know the new codes. There are a wide variety of training opportunities and materials available through professional associations, online courses, webinars, and onsite training. If you have a small practice, think about teaming up with other local providers. You might be able, for example, to provide training for a staff person from one practice, who can in turn train staff members in other practices. Coding professionals recommend that training take place approximately 6 months prior to the October 1, 2013, compliance date.

☑ **Budget for time and costs related to ICD-10 implementation, including expenses for system changes, resource materials, and training.**

Assess the costs of any necessary software updates, reprinting of superbills, training and related expenses.

☑ **Conduct test transactions using Version 5010/ICD-10 codes with your payers and clearinghouses.**

Testing is critical. Allow yourself enough time to first test that your Version 5010 transactions, and subsequently, claims containing ICD-10 codes are being successfully transmitted and received by your payers and billing service or clearinghouse. Check to see when they will begin testing, and the test days they have scheduled. If you submit electronic claims, you need to have completed internal testing of Version 5010 systems in time to begin external testing with your payers, clearinghouses, billing services, and other business partners by **January 1, 2011**.

PARTIAL CODE FREEZE FOR ICD-9-CM AND ICD-10

The ICD-9-CM Coordination and Maintenance Committee will implement a partial freeze of the ICD-9-CM and ICD-10 (ICD-10-CM and ICD-10-PCS) codes prior to the implementation of ICD-10 on October 1, 2013. The partial freeze will be implemented as follows:

- The last regular, annual updates to both ICD-9-CM and ICD-10 code sets will be made on October 1, 2011.

- On October 1, 2012, there will be only limited code updates to both the ICD-9-CM and ICD-10 code sets to capture new technologies and diseases as required by section 503(a) of Pub. L. 108-173.

- On October 1, 2013, there will be only limited code updates to ICD-10 code sets to capture new technologies and diagnoses as required by section 503(a) of Pub. L. 108-173. There will be no updates to ICD-9-CM, as it will no longer be used for reporting.

- On October 1, 2014, regular updates to ICD-10 will begin.

The ICD-9-CM Coordination and Maintenance Committee will continue to meet twice a year during the partial freeze. At these meetings, the public will be asked to comment on whether or not requests for new diagnosis or procedure codes should be created based on the criteria of the need to capture a new technology or disease. Any code requests that do not meet the criteria will be evaluated for implementation within ICD-10 on and after October 1, 2014 once the partial freeze has ended.

Because their will be changes to ICD-9-CM for the 2012 (October 1, 2011 – September 30, 2012) and 2013 (October 1, 2012 – September 30, 2013) reporting periods, you will need to update your ICD-9-CM coding references for both those years in addition to planning for the transition to ICD-10.

YOU NEED 2012 AND 2013 ICD-9-CM CODE BOOKS

Because of the phrase "partial coding freeze" you may be tempted to skip buying ICD-9-CM code books for 2012 and 2013. The ICD-9-CM 2012, effective October 1, 2011 includes hundreds of revisions. The "limited changes" to ICD-9-CM 2013, effective October 1, 2012 may have a significant effect on your reimbursement, depending on changes made in your specialty area. Missing a single significant code change could cost your practice hundreds or thousands of dollars due to delayed or denied claims.

ICD-10-CM OVERVIEW

WHAT IS ICD-10-CM?

ICD-10-CM is an acronym for *__International Classification of Diseases, 10th Revision, Clinical Modification__*, published under different names since 1900. ICD-10-CM is a statistical classification system that arranges diseases and injuries into groups according to established criteria. Most ICD-9-CM codes are numeric and consist of three seven digits and a description. The codes are revised approximately every 10 years by the World Health Organization and annual updates are published by Center for Medicare and Medicaid Services (CMS).

KEY POINTS REGARDING ICD-10-CM

1. ICD-10-CM codes are three (3) to seven (7) digit alphanumeric codes.

2. ICD-10-CM codes describe illnesses, injuries, signs and symptoms, and procedures.

3. ICD-10-CM codes must be used on all health insurance claims as of October 1, 2013.

4. Most ICD-10-CM codes have a specific definition; however, some ICD-10-CM codes have more than one definition.

5. Correct ICD-10-CM coding can make a significant difference in your reimbursement.

6. Accurate ICD-10-CM coding puts you in control of the reimbursement process.

BENEFITS OF ICD-10-CM

The transition to the ICD-10-CM classification system will provide better data for:

*   Measuring the quality, safety, and efficacy of care
*   Designing payment systems and processing claims for reimbursement
*   Conducting research, epidemiological studies, and clinical trials
*   Setting health policy
*   Operational and strategic planning and designing healthcare delivery systems
*   Monitoring resource utilization
*   Improving clinical, financial, and administrative performance
*   Preventing and detecting healthcare fraud and abuse
*   Tracking public health and risks

Non-specific codes still exist for use when the medical record documentation does not support a more specific code.

STRUCTURE OF ICD-10-CM COMPARED TO ICD-9-CM

The easiest way to understand the structural difference between ICD-9-CM and ICD-10-CM is with a comparative visual representation of the two coding systems. The illustrations below clearly show the differences in structure and length.

STRUCTURE OF AN ICD-9-CM CODE

414.00   **Coronary atherosclerosis of unspecified type of vessel, native or graft**

Number or Letter (V/E)	Numbers Only				
1st Digit	2nd Digit	3rd Digit		4th Digit	5th Digit
4	**1**	**4 .**		**0**	**0**
	Category			Etiology, anatomic site, manifestation	

Length:	3-5 digits
First character:	Number or Letter (E or V)
Characters 2-5:	Numbers only
Minimum length:	3 characters
Decimal:	After 3rd character

STRUCTURE OF AN ICD-10-CM CODE

S32.010A   **Wedge compression fracture of first lumbar vertebra, initial encounter for closed fracture**

Letter	Number or Letter					
1ST Digit	2nd Digit	3rd Digit	4th Digit	5th Digit	6th Digit	7th Digit
S	**3**	**2 .**	**0**	**1**	**0**	**A**
	Category		Etiology, anatomic site, severity			Added code extensions for obstetrics, injuries and external causes of injury

Length:	3-7 digits
First character:	Letter only (all letters except U are used)
Character 2:	Number only
Characters 3-7:	Numbers or letter
Decimal:	After 3rd character
Placeholder:	Use of "x" as a dummy placeholder
Letter format:	Letters are case-sensitive

SIMILARITY OF ICD-10-CM TO ICD-9-CM

While there are more codes in the ICD-10-CM coding system than the ICD-9-CM coding system and the coding is a bit more complex, there are many similarities between the two systems. Experienced coders should be able to use the ICD-10-CM system relatively quickly due in part to these similarities.

1. Format – Both ICD-10-CM and ICD-9-CM have a Tabular List and Index.

2. Chapters in the ICD-10-CM Tabular list are structured similarly to ICD-9-CM, with minor exceptions.

   - A few chapters have been restructured
   - Sense organs (eye and ear) separated from Nervous System chapter and moved to their own Chapters

3. Index of ICD-10-CM is structured the same as ICD-9-CM.

   - Alphabetic Index of Diseases and Injuries
   - Alphabetic Index of External Causes
   - Table of Neoplasms
   - Table of Drugs and Chemicals

4. Divided into Alphabetic Index and Tabular List.

   - Structure and format are the same
   - Index is alphabetical list of terms and their corresponding codes

5. Alphabetic Index lists main terms in alphabetical order with indented subterms under main terms.

6. The Alphabetic Index is divided into 2 parts: Index to Diseases and Injuries and Index to External Causes.

7. The Tabular List is a chronological list of codes divided into chapters based on body system or condition.

8. The Tabular List is presented in code number order.

9. ICD-10-CM and ICD-9-CM have the same hierarchical structure.

10. Codes are invalid in both ICD-10-CM and ICD-9-CM if they are missing an applicable character.

11. ICD-10-CM and ICD-9-CM codes are looked up the same way.

    - Look up diagnostic terms in Alphabetic Index
    - Then verify code number in Tabular List

12. Many conventions have same meaning in ICD-10-CM and ICD-9-CM.

- Abbreviations, punctuation, symbols, notes such as "code first" and "use additional code"

13. Nonspecific codes ("unspecified" or "not otherwise specified") are available to use when detailed documentation to support more specific code is not available.

14. ICD-10-CM Official Guidelines for Coding and Reporting accompany and complement ICD-10-CM conventions and instructions.

15. Adherence to the official coding guidelines in all healthcare settings is required under the Health Insurance Portability and Accountability Act.

DIFFERENCES BETWEEN ICD-10-CM AND ICD-9-CM

While there are more similarities than differences between the ICD-10-CM and ICD-9-CM, the differences are significant. Understanding the differences will be the key to a successful transition to the new coding system.

1. All ICD-10-CM codes are alphanumeric (letter and numbers).

   - 1st character is always alpha and alpha characters may appear elsewhere in the code as well

2. ICD-10-CM codes can be up to 7 characters in length.

3. ICD-10-CM codes are more specific than ICD-9-CM codes.

4. ICD-10-CM code titles are more complete (no need to refer back to a category, subcategory, or subclassification level to determine complete meaning of code).

5. Laterality (side of the body affected) has been added to relevant ICD-10-CM codes.

6. ICD-10-CM features an expanded use of combination codes.

   - Certain conditions and associated common symptoms or manifestations
   - Poisonings and associated external cause

7. Injuries grouped by anatomical site rather than type of injury.

8. Codes reflect modern medicine and updated medical terminology.

9. Addition of 7th character

   - Used in certain chapters to provide information about the characteristic of the encounter
   - Must always be used in the 7th character position
   - If a code has an applicable 7th character, the code must be reported with an appropriate 7th character value in order to be valid

   Valid 7th Digit Character for Injuries and External Causes

   A   Initial encounter
   D   Subsequent encounter

S   Sequela

Note: For aftercare of an injury, assign acute injury code with 7th character "D"

Valid 7th Digit Character for Fractures

A   Initial encounter for closed fracture
B   Initial encounter for open fracture
D   Subsequent encounter for fracture with routine healing
G   Subsequent encounter for fracture with delayed healing
K   Subsequent encounter for fracture with nonunion
P   Subsequent encounter for fracture with malunion
S   Sequela

10. Addition of dummy placeholder "X" is used in certain codes to:

- Allow for future expansion
- Fill out empty characters when a code contains fewer than 6 characters and a 7th character applies

When placeholder character applies, it must be used in order for the code to be considered valid.

11. ICD-10-CM includes two types of Excludes Notes.

- **Excludes1 Note**

    Indicates that code identified in the note and code where the note appears cannot be reported together because the 2 conditions cannot occur together.

    Examples:

    E10   Type 1 Diabetes mellitus

        Excludes1:   diabetes mellitus due to underlying condition (E08.-)
                        drug or chemical induced diabetes mellitus (E09.-)
                        gestational diabetes (O24.4-)
                        hyperglycemia NOS (R73.9)
                        neonatal diabetes mellitus (P70.2)
                        type 2 diabetes mellitus (E11.-)

    M21   Other acquired deformities of limbs

        Excludes1:   acquired absence of limb (Z89.-)
                        congenital absence of limbs (Q71-Q73)

- **Excludes2 Note**

    Indicates that condition identified in the note is not part of the condition represented by the code where the note appears, so both codes may be reported together if the patient has both conditions

Examples:

L89   Pressure ulcer

Excludes2:   diabetic ulcers (E08.621, E08.622, E09.621, E09.622, E10.621, E10.622, E11.621, E11.622, E13.621, E13.622)
non-pressure chronic ulcer of skin (L97.-)
skin infections (L00-L08)
varicose ulcer (I83.0, I83.2)

I70.2   Atherosclerosis of native arteries of the extremities

Excludes2:   atherosclerosis of bypass graft of extremities (I70.30-I70.79)

12. ICD-10-CM provides for increased specificity in comparison to ICD-9-CM.

Examples

S72.044G   Nondisplaced fracture of base of neck of right femur, subsequent encounter for closed fracture with delayed healing

I69.351   Sequelae of cerebral infarction, Hemiplegia and hemiparesis following cerebral infarction affecting right dominant side

Z47.81   Encounter for orthopedic aftercare following surgical amputation

Z48.21   Encounter for aftercare following heart transplant

13. ICD-10-CM provides specific codes to identify laterality, i.e. left, right, unspecified. This applies to extremities as well as many organ systems; i.e. eyes, ears, shoulders, arms, hands, hips, legs, feet, lungs, kidneys, ovaries, testicles, etc.

Examples

C50.511   Malignant neoplasm of lower-outer quadrant of <u>right</u> female breast

C50.512   Malignant neoplasm of lower-outer quadrant of <u>left</u> female breast

C50.519   Malignant neoplasm of lower-outer quadrant of <u>unspecified</u> female breast

ICD-10-CM CODING EXAMPLES

HYPERTENSION

Step 1: **Look up term in Alphabetic Index:**

Hypertension, hypertensive (accelerated) (benign) (essential) (idiopathic) (malignant)(systemic) I10

Step 2: **Verify code in Tabular:**

I10   Essential (primary) hypertension

        Includes: high blood pressure
                     hypertension (arterial) (benign) (essential)(malignant) (primary) (systemic)

        Excludes1: hypertensive disease complicating pregnancy, childbirth and the puerperium (O10-O11, O13-O16)
        Excludes2: essential (primary) hypertension involving vessels of brain (I60-I69)
                     essential (primary) hypertension involving vessels of eye (H35.0)

TYPE I DIABETES MELLITUS WITH DIABETIC NEPHROPATHY

Step 1: **Look up term in Alphabetic Index:**

Diabetes, diabetic (mellitus) (sugar) E11.9
type 1 E10.9
with nephropathy E10.21

Step 2: **Verify code in Tabular List:**

E10   Type 1 diabetes mellitus
    E10.2   Type 1 diabetes mellitus with kidney complications
        E10.21   Type 1 diabetes mellitus with diabetic nephropathy

Type 1 diabetes mellitus with intercapillary glomerulosclerosis
Type 1 diabetes mellitus with intracapillary glomerulonephritis
Type 1 diabetes mellitus with Kimmelstiel-Wilson disease

STAGE III DECUBITUS ULCER OF COCCYX

Step 1: **Look up term in Alphabetic Index:**

Ulcer, ulcerated, ulcerating, ulceration, ulcerative decubitus -
see Ulcer, pressure, by site
pressure (pressure area) L89.9-
coccyx L89.15-

OR

stage III (healing) (full thickness skin loss involving damage or necrosis of
subcutaneous tissue)
coccyx L89.15-

Step 2: **Verify code in Tabular List**

L89   Pressure ulcer
         Includes: bed sore
         decubitus ulcer

   L89.15   Pressure ulcer of sacral region
               Pressure ulcer of coccyx
               Pressure ulcer of tailbone

      L89.153   Pressure ulcer of sacral region, stage III

Healing pressure ulcer of sacral region, stage III
Pressure ulcer with full thickness skin loss involving damage or necrosis of subcutaneous tissue,
sacral region

LATE EFFECT OF STROKE WITH FACIAL DROOP

Step 1: Look up term in Alphabetic Index

Late effect(s) - see Sequelae

Sequelae (of) - see also condition
 stroke NOS I69.30
 facial droop I69.392

Step 2: Verify code in Tabular List:

I69 Sequelae of cerebrovascular disease
   I69.3   Sequelae of cerebral infarction
               Sequelae of stroke NOS
      I69.392 Facial weakness following cerebral infarction
                  Facial droop following cerebral infarction

POSTMENOPAUSAL OSTEOPOROSIS WITH CURRENT PATHOLOGICAL FRACTURE, VERTEBRA, INITIAL ENCOUNTER FOR FRACTURE

Step 1: **Look up term in Alphabetic Index**

Osteoporosis (female) (male) M81.0
 postmenopausal M81.0
 vertebra M80.08

Step 2: **Verify code in Tabular List**

M80 Osteoporosis with current pathological fracture

The appropriate 7th character is to be added to each code from category M80:

A   initial encounter for fracture
D   subsequent encounter for fracture with routine healing
G   subsequent encounter for fracture with delayed healing
K   subsequent encounter for fracture with nonunion
P   subsequent encounter for fracture with malunion
S   sequela

M80.08 Age-related osteoporosis with current pathological fracture, vertebra(e)

Report code M80.08xA because code is only 5 characters long and it requires a 7th character, so the placeholder "x" is needed in 6th character position

AFTERCARE FOLLOWING HIP REPLACEMENT (NOT FOR FRACTURE)

Step 1: **Look up term in Alphabetic Index**

Aftercare (see also Care) Z51.89
 following surgery (for) (on)
 joint replacement Z47.1

Step 2: **Verify code in Tabular List**

Z47   Orthopedic aftercare
        Excludes1: aftercare for healing fracture-code to fracture with 7th
        character D
   Z47.1   Aftercare following joint replacement surgery

Use additional code to identify the joint (Z96.6-)

DISLOCATION, JAW, SUBSEQUENT ENCOUNTER

Step 1: Look up term in Alphabetic Index

Dislocation (articular)
 jaw (cartilage) (meniscus) S03.0

Step 2: Verify code in Tabular List

S03   Dislocation and sprain of joints and ligaments of head

The appropriate 7th character is to be added to each code from category S03:

A   initial encounter
D   subsequent encounter
S   sequela

S03.0   Dislocation of jaw

Dislocation of jaw (cartilage) (meniscus)
Dislocation of mandible
Dislocation of temporomandibular (joint)

Report code S03.0xxD because code is only 4 characters long and it requires a 7th character, so the placeholder "x" is needed in the 5th and 6th character positions

ICD-10 MYTHS VERSUS FACTS

| MYTH | The October 1, 2013 compliance date for implementation of ICD-10-CM/PCS should be considered a flexible date. |

| FACT | All HIPAA covered entities MUST report ICD-10 codes on all health insurance claims filed on or after October 1, 2013. |

| MYTH | ICD-10 coding is much more difficult than ICD-9 coding. |

| FACT | If you know how to code using ICD-9 then you already know how to code using ICD-10. The process is the same…the codes are different. There ARE many more codes in ICD-10 than ICD-9, but that only means that you have more choices, not that the coding process is more difficult. AHIMA and the AAPC have stated that most coders will be able to grasp ICD-10 coding with little difficulty. |

| MYTH | You don't need to update ICD-9-CM for 2012 and 2013. |

| FACT | There WILL be revisions to ICD-9-CM for both 2012 and 2013. ICD-9-CM is required for all health insurance claims filed up to and including September 30, 2013. Using the most current codes maximizes your reimbursement and protects you from audit liability. |

| MYTH | Unnecessarily detailed medical record documentation will be required. |

| FACT | As with ICD-9-CM, ICD-10-CM codes should be based on medical record documentation. While documentation supporting accurate and specific codes will result in higher-quality data, nonspecific codes are still available for use when documentation doesn't support a higher level of specificity. As demonstrated by the American Hospital Association/ AHIMA field testing study, much of the detail contained in ICD-10-CM is already in medical record documentation but is not currently needed for ICD-9-CM coding. |

| MYTH | The increased number of codes will make ICD-10-CM impossible to use. |

| FACT | Just as the size of a dictionary doesn't make it more difficult to use, a higher number of codes doesn't necessarily increase the complexity of the coding system – in fact, it makes it easier to find the right code. |

Greater specificity and clinical accuracy make ICD-10-CM easier to use than ICD-9-CM. Because ICD-10-CM is much more specific, is more clinically accurate, and uses a more logical structure, it is much easier to use than ICD-9-CM.

The improved structure and specificity of ICD-10-CM will facilitate the development of increasingly sophisticated electronic coding tools that will assist in faster code selection.

ICD-10-CM IMPACT ON CODING, DOCUMENTATION, PLANNING AND TRAINING

IMPACT ON CODING AND DOCUMENTATION

- Increased detail in new coding systems will allow improved coding specificity.

- Improvements in ICD-10-CM facilitate coding process (more complete and specific code titles, updated medical terminology, expanded and clearer instructional notes).

- While detailed medical record documentation would result in higher coding specificity and higher data quality, non-specific codes are still available when detailed documentation is unavailable.

IMPLEMENTATION PLANNING

- Identify medical record documentation improvement opportunities.

  - ICD-10-CM does not require improvements in documentation, but high-quality documentation would increase the benefits of a new coding system and is increasingly being demanded by other initiatives.

- Start by reviewing medical record documentation on the most frequently- coded conditions.

TRAINING NEEDS FOR CODING PERSONNEL

- Intensive coder training should not be provided until 6 - 9 months prior to implementation.

- 16 hours of ICD-10-CM training will likely be adequate for most coders, and very proficient ICD-9-CM coders may not need that much.

- Additional training may be needed to refresh or expand knowledge in the biomedical sciences (anatomy, physiology, pathophysiology, pharmacology, and medical terminology).

ICD-10-CM OFFICIAL GUIDELINES

The Centers for Medicare and Medicaid Services (CMS) and the National Center for Health Statistics (NCHS), two departments within the U.S. Federal Government's Department of Health and Human Services (DHHS) provide the following guidelines for coding and reporting using the International Classification of Diseases, 10th Revision, Clinical Modification (ICD-10-CM). These guidelines should be used as a companion document to the official version of the ICD-10- CM as published on the NCHS website. The ICD-10-CM is a morbidity classification published by the United States for classifying diagnoses and reason for visits in all health care settings. The ICD-10-CM is based on the ICD-10, the statistical classification of disease published by the World Health Organization (WHO).

These guidelines have been approved by the four organizations that make up the Cooperating Parties for the ICD-10-CM: the American Hospital Association (AHA), the American Health Information Management Association (AHIMA), CMS, and NCHS.

These guidelines are a set of rules that have been developed to accompany and complement the official conventions and instructions provided within the ICD-10-CM itself. The instructions and conventions of the classification take precedence over guidelines. These guidelines are based on the coding and sequencing instructions in the Tabular List and Alphabetic Index of ICD-10-CM, but provide additional instruction. Adherence to these guidelines when assigning ICD-10-CM diagnosis codes is required under the Health Insurance Portability and Accountability Act (HIPAA). The diagnosis codes (Tabular List and Alphabetic Index) have been adopted under HIPAA for all healthcare settings. A joint effort between the healthcare provider and the coder is essential to achieve complete and accurate documentation, code assignment, and reporting of diagnoses and procedures. These guidelines have been developed to assist both the healthcare provider and the coder in identifying those diagnoses and procedures that are to be reported. The importance of consistent, complete documentation in the medical record cannot be overemphasized. Without such documentation accurate coding cannot be achieved. The entire record should be reviewed to determine the specific reason for the encounter and the conditions treated.

The term encounter is used for all settings, including hospital admissions. In the context of these guidelines, the term provider is used throughout the guidelines to mean physician or any qualified health care practitioner who is legally accountable for establishing the patient's diagnosis. Only this set of guidelines, approved by the Cooperating Parties, is official.

The guidelines are organized into sections. Section I includes the structure and conventions of the classification and general guidelines that apply to the entire classification, and chapter- specific guidelines that correspond to the chapters as they are arranged in the classification. Section II includes guidelines for selection of principal diagnosis for non-outpatient settings. Section III includes guidelines for reporting additional diagnoses in non-outpatient settings. Section IV is for outpatient coding and reporting. It is necessary to review all sections of the guidelines to fully understand all of the rules and instructions needed to code properly.

SECTION I: CONVENTIONS, GENERAL CODING GUIDELINES AND CHAPTER SPECIFIC GUIDELINES

The conventions, general guidelines and chapter-specific guidelines are applicable to all health care settings unless otherwise indicated. The conventions and instructions of the classification take precedence over guidelines.

CONVENTIONS FOR THE ICD-10-CM

The conventions for the ICD-10-CM are the general rules for use of the classification independent of the guidelines. These conventions are incorporated within the Alphabetic Index and Tabular List of the ICD-10-CM as instructional notes.

1. THE ALPHABETIC INDEX AND TABULAR LIST

The ICD-10-CM is divided into the Alphabetic Index, an alphabetical list of terms and their corresponding code, and the Tabular List, a chronological list of codes divided into chapters based on body system or condition. The Alphabetic Index consists of the following parts: the Index of Diseases and Injury, the Index of External Causes of Injury, the Table of Neoplasms and the Table of Drugs and Chemicals.

2. FORMAT AND STRUCTURE:

The ICD-10-CM Tabular List contains categories, subcategories and codes. Characters for categories, subcategories and codes may be either a letter or a number. All categories are 3 characters. A three-character category that has no further subdivision is equivalent to a code. Subcategories are either 4 or 5 characters. Codes may be 3, 4, 5, 6 or 7 characters. That is, each level of subdivision after a category is a subcategory. The final level of subdivision is a code. Codes that have applicable 7th characters are still referred to as codes, not subcategories. A code that has an applicable 7th character is considered invalid without the 7th character.

The ICD-10-CM uses an indented format for ease in reference.

3. USE OF CODES FOR REPORTING PURPOSES

For reporting purposes only codes are permissible, not categories or subcategories, and any applicable 7th character is required.

4. PLACEHOLDER CHARACTER

The ICD-10-CM utilizes a placeholder character "X". The "X" is used as a placeholder at certain codes to allow for future expansion. An example of this is at the poisoning, adverse effect and underdosing codes, categories T36-T50.

Where a placeholder exists, the X must be used in order for the code to be considered a valid code.

5.   7TH CHARACTERS

Certain ICD-10-CM categories have applicable 7th characters. The applicable 7th character is required for all codes within the category, or as the notes in the Tabular List instruct. The 7th character must always be the 7th character in the data field. If a code that requires a 7th character is not 6 characters, a placeholder X must be used to fill in the empty characters.

6.   ABBREVIATIONS

a.   Alphabetic Index abbreviations

NEC   "Not elsewhere classifiable"

This abbreviation in the Alphabetic Index represents "other specified". When a specific code is not available for a condition, the Alphabetic Index directs the coder to the "other specified" code in the Tabular List.

NOS   "Not otherwise specified"

This abbreviation is the equivalent of unspecified.

b.   Tabular List abbreviations

NEC   "Not elsewhere classifiable"

This abbreviation in the Tabular List represents "other specified". When a specific code is not available for a condition the Tabular List includes an NEC entry under a code to identify the code as the "other specified" code.

NOS   "Not otherwise specified"

This abbreviation is the equivalent of unspecified.

7.   PUNCTUATION

[ ]   Brackets are used in the Tabular List to enclose synonyms, alternative wording or explanatory phrases. Brackets are used in the Alphabetic Index to identify manifestation codes.

( )   Parentheses are used in both the Alphabetic Index and Tabular List to enclose supplementary words that may be present or absent in the statement of a disease or procedure without affecting the code number to which it is assigned. The terms within the parentheses are referred to as nonessential modifiers.

:   Colons are used in the Tabular List after an incomplete term which needs one or more of the modifiers following the colon to make it assignable to a given category.

8.   USE OF "AND"

When the term "and" is used in a narrative statement it represents and/or.

9. OTHER AND UNSPECIFIED CODES

a. "Other" codes

Codes titled "other" or "other specified" are for use when the information in the medical record provides detail for which a specific code does not exist. Alphabetic Index entries with NEC in the line designate "other" codes in the Tabular List. These Alphabetic Index entries represent specific disease entities for which no specific code exists so the term is included within an "other" code.

b. "Unspecified" codes

Codes titled "unspecified" are for use when the information in the medical record is insufficient to assign a more specific code. For those categories for which an unspecified code is not provided, the "other specified" code may represent both other and unspecified.

10. INCLUDES NOTES

This note appears immediately under a three character code title to further define, or give examples of, the content of the category.

11. INCLUSION TERMS

List of terms is included under some codes. These terms are the conditions for which that code is to be used. The terms may be synonyms of the code title, or, in the case of "other specified" codes, the terms are a list of the various conditions assigned to that code. The inclusion terms are not necessarily exhaustive. Additional terms found only in the Alphabetic Index may also be assigned to a code.

12. EXCLUDES NOTES

The ICD-10-CM has two types of excludes notes. Each type of note has a different definition for use but they are all similar in that they indicate that codes excluded from each other are independent of each other.

a. *Excludes1*

A type 1 Excludes note is a pure excludes note. It means "NOT CODED HERE!" An Excludes1 note indicates that the code excluded should never be used at the same time as the code above the Excludes1 note. An Excludes1 is used when two conditions cannot occur together, such as a congenital form versus an acquired form of the same condition.

b. *Excludes2*

A type 2 excludes note represents "Not included here". An excludes2 note indicates that the condition excluded is not part of the condition represented by the code, but a patient may have both conditions at the same time. When an Excludes2 note appears under a code, it is acceptable to use both the code and the excluded code together, when appropriate.

13. ETIOLOGY/MANIFESTATION CONVENTION ("CODE FIRST", "USE ADDITIONAL CODE" AND "IN DISEASES CLASSIFIED ELSEWHERE" NOTES)

Certain conditions have both an underlying etiology and multiple body system manifestations due to the underlying etiology. For such conditions, the ICD- 10-CM has a coding convention that requires the underlying condition be sequenced first followed by the manifestation. Wherever such a combination exists, there is a "use additional code" note at the etiology code, and a "code first" note at the manifestation code. These instructional notes indicate the proper sequencing order of the codes, etiology followed by manifestation.

In most cases the manifestation codes will have in the code title, "in diseases classified elsewhere." Codes with this title are a component of the etiology/ manifestation convention. The code title indicates that it is a manifestation code. "In diseases classified elsewhere" codes are never permitted to be used as first-listed or principal diagnosis codes. They must be used in conjunction with an underlying condition code and they must be listed following the underlying condition. See category F02, Dementia in other diseases classified elsewhere, for an example of this convention.

There are manifestation codes that do not have "in diseases classified elsewhere" in the title. For such codes a "use additional code" note will still be present and the rules for sequencing apply.

In addition to the notes in the Tabular List, these conditions also have a specific Alphabetic Index entry structure. In the Alphabetic Index both conditions are listed together with the etiology code first followed by the manifestation codes in brackets. The code in brackets is always to be sequenced second.

An example of the etiology/manifestation convention is dementia in Parkinson's disease. In the Alphabetic Index, code G20 is listed first, followed by code F02.80 or F02.81 in brackets. Code G20 represents the underlying etiology, Parkinson's disease, and must be sequenced first, whereas codes F02.80 and F02.81 represent the manifestation of dementia in diseases classified elsewhere, with or without behavioral disturbance.

"Code first" and "Use additional code" notes are also used as sequencing rules in the classification for certain codes that are not part of an etiology/ manifestation combination.

14. "AND"

The word "and" should be interpreted to mean either "and" or "or" when it appears in a title.

15. "WITH"

The word "with" should be interpreted to mean "associated with" or "due to" when it appears in a code title, the Alphabetic Index, or an instructional note in the Tabular List.

The word "with" in the Alphabetic Index is sequenced immediately following the main term, not in alphabetical order.

16. "SEE" AND "SEE ALSO"

The "see" instruction following a main term in the Alphabetic Index indicates that another term should be referenced. It is necessary to go to the main term referenced with the "see" note to locate the correct code.

A "see also" instruction following a main term in the Alphabetic Index instructs that there is another main term that may also be referenced that may provide additional Alphabetic Index entries that may be useful. It is not necessary to follow the "see also" note when the original main term provides the necessary code.

17. "CODE ALSO NOTE"

A "code also" note instructs that two codes may be required to fully describe a condition, but this note does not provide sequencing direction.

18. DEFAULT CODES

A code listed next to a main term in the ICD-10-CM Alphabetic Index is referred to as a default code. The default code represents that condition that is most commonly associated with the main term, or is the unspecified code for the condition. If a condition is documented in a medical record (for example, appendicitis) without any additional information, such as acute or chronic, the default code should be assigned.

19. SYNDROMES

Follow the Alphabetic Index guidance when coding syndromes. In the absence of Alphabetic Index guidance, assign codes for the documented manifestations of the syndrome.

GENERAL CODING GUIDELINES

1. LOCATING A CODE IN THE ICD-10-CM

To select a code in the classification that corresponds to a diagnosis or reason for visit documented in a medical record, first locate the term in the Alphabetic Index, and then verify the code in the Tabular List. Read and be guided by instructional notations that appear in both the Alphabetic Index and the Tabular List.

It is essential to use both the Alphabetic Index and Tabular List when locating and assigning a code. The Alphabetic Index does not always provide the full code. Selection of the full code, including laterality and any applicable 7th character can only be done in the Tabular List. A dash (-) at the end of an Alphabetic Index entry indicates that additional characters are required. Even if a dash is not included at the Alphabetic Index entry, it is necessary to refer to the Tabular List to verify that no 7th character is required.

2. LEVEL OF DETAIL IN CODING

Diagnosis codes are to be used and reported at their highest number of characters available.

ICD-10-CM diagnosis codes are composed of codes with 3, 4, 5, 6 or 7 characters. Codes with three characters are included in ICD-10-CM as the heading of a category of codes that may be further subdivided by the use of fourth and/or fifth characters and/or sixth characters, which provide greater detail.

A three-character code is to be used only if it is not further subdivided. A code is invalid if it has not been coded to the full number of characters required for that code, including the 7th character, if applicable.

3. CODE OR CODES FROM A00.0 THROUGH T88.9, Z00-Z99.8

The appropriate code or codes from A00.0 through T88.9, Z00-Z99.8 must be used to identify diagnoses, symptoms, conditions, problems, complaints or other reason(s) for the encounter/ visit.

4. SIGNS AND SYMPTOMS

Codes that describe symptoms and signs, as opposed to diagnoses, are acceptable for reporting purposes when a related definitive diagnosis has not been established (confirmed) by the provider. Chapter 18 of ICD-10-CM, Symptoms, Signs, and Abnormal Clinical and Laboratory Findings, Not Elsewhere Classified (codes R00.0 - R99) contains many, but not all codes for symptoms.

5. CONDITIONS THAT ARE AN INTEGRAL PART OF A DISEASE PROCESS

Signs and symptoms that are associated routinely with a disease process should not be assigned as additional codes, unless otherwise instructed by the classification.

6. CONDITIONS THAT ARE NOT AN INTEGRAL PART OF A DISEASE PROCESS

Additional signs and symptoms that may not be associated routinely with a disease process should be coded when present.

7. MULTIPLE CODING FOR A SINGLE CONDITION

In addition to the etiology/manifestation convention that requires two codes to fully describe a single condition that affects multiple body systems, there are other single conditions that also require more than one code. "Use additional code" notes are found in the Tabular List at codes that are not part of an etiology/manifestation pair where a secondary code is useful to fully describe a condition. The sequencing rule is the same as the etiology/manifestation pair, "use additional code" indicates that a secondary code should be added.

For example, for bacterial infections that are not included in chapter 1, a secondary code from category B95, Streptococcus, Staphylococcus, and Enterococcus, as the cause of diseases classified elsewhere, or B96, Other bacterial agents as the cause of diseases classified elsewhere, may be required to identify the bacterial organism causing the infection. A "use additional code" note will normally be found at the infectious disease code, indicating a need for the organism code to be added as a secondary code.

"Code first" notes are also under certain codes that are not specifically manifestation codes but may be due to an underlying cause. When there is a "code first" note and an underlying condition is present, the underlying condition should be sequenced first.

"Code, if applicable, any causal condition first", notes indicate that this code may be assigned as a principal diagnosis when the causal condition is unknown or not applicable. If a causal condition is known, then the code for that condition should be sequenced as the principal or first-listed diagnosis.

Multiple codes may be needed for late effects, complication codes and obstetric codes to more fully describe a condition. See the specific guidelines for these conditions for further instruction.

8. ACUTE AND CHRONIC CONDITIONS

If the same condition is described as both acute (subacute) and chronic, and separate subentries exist in the Alphabetic Index at the same indentation level, code both and sequence the acute (subacute) code first.

9. COMBINATION CODE

A combination code is a single code used to classify:

- Two diagnoses, or
- A diagnosis with an associated secondary process (manifestation)
- A diagnosis with an associated complication

Combination codes are identified by referring to subterm entries in the Alphabetic Index and by reading the inclusion and exclusion notes in the Tabular List.

Assign only the combination code when that code fully identifies the diagnostic conditions involved or when the Alphabetic Index so directs. Multiple coding should not be used when the classification provides a combination code that clearly identifies all of the elements documented in the diagnosis. When the combination code lacks necessary specificity in describing the manifestation or complication, an additional code should be used as a secondary code.

10. LATE EFFECTS (SEQUELA)

A late effect is the residual effect (condition produced) after the acute phase of an illness or injury has terminated. There is no time limit on when a late effect code can be used. The residual may be apparent early, such as in cerebral infarction, or it may occur months or years later, such as that due to a previous injury. Coding of late effects generally requires two codes sequenced in the following order: The condition or nature of the late effect is sequenced first. The late effect code is sequenced second.

An exception to the above guidelines are those instances where the code for late effect is followed by a manifestation code identified in the Tabular List and title, or the late effect code has been expanded (at the fourth, fifth or sixth character levels) to include the manifestation(s). The code for the acute phase of an illness or injury that led to the late effect is never used with a code for the late effect.

11. IMPENDING OR THREATENED CONDITION

Code any condition described at the time of discharge as "impending" or "threatened" as follows:

- If it did occur, code as confirmed diagnosis.

- If it did not occur, reference the Alphabetic Index to determine if the condition has a subentry term for "impending" or "threatened" and also reference main term entries for "Impending" and for "Threatened."

- If the subterms are listed, assign the given code.

- If the subterms are not listed, code the existing underlying condition(s) and not the condition described as impending or threatened.

12. REPORTING SAME DIAGNOSIS CODE MORE THAN ONCE

Each unique ICD-10-CM diagnosis code may be reported only once for an encounter. This applies to bilateral conditions when there are no distinct codes identifying laterality or two different conditions classified to the same ICD-10-CM diagnosis code.

13. LATERALITY

For bilateral sites, the final character of the codes in the ICD-10-CM indicates laterality. An unspecified side code is also provided should the side not be identified in the medical record. If no bilateral code is provided and the condition is bilateral, assign separate codes for both the left and right side.

14. DOCUMENTATION FOR BMI AND PRESSURE ULCER STAGES

For the Body Mass Index (BMI) and pressure ulcer stage codes, code assignment may be based on medical record documentation from clinicians who are not the patient's provider (i.e., physician or other qualified healthcare practitioner legally accountable for establishing the patient's diagnosis), since this information is typically documented by other clinicians involved in the care of the patient (e.g., a dietitian often documents the BMI and nurses often documents the pressure ulcer stages). However, the associated diagnosis (such as overweight, obesity, or pressure ulcer) must be documented by the patient's provider. If there is conflicting medical record documentation, either from the same clinician or different clinicians, the patient's attending provider should be queried for clarification.

The BMI codes should only be reported as secondary diagnoses. As with all other secondary diagnosis codes, the BMI codes should only be assigned when they meet the definition of a reportable additional diagnosis (see Section III, Reporting Additional Diagnoses).

GENERAL EQUIVALENCE MAPPINGS (GEM)

The Centers for Medicare & Medicaid Services (CMS) and the Centers for Disease Control and Prevention created the national version of the General Equivalence Mappings (GEM) to ensure that consistency in national data is maintained. They have made a commitment to update the

GEMs annually along with the updates to International Classification of Diseases, 10th Edition, Clinical Modification (ICD-10-CM) and Procedure Coding System (PCS) during the transition period prior to ICD-10 implementation. CMS and CDC will maintain the GEMs for at least three years beyond October 1, 2013, which is the compliance date for implementation of ICD-10 for all covered entities.

WHAT ARE THE GENERAL EQUIVALENCE MAPPINGS?

The GEMs are a tool that can be used to convert data from ICD-9-CM to ICD-10-CM and ICD-10-PCS and vice versa. Mapping from ICD-10-CM and ICD-10-PCS codes back to ICD-9-CM codes is referred to as backward mapping. Mapping from ICD-9-CM codes to ICD-10-CM and ICD-10-PCS codes is referred to as forward mapping. The GEMs are a comprehensive translation dictionary that can be used to accurately and effectively translate any ICD-9-CM-based data, including data for:

- Tracking quality;
- Recording morbidity/mortality;
- Calculating reimbursement; or
- Converting any ICD-9-CM-based application to ICD-10-CM/PCS.

The Centers for Medicare & Medicaid Services (CMS) and the Centers for Disease Control and Prevention (CDC) created the national version of the General Equivalence Mappings (GEM) to ensure that consistency in national data is maintained. They have made a commitment to update the GEMs annually along with the updates to International Classification of Diseases, 10th Edition, Clinical Modification (ICD-10-CM) and Procedure Coding System (PCS) during the transition period prior to ICD-10 implementation. CMS and CDC will maintain the GEMs for at least three years beyond October 1, 2013, which is the compliance date for implementation of ICD-10 for all covered entities.

GENERAL EQUIVALENCE MAPPINGS

The GEMs are complete in their description of all the mapping possibilities as well as when there are new concepts in ICD-10 that are not found in ICD-9-CM. *All* ICD-9-CM codes and *all* ICD-10-CM/ ICD-10-PCS codes are included in the collective GEMs:

- All ICD-10-CM codes are in the ICD-10-CM to ICD-9-CM GEM;
- All ICD-9-CM Diagnosis Codes are in the ICD-9-CM to ICD-10-CM GEM;
- All ICD-10-PCS codes are in the ICD-10-PCS to ICD-9-CM GEM; and
- All ICD-9-CM Procedure Codes are in the ICD-9-CM to ICD-10-PCS GEM.

ARE THE GENERAL EQUIVALENCE MAPPINGS A SUBSTITUTE FOR LEARNING TO USE THE ICD-10-CM AND ICD-10-PCS?

No. The GEMs are not a substitute for learning how to use the ICD-10-CM and ICD-10-PCS. Providers' coding staff will assign codes describing the patients' encounters from the ICD-10-CM and ICD-10-PCS code books or encoder systems. In coding individual claims, it will be more efficient and accurate to work from the medical record documentation and then select the appropriate code(s) from the coding book or encoder system. The GEMs are a tool to assist with converting larger International Classification of Diseases, 9th Edition, Clinical Modification (ICD-9-CM) databases to ICD-10-CM and ICD-10-PCS.

WHO CAN USE THE GENERAL EQUIVALENCE MAPPINGS?

The GEMs can be used by anyone who wants to convert coded data. Possible users of the GEMs include the following:

- All payers;
- All providers;
- Medical researchers;
- Informatics professionals;
- Coding professionals—to convert large data sets;
- Software vendors—to use within their own products;
- Organizations—to make mappings that suit their internal purposes or that are based on their own historical data; and
- Others who use coded data.

MAPPING DIRECTION

Mapping is done in two directions; forward and backward. Forward mapping is the process of mapping from an older coding system to a newer coding system. Backward mapping is the process of mapping from a new coding system to an older coding system.

NOTE: This detailed explanation of mapping is not repeated in subsequent chapters.

CHAPTER-SPECIFIC ICD-10-CM CODING GUIDELINES

In addition to general coding guidelines, there are guidelines for specific diagnoses and/or conditions in the classification. Unless otherwise indicated, these guidelines apply to all health care settings. Please refer to Section II for guidelines on the selection of principal diagnosis.

CHAPTER 1: CERTAIN INFECTIOUS AND PARASITIC DISEASES (A00- B99)

GENERAL GUIDELINES

HUMAN IMMUNODEFICIENCY VIRUS (HIV) INFECTIONS

1) **Code only confirmed cases**

    Code only confirmed cases of HIV infection/illness. This is an exception to the hospital inpatient guideline Section II, H.

    In this context, "confirmation" does not require documentation of positive serology or culture for HIV; the provider's diagnostic statement that the patient is HIV positive, or has an HIV-related illness is sufficient.

2) **Selection and sequencing of HIV codes**

    (a) Patient admitted for HIV-related condition

    If a patient is admitted for an HIV-related condition, the principal diagnosis should be B20, followed by additional diagnosis codes for all reported HIV-related conditions.

    (b) Patient with HIV disease admitted for unrelated condition

    If a patient with HIV disease is admitted for an unrelated condition (such as a traumatic injury), the code for the unrelated condition (e.g., the nature of injury code) should be the principal diagnosis. Other diagnoses would be B20 followed by additional diagnosis codes for all reported HIV-related conditions.

    (c) Whether the patient is newly diagnosed

    Whether the patient is newly diagnosed or has had previous admissions/encounters for HIV conditions is irrelevant to the sequencing decision.

    (d) Asymptomatic human immunodeficiency virus

    Z21, Asymptomatic human immunodeficiency virus [HIV] infection status, is to be applied when the patient without any documentation of symptoms is listed as being "HIV positive," "known HIV," "HIV test positive," or similar terminology. Do not use this code if the term "AIDS" is used or if the patient is treated for any HIV-related illness or is described as having any condition(s) resulting from his/her HIV positive status; use B20 in these cases.

(e) Patients with inconclusive HIV serology

Patients with inconclusive HIV serology, but no definitive diagnosis or manifestations of the illness, may be assigned code R75, Inconclusive laboratory evidence of human immunodeficiency virus [HIV].

(f) Previously diagnosed HIV-related illness

Patients with any known prior diagnosis of an HIV-related illness should be coded to B20. Once a patient has developed an HIV-related illness, the patient should always be assigned code B20 on every subsequent admission/encounter. Patients previously diagnosed with any HIV illness (B20) should never be assigned to R75 or Z21, Asymptomatic human immuno-deficiency virus [HIV] infection status.

(g) HIV Infection in Pregnancy, Childbirth and the Puerperium

During pregnancy, childbirth or the puerperium, a patient admitted (or presenting for a health care encounter) because of an HIV-related illness should receive a principal diagnosis code of O98.7-, Human immunodeficiency [HIV] disease complicating pregnancy, childbirth and the puerperium, followed by B20 and the code(s) for the HIV-related illness(es). Codes from Chapter 15 always take sequencing priority.

Patients with asymptomatic HIV infection status admitted (or presenting for a health care encounter) during pregnancy, childbirth, or the puerperium should receive codes of O98.7- and Z21.

(h) Encounters for testing for HIV

If a patient is being seen to determine his/her HIV status, use code Z11.4, Encounter for screening for human immunodeficiency virus [HIV]. Use additional codes for any associated high risk behavior.

If a patient with signs or symptoms is being seen for HIV testing, code the signs and symptoms. An additional counseling code Z71.7, Human immunodeficiency virus [HIV] counseling, may be used if counseling is provided during the encounter for the test.

When a patient returns to be informed of his/her HIV test results and the test result is negative, use code Z71.7, Human immunodeficiency virus [HIV] counseling.

If the results are positive, see previous guidelines and assign codes as appropriate.

INFECTIOUS AGENTS AS THE CAUSE OF DISEASES CLASSIFIED TO OTHER CHAPTERS

Certain infections are classified in chapters other than Chapter 1 and no organism is identified as part of the infection code. In these instances, it is necessary to use an additional code from Chapter 1 to identify the organism. A code from category B95, Streptococcus, Staphylococcus, and Enterococcus as the cause of diseases classified to other chapters, B96, Other bacterial agents as the cause of diseases classified to other chapters, or B97, Viral agents as the cause of diseases classified to other chapters, is to be used as an additional code to identify the organism. An instructional note will be found at the infection code advising that an additional organism code is required.

INFECTIONS RESISTANT TO ANTIBIOTICS

Many bacterial infections are resistant to current antibiotics. It is necessary to identify all infections documented as antibiotic resistant. Assign code Z16, Infection with drug resistant microorganisms, following the infection code for these cases.

SEPSIS, SEVERE SEPSIS, AND SEPTIC SHOCK 1) CODING OF SEPSIS AND SEVERE SEPSIS

1) **Coding of Sepsis and Severe Sepsis**

   (a) **Sepsis**

   For a diagnosis of sepsis, assign the appropriate code for the underlying systemic infection. If the type of infection or causal organism is not further specified, assign code A41.9, Sepsis, unspecified.

   A code from subcategory R65.2, Severe sepsis, should not be assigned unless severe sepsis or an associated acute organ dysfunction is documented.

   (i) Negative or inconclusive blood cultures and sepsis

   Negative or inconclusive blood cultures do not preclude a diagnosis of sepsis in patients with clinical evidence of the condition, however, the provider should be queried.

   (ii) Urosepsis

   The term urosepsis is a nonspecific term. It is not to be considered synonymous with sepsis. It has no default code in the Alphabetic Index. Should a provider use this term, he/she must be queried for clarification.

   (iii) Sepsis with organ dysfunction

   If a patient has sepsis and associated acute organ dysfunction or multiple organ dysfunction (MOD), follow the instructions for coding severe sepsis.

   (iv) Acute organ dysfunction that is not clearly associated with the sepsis

   If a patient has sepsis and an acute organ dysfunction, but the medical record documentation indicates that the acute organ dysfunction is related to a medical condition other than the sepsis, do not assign a code from subcategory R65.2, Severe sepsis. An acute organ dysfunction must be associated with the sepsis in order to assign the severe sepsis code. If the documentation is not clear as to whether an acute organ dysfunction is related to the sepsis or another medical condition, query the provider.

(b) **Severe sepsis**

The coding of severe sepsis requires a minimum of 2 codes: first a code for the underlying systemic infection, followed by a code from subcategory R65.2, Severe sepsis. If the causal organism is not documented, assign code A41.9, Sepsis, unspecified, for the infection. Additional code(s) for the associated acute organ dysfunction are also required.

Due to the complex nature of severe sepsis, some cases may require querying the provider prior to assignment of the codes.

2) Septic shock

Septic shock is circulatory failure associated with severe sepsis, and therefore, it represents a type of acute organ dysfunction. For all cases of septic shock, the code for the underlying systemic infection should be sequenced first, followed by code R65.21, Severe sepsis with septic shock. Any additional codes for the other acute organ dysfunctions should also be assigned.

Septic shock indicates the presence of severe sepsis. Code R65.21, Severe sepsis with septic shock, must be assigned if septic shock is documented in the medical record, even if the term severe sepsis is not documented.

3) Sequencing of severe sepsis

If severe sepsis is present on admission, and meets the definition of principal diagnosis, the underlying systemic infection should be assigned as principal diagnosis followed by the appropriate code from subcategory R65.2 as required by the sequencing rules in the Tabular List. A code from subcategory R65.2 can never be assigned as a principal diagnosis.

When severe sepsis develops during an encounter (it was not present on admission) the underlying systemic infection and the appropriate code from subcategory R65.2 should be assigned as secondary diagnoses.

Severe sepsis may be present on admission but the diagnosis may not be confirmed until sometime after admission. If the documentation is not clear whether severe sepsis was present on admission, the provider should be queried.

4) Sepsis and severe sepsis with a localized infection

If the reason for admission is both sepsis or severe sepsis and a localized infection, such as pneumonia or cellulitis, a code(s) for the underlying systemic infection should be assigned first and the code for the localized infection should be assigned as a secondary diagnosis. If the patient has severe sepsis, a code from subcategory R65.2 should also be assigned as a secondary diagnosis. If the patient is admitted with a localized infection, such as pneumonia, and sepsis/severe sepsis doesn't develop until after admission, the localized infection should be assigned first, followed by the appropriate sepsis/severe sepsis codes.

5) Sepsis due to a postprocedural infection

Sepsis resulting from a postprocedural infection is a complication of medical care. For such cases, the postprocedural infection code, such as, T80.2, Infections following infusion, transfusion, and therapeutic injection, T81.4, Infection following a procedure, T88.0, Infection following immunization, or O86.0, Infection of obstetric surgical wound, should be coded first, followed by the code for the specific infection. If the patient has severe sepsis the appropriate code from subcategory R65.2 should also be assigned with the additional code(s) for any acute organ dysfunction.

6) Sepsis and severe sepsis associated with a noninfectious process (condition)

In some cases a noninfectious process (condition), such as trauma, may lead to an infection which can result in sepsis or severe sepsis. If sepsis or severe sepsis is documented as associated with a noninfectious condition, such as a burn or serious injury, and this condition meets the definition for principal diagnosis, the code for the noninfectious condition should be sequenced first, followed by the code for the resulting infection. If severe sepsis, is present a code from subcategory R65.2 should also be assigned with any associated organ dysfunction(s) codes. It is not necessary to assign a code from subcategory R65.1, Systemic inflammatory response syndrome (SIRS) of non-infectious origin, for these cases.

If the infection meets the definition of principal diagnosis it should be sequenced before the non-infectious condition. When both the associated non-infectious condition and the infection meet the definition of principal diagnosis either may be assigned as principal diagnosis.

Only one code from category R65, Symptoms and signs specifically associated with systemic inflammation and infection, should be assigned. Therefore, when a non-infectious condition leads to an infection resulting in severe sepsis, assign the appropriate code from subcategory R65.2, Severe sepsis. Do not additionally assign a code from subcategory R65.1, Systemic inflammatory response syndrome (SIRS) of noninfectious origin.

SAMPLE ICD-10-CM CODES FROM THIS CHAPTER

Use additional code for any associated drug resistance (Z16)

Excludes1: carrier or suspected carrier of infectious disease (Z22.-)
certain localized infections - see body system-related chapters
infectious and parasitic diseases complicating pregnancy, childbirth and the puerperium (O98.-)
influenza and other acute respiratory infections (J00-J22)
infectious and parasitic diseases specific to the perinatal period (P35-P39)

This chapter includes the following blocks:	
A00-A09	Intestinal infectious diseases
A15-A19	Tuberculosis
A20-A28	Certain zoonotic bacterial diseases
A30-A49	Other bacterial diseases
A50-A64	Infections with a predominantly sexual mode of transmission
A65-A69	Other spirochetal diseases

A70-A74	Other diseases caused by chlamydiae
A75-A79	Rickettsioses
A80-A89	Viral and prion infections of the central nervous system
A90-A99	Arthropod-borne viral fevers and viral hemorrhagic fevers
B00-B09	Viral infections characterized by skin and mucous membrane lesions
B10	Other human herpesviruses
B15-B19	Viral hepatitis
B20	Human immunodeficiency virus [HIV] disease
B25-B34	Other viral diseases
B35-B49	Mycoses
B50-B64	Protozoal diseases
B65-B83	Helminthiases
B85-B89	Pediculosis, acariasis and other infestations
B90-B94	Sequelae of infectious and parasitic diseases
B95-B97	Bacterial and viral infectious agents
B99	Other infectious diseases

INTESTINAL INFECTIOUS DISEASES (A00-A09)

A00   Cholera

    A00.0   Cholera due to Vibrio cholerae 01, biovar cholerae
    Classical cholera

    A00.1   Cholera due to Vibrio cholerae 01, biovar eltor
    Cholera eltor

    A00.9   Cholera, unspecified

A01   Typhoid and paratyphoid fevers

    A01.0   Typhoid fever
    Infection due to Salmonella typhi

        A01.00   Typhoid fever, unspecified

        A01.01   Typhoid meningitis

        A01.02   Typhoid fever with heart involvement
        Typhoid endocarditis
        Typhoid myocarditis

        A01.03   Typhoid pneumonia

        A01.04   Typhoid arthritis

A01.05   Typhoid osteomyelitis

A01.09   Typhoid fever with other complications

A01.1   Paratyphoid fever A

A01.2   Paratyphoid fever B

A01.3   Paratyphoid fever C

A01.4   Paratyphoid fever, unspecified
Infection due to Salmonella paratyphi NOS

A02   Other salmonella infections

Includes: infection or foodborne intoxication due to any Salmonella species other than S. typhi and S. paratyphi

A02.0   Salmonella enteritis
Salmonellosis

A02.1   Salmonella sepsis

A02.2   Localized salmonella infections

A02.20   Localized salmonella infection, unspecified

A02.21   Salmonella meningitis

A02.22   Salmonella pneumonia

A02.23   Salmonella arthritis

A02.24   Salmonella osteomyelitis

A02.25   Salmonella pyelonephritis
Salmonella tubulo-interstitial nephropathy

A02.29   Salmonella with other localized infection

A02.8   Other specified salmonella infections

A02.9   Salmonella infection, unspecified

A03   Shigellosis

A03.0   Shigellosis due to Shigella dysenteriae
Group A shigellosis [Shiga-Kruse dysentery]

A03.1   Shigellosis due to Shigella flexneri
Group B shigellosis

A03.2 Shigellosis due to Shigella boydii
Group C shigellosis

A03.3 Shigellosis due to Shigella sonnei
Group D shigellosis

A03.8 Other shigellosis

A03.9 Shigellosis, unspecified
Bacillary dysentery NOS

A04 Other bacterial intestinal infections

Excludes 1: bacterial foodborne intoxications, NEC (A05.-)
tuberculous enteritis (A18.32)

A04.0 Enteropathogenic Escherichia coli infection

A04.1 Enterotoxigenic Escherichia coli infection

A04.2 Enteroinvasive Escherichia coli infection

A04.3 Enterohemorrhagic Escherichia coli infection

A04.4 Other intestinal Escherichia coli infections
Escherichia coli enteritis NOS

A04.5 Campylobacter enteritis

A04.6 Enteritis due to Yersinia enterocolitica
Excludes 1: extraintestinal yersiniosis (A28.2)

A04.7 Enterocolitis due to Clostridium difficile
Foodborne intoxication by Clostridium difficile
Pseudomembranous colitis

A04.8 Other specified bacterial intestinal infections

A04.9 Bacterial intestinal infection, unspecified
Bacterial enteritis NOS

FORWARD MAPPING SAMPLE (ICD-9-CM ➡ ICD-10-CM)			
ICD-9-CM CODE & DESCRIPTION		ICD-10-CM CODE & DESCRIPTION	
001.0	Cholera due to vibrio cholerae	A00.0	Cholera due to Vibrio cholerae 01 biovar cholerae
001.1	Cholera due to vibrio cholerae el tor	A00.1	Cholera due to Vibrio cholerae 01 biovar eltor
001.9	Cholera unspecified	A00.9	Cholera unspecified
002.0	Typhoid fever	A01.00	Typhoid fever unspecified

002.1	Paratyphoid fever a	A01.1	Paratyphoid fever A
002.2	Paratyphoid fever b	A01.2	Paratyphoid fever B
002.3	Paratyphoid fever c	A01.3	Paratyphoid fever C
002.9	Paratyphoid fever unspecified	A01.4	Paratyphoid fever unspecified
003.0	Salmonella gastroenteritis	A02.0	Salmonella enteritis
003.1	Salmonella septicemia	A02.1	Salmonella sepsis
003.20	Localized salmonella infection unspecified	A02.20	Localized salmonella infection unspecified
003.21	Salmonella meningitis	A02.21	Salmonella meningitis
003.22	Salmonella pneumonia	A02.22	Salmonella pneumonia
003.23	Salmonella arthritis	A02.23	Salmonella arthritis
003.24	Salmonella osteomyelitis	A02.24	Salmonella osteomyelitis
003.29	Other localized salmonella infections	A02.29	Salmonella with other localized infection
003.8	Other specified salmonella infections	A02.8	Other specified salmonella infections
003.9	Salmonella infection unspecified	A02.9	Salmonella infection unspecified
004.0	Shigella dysenteriae	A03.0	Shigellosis due to Shigella dysenteriae
004.1	Shigella flexneri	A03.1	Shigellosis due to Shigella flexneri
004.2	Shigella boydii	A03.2	Shigellosis due to Shigella boydii
004.3	Shigella sonnei	A03.3	Shigellosis due to Shigella sonnei
004.8	Other specified shigella infections	A03.8	Other shigellosis
004.9	Shigellosis unspecified	A03.9	Shigellosis unspecified
005.0	Staphylococcal food poisoning	A05.0	Foodborne staphylococcal intoxication
005.1	Botulism food poisoning	A05.1	Botulism food poisoning
005.2	Food poisoning due to clostridium perfringens (c. welchii)	A05.2	Foodborne Clostridium perfringens [Clostridium welchii] intoxication
005.3	Food poisoning due to other clostridia	A05.8	Other specified bacterial foodborne intoxications
005.4	Food poisoning due to vibrio parahaemolyticus	A05.3	Foodborne Vibrio parahaemolyticus intoxication
005.81	Food poisoning due to vibrio vulnificus	A05.5	Foodborne Vibrio vulnificus intoxication
005.89	Other bacterial food poisoning	A05.8	Other specified bacterial foodborne intoxications
005.9	Food poisoning unspecified	A05.9	Bacterial foodborne intoxication unspecified
006.0	Acute amebic dysentery without abscess	A06.0	Acute amebic dysentery

006.1	Chronic intestinal amebiasis without abscess	A06.1	Chronic intestinal amebiasis
006.2	Amebic nondysenteric colitis	A06.2	Amebic nondysenteric colitis
006.3	Amebic liver abscess	A06.4	Amebic liver abscess
006.4	Amebic lung abscess	A06.5	Amebic lung abscess
006.5	Amebic brain abscess	A06.6	Amebic brain abscess
006.6	Amebic skin ulceration	A06.7	Cutaneous amebiasis
006.8	Amebic infection of other sites	A06.89	Other amebic infections

BACKWARD MAPPING SAMPLE (ICD-10-CM ➡ ICD-9-CM)

ICD-9-CM CODE & DESCRIPTION		ICD-10-CM CODE & DESCRIPTION	
A00.0	Cholera due to Vibrio cholerae 01 biovar cholerae	001.0	Cholera due to vibrio cholerae
A00.1	Cholera due to Vibrio cholerae 01 biovar eltor	001.1	Cholera due to vibrio cholerae el tor
A00.9	Cholera unspecified	001.9	Cholera unspecified
A01.00	Typhoid fever unspecified	002.0	Typhoid fever
A01.01	Typhoid meningitis	002.0	Typhoid fever
A01.02	Typhoid fever with heart involvement	002.0	Typhoid fever
A01.03	Typhoid pneumonia	002.0	Typhoid fever
A01.04	Typhoid arthritis	002.0	Typhoid fever
A01.05	Typhoid osteomyelitis	002.0	Typhoid fever
A01.09	Typhoid fever with other complications	002.0	Typhoid fever
A01.1	Paratyphoid fever A	002.1	Paratyphoid fever a
A01.2	Paratyphoid fever B	002.2	Paratyphoid fever b
A01.3	Paratyphoid fever C	002.3	Paratyphoid fever c
A01.4	Paratyphoid fever unspecified	002.9	Paratyphoid fever unspecified
A02.0	Salmonella enteritis	003.0	Salmonella gastroenteritis
A02.1	Salmonella sepsis	003.1	Salmonella septicemia
A02.20	Localized salmonella infection unspecified	003.20	Localized salmonella infection unspecified
A02.21	Salmonella meningitis	003.21	Salmonella meningitis
A02.22	Salmonella pneumonia	003.22	Salmonella pneumonia
A02.23	Salmonella arthritis	003.23	Salmonella arthritis
B00.0	Eczema herpeticum	054.0	Eczema herpeticum
B00.1	Herpesviral vesicular dermatitis	054.73	Herpes simplex otitis externa
B00.2	Herpesviral gingivostomatitis and pharyngotonsillitis	054.2	Herpetic gingivostomatitis

B00.3	Herpesviral meningitis	054.72	Herpes simplex meningitis
B00.4	Herpesviral encephalitis	058.29	Other human herpesvirus encephalitis
B00.50	Herpesviral ocular disease unspecified	054.40	Herpes simplex with unspecified ophthalmic complication
B00.51	Herpesviral iridocyclitis	054.44	Herpes simplex iridocyclitis
B00.52	Herpesviral keratitis	054.42	Dendritic keratitis
B00.52	Herpesviral keratitis	054.43	Herpes simplex disciform keratitis
B00.53	Herpesviral conjunctivitis	054.49	Herpes simplex with other ophthalmic complications
B00.59	Other herpesviral disease of eye	054.41	Herpes simplex dermatitis of eyelid
B00.59	Other herpesviral disease of eye	054.49	Herpes simplex with other ophthalmic complications
B00.7	Disseminated herpesviral disease	054.5	Herpetic septicemia
B00.81	Herpesviral hepatitis	054.71	Visceral herpes simplex
B00.82	Herpes simplex myelitis	054.74	Herpes simplex myelitis
B00.89	Other herpesviral infection	054.6	Herpetic whitlow
B00.89	Other herpesviral infection	054.79	Herpes simplex with other specified complications
B00.9	Herpesviral infection unspecified	054.8	Herpes simplex with unspecified complication
B00.9	Herpesviral infection unspecified	054.9	Herpes simplex without complication
B01.0	Varicella meningitis	047.8	Other specified viral meningitis

CHAPTER 2: NEOPLASMS (C00-D49)

GENERAL GUIDELINES

Chapter 2 of the ICD-10-CM contains the codes for most benign and all malignant neoplasms. Certain benign neoplasms, such as prostatic adenomas, may be found in the specific body system chapters. To properly code a neoplasm it is necessary to determine from the record if the neoplasm is benign, in-situ, malignant, or of uncertain histologic behavior. If malignant, any secondary (metastatic) sites should also be determined.

The neoplasm table in the Alphabetic Index should be referenced first. However, if the histological term is documented, that term should be referenced first, rather than going immediately to the Neoplasm Table, in order to determine which column in the Neoplasm Table is appropriate. For example, if the documentation indicates "adenoma," refer to the term in the Alphabetic Index to review the entries under this term and the instructional note to "see also neoplasm, by site, benign." The table provides the proper code based on the type of neoplasm and the site. It is important to select the proper column in the table that corresponds to the type of neoplasm. The Tabular List should then be referenced to verify that the correct code has been selected from the table and that a more specific site code does not exist.

TREATMENT DIRECTED AT THE MALIGNANCY

If the treatment is directed at the malignancy, designate the malignancy as the principal diagnosis. The only exception to this guideline is if a patient admission/encounter is solely for the administration of chemotherapy, immunotherapy or radiation therapy, assign the appropriate Z51.-- code as the first-listed or principal diagnosis, and the diagnosis or problem for which the service is being performed as a secondary diagnosis.

TREATMENT OF SECONDARY SITE

When a patient is admitted because of a primary neoplasm with metastasis and treatment is directed toward the secondary site only, the secondary neoplasm is designated as the principal diagnosis even though the primary malignancy is still present.

CODING AND SEQUENCING OF COMPLICATIONS

Coding and sequencing of complications associated with the malignancies or with the therapy thereof are subject to the following guidelines:

1) **Anemia associated with malignancy**

   When admission/encounter is for management of an anemia associated with the malignancy, and the treatment is only for anemia, the appropriate code for the malignancy is sequenced as the principal or first-listed diagnosis followed by code D63.0, Anemia in neoplastic disease.

2) **Anemia associated with chemotherapy, immunotherapy and radiation therapy**

   When the admission/encounter is for management of an anemia associated with an adverse effect of chemotherapy or immuno-therapy and the only treatment is for the anemia, the appropriate adverse effect code should be sequenced first, followed by the appropriate codes for the anemia and neoplasm.

   When the admission/encounter is for management of an anemia associated with an adverse effect of radiotherapy, the anemia code should be sequenced first, followed by the appropriate neoplasm code and code Y84.2, Radiological procedure and radiotherapy as the cause of abnormal reaction of the patient, or of later complication, without mention of misadventure at the time of the procedure.

3) **Management of dehydration due to the malignancy**

   When the admission/encounter is for management of dehydration due to the malignancy and only the dehydration is being treated (intravenous rehydration), the dehydration is sequenced first, followed by the code(s) for the malignancy.

4) **Treatment of a complication resulting from a surgical procedure**

   When the admission/encounter is for treatment of a complication resulting from a surgical procedure, designate the complication as the principal or first-listed diagnosis if treatment is directed at resolving the complication.

PRIMARY MALIGNANCY PREVIOUSLY EXCISED

When a primary malignancy has been previously excised or eradicated from its site and there is no further treatment directed to that site and there is no evidence of any existing primary malignancy, a code from category Z85, Personal history of malignant neoplasm, should be used to indicate the former site of the malignancy. Any mention of extension, invasion, or metastasis to another site is coded as a secondary malignant neoplasm to that site. The secondary site may be the principal or first-listed with the Z85 code used as a secondary code.

ADMISSIONS/ENCOUNTERS INVOLVING CHEMOTHERAPY, IMMUNOTHERAPY AND RADIATION THERAPY

1) Episode of care involves surgical removal of neoplasm

When an episode of care involves the surgical removal of a neoplasm, primary or secondary site, followed by adjunct chemotherapy or radiation treatment during the same episode of care, the code for the neoplasm should be assigned as principal or first-listed diagnosis.

2) Patient admission/encounter solely for administration of chemotherapy, immunotherapy and radiation therapy

If a patient admission/encounter is solely for the administration of chemotherapy, immunotherapy or radiation therapy assign code Z51.0, Encounter for antineoplastic radiation therapy, or Z51.11, Encounter for antineoplastic chemotherapy, or Z51.12, Encounter for antineoplastic immunotherapy as the first-listed or principal diagnosis. If a patient receives more than one of these therapies during the same admission more than one of these codes may be assigned, in any sequence.

The malignancy for which the therapy is being administered should be assigned as a secondary diagnosis.

3) Patient admitted for radiation therapy, chemotherapy or immunotherapy and develops complications

When a patient is admitted for the purpose of radiotherapy, immunotherapy or chemotherapy and develops complications such as uncontrolled nausea and vomiting or dehydration, the principal or first-listed diagnosis is Z51.0, Encounter for antineoplastic radiation therapy, or Z51.11, Encounter for antineoplastic chemotherapy, or Z51.12, Encounter for antineoplastic immunotherapy followed by any codes for the complications.

ADMISSION/ENCOUNTER TO DETERMINE EXTENT OF MALIGNANCY

When the reason for admission/encounter is to determine the extent of the malignancy, or for a procedure such as paracentesis or thoracentesis, the primary malignancy or appropriate metastatic site is designated as the principal or first-listed diagnosis, even though chemotherapy or radiotherapy is administered.

SYMPTOMS, SIGNS, AND ABNORMAL FINDINGS LISTED IN CHAPTER 18 ASSOCIATED WITH NEOPLASMS

Symptoms, signs, and ill-defined conditions listed in Chapter 18 characteristic of, or associated with, an existing primary or secondary site malignancy cannot be used to replace the malignancy as principal or first-listed diagnosis, regardless of the number of admissions or encounters for treatment and care of the neoplasm.

MALIGNANCY IN TWO OR MORE NONCONTIGUOUS SITES

A patient may have more than one malignant tumor in the same organ. These tumors may represent different primaries or metastatic disease, depending on the site. Should the documentation be unclear, the provider should be queried as to the status of each tumor so that the correct codes can be assigned.

DISSEMINATED MALIGNANT NEOPLASM, UNSPECIFIED

Code C80.0, Disseminated malignant neoplasm, unspecified, is for use only in those cases where the patient has advanced metastatic disease and no known primary or secondary sites are specified. It should not be used in place of assigning codes for the primary site and all known secondary sites.

MALIGNANT NEOPLASM WITHOUT SPECIFICATION OF SITE

Code C80.1, Malignant (primary) neoplasm, unspecified, equates to Cancer, unspecified. This code should only be used when no determination can be made as to the primary site of a malignancy. This code should rarely be used in the inpatient setting.

SEQUENCING OF NEOPLASM CODES

1) **Encounter for treatment of primary malignancy**

   If the reason for the encounter is for treatment of a primary malignancy, assign the malignancy as the principal/first-listed diagnosis. The primary site is to be sequenced first, followed by any metastatic sites.

2) **Encounter for treatment of secondary malignancy**

   When an encounter is for a primary malignancy with metastasis and treatment is directed toward the metastatic (secondary) site(s) only, the metastatic site(s) is designated as the principal/first-listed diagnosis. The primary malignancy is coded as an additional code.

3) **Malignant neoplasm in a pregnant patient**

   When a pregnant woman has a malignant neoplasm, a code from subcategory O9A.1-, Malignant neoplasm complicating pregnancy, childbirth, and the puerperium, should be sequenced first, followed by the appropriate code from Chapter 2 to indicate the type of neoplasm.

4) **Encounter for complication associated with a neoplasm**

When an encounter is for management of a complication associated with a neoplasm, such as dehydration, and the treatment is only for the complication, the complication is coded first, followed by the appropriate code(s) for the neoplasm.

The exception to this guideline is anemia. When the admission/encounter is for management of an anemia associated with the malignancy, and the treatment is only for anemia, the appropriate code for the malignancy is sequenced as the principal or first-listed diagnosis followed by code D63.0, Anemia in neoplastic disease.

5) Complication from surgical procedure for treatment of a neoplasm

When an encounter is for treatment of a complication resulting from a surgical procedure performed for the treatment of the neoplasm, designate the complication as the principal/first-listed diagnosis. See guideline regarding the coding of a current malignancy versus personal history to determine if the code for the neoplasm should also be assigned.

6) Pathologic fracture due to a neoplasm

When an encounter is for a pathological fracture due to a neoplasm, if the focus of treatment is the fracture, a code from subcategory M84.5, Pathological fracture in neoplastic disease, should be sequenced first, followed by the code for the neoplasm.

If the focus of treatment is the neoplasm with an associated pathological fracture, the neoplasm code should be sequenced first, followed by a code from M84.5 for the pathological fracture.

CURRENT MALIGNANCY VERSUS PERSONAL HISTORY OF MALIGNANCY

When a primary malignancy has been excised but further treatment, such as an additional surgery for the malignancy, radiation therapy or chemotherapy is directed to that site, the primary malignancy code should be used until treatment is completed.

When a primary malignancy has been previously excised or eradicated from its site, there is no further treatment (of the malignancy) directed to that site, and there is no evidence of any existing primary malignancy, a code from category Z85, Personal history of malignant neoplasm, should be used to indicate the former site of the malignancy.

Leukemia, Multiple Myeloma, and Malignant Plasma Cell Neoplasms in remission versus personal history

The categories for leukemia, and category C90, Multiple myeloma and malignant plasma cell neoplasms, have codes for in remission. There are also codes Z85.6, Personal history of leukemia, and Z85.79, Personal history of other malignant neoplasms of lymphoid, hematopoietic and related tissues. If the documentation is unclear, as to whether the patient is in remission, the provider should be queried.

Malignant Neoplasm Associated With Transplanted Organ

A malignant neoplasm of a transplanted organ should be coded as a transplant complication. Assign first the appropriate code from category T86.-, Complications of transplanted organs and tissue, followed by code C80.2, Malignant neoplasm associated with transplanted organ. Use an additional code for the specific malignancy.

SAMPLE ICD-10-CM CODES FROM THIS CHAPTER

NEOPLASMS (C00-D49)

NOTE: FUNCTIONAL ACTIVITY

All neoplasms are classified in this chapter, whether they are functionally active or not. An additional code from Chapter 4 may be used, to identify functional activity associated with any neoplasm.

MORPHOLOGY [HISTOLOGY]

Chapter 2 classifies neoplasms primarily by site (topography), with broad groupings for behavior, malignant, in situ, benign, etc. The Table of Neoplasms should be used to identify the correct topography code. In a few cases, such as for malignant melanoma and certain neuroendocrine tumors, the morphology (histologic type) is included in the category and codes. To identify the morphology for the majority of Chapter 2 codes that do not include the histologic type, comprehensive separate morphology codes are provided. These morphology codes are derived from the International Classification of Diseases for Oncology (ICD-O).

PRIMARY MALIGNANT NEOPLASMS OVERLAPPING SITE BOUNDARIES

A primary malignant neoplasm that overlaps two or more contiguous (next to each other) sites should be classified to the subcategory/code .8 ('overlapping lesion'), unless the combination is specifically indexed elsewhere. For multiple neoplasms of the same site that are not contiguous, such as tumors in different quadrants of the same breast, codes for each site should be assigned.

MALIGNANT NEOPLASM OF ECTOPIC TISSUE

Malignant neoplasms of ectopic tissue are to be coded to the site mentioned, e.g., ectopic pancreatic malignant neoplasms are coded to pancreas, unspecified (C25.9).

This chapter contains the following blocks:	
C00-C14	Malignant neoplasm of lip, oral cavity and pharynx
C15-C26	Malignant neoplasm of digestive organs
C30-C39	Malignant neoplasm of respiratory and intrathoracic organs
C40-C41	Malignant neoplasm of bone and articular cartilage
C43-C44	Melanoma and other malignant neoplasms of skin
C45-C49	Malignant neoplasms of mesothelial and soft tissue
C50	Malignant neoplasm of breast
C51-C58	Malignant neoplasm of female genital organs
C60-C63	Malignant neoplasms of male genital organs
C64-C68	Malignant neoplasm of urinary tract
C69-C72	Malignant neoplasms of eye, brain and other parts of central nervous system
C73-C75	Malignant neoplasm of thyroid and other endocrine glands
C7A	Malignant neuroendocrine tumors

C7B	Secondary neuroendocrine tumors
C76-C80	Malignant neoplasms of ill-defined, other secondary and unspecified sites
C81-C96	Malignant neoplasms of lymphoid, hematopoietic and related tissue
D00-D09	In situ neoplasms
D10-D36	Benign neoplasms, except benign neuroendocrine tumors
D3A	Benign neuroendocrine tumors
D37-D48	Neoplasms of uncertain behavior, polycythemia vera and myelodysplastic syndromes
D49	Neoplasms of unspecified behavior

C40 MALIGNANT NEOPLASM OF BONE AND ARTICULAR CARTILAGE OF LIMBS

Use additional code to identify major osseous defect, if applicable (M89.7-)

C40.0 Malignant neoplasm of scapula and long bones of upper limb

C40.00   Malignant neoplasm of scapula and long bones of unspecified upper limb

C40.01   Malignant neoplasm of scapula and long bones of right upper limb

C40.02   Malignant neoplasm of scapula and long bones of left upper limb

C40.1 Malignant neoplasm of short bones of upper limb

C40.10   Malignant neoplasm of short bones of unspecified upper limb

C40.11   Malignant neoplasm of short bones of right upper limb

C40.12   Malignant neoplasm of short bones of left upper limb

C40.2 Malignant neoplasm of long bones of lower limb

C40.20   Malignant neoplasm of long bones of unspecified lower limb

C40.21   Malignant neoplasm of long bones of right lower limb

C40.22   Malignant neoplasm of long bones of left lower limb

C40.3 Malignant neoplasm of short bones of lower limb

C40.30   Malignant neoplasm of short bones of unspecified lower limb

C40.31   Malignant neoplasm of short bones of right lower limb

C40.32   Malignant neoplasm of short bones of left lower limb

C40.8 Malignant neoplasm of overlapping sites of bone and articular cartilage of limb

C40.80   Malignant neoplasm of overlapping sites of bone and articular cartilage of unspecified limb

C40.81   Malignant neoplasm of overlapping sites of bone and articular cartilage of right limb

C40.82   Malignant neoplasm of overlapping sites of bone and articular cartilage of left limb

C40.9 Malignant neoplasm of unspecified bones and articular cartilage of limb

C40.90   Malignant neoplasm of unspecified bones and articular cartilage of unspecified limb
C40.91   Malignant neoplasm of unspecified bones and articular cartilage of right limb
C40.92   Malignant neoplasm of unspecified bones and articular cartilage of left limb

C41 Malignant neoplasm of bone and articular cartilage of other and unspecified sites

Excludes 1: malignant neoplasm of bones of limbs (C40.-)
malignant neoplasm of cartilage of:
ear (C49.0)
eyelid (C49.0)
larynx (C32.3)
limbs (C40.-)
nose (C30.0)

C41.0 Malignant neoplasm of bones of skull and face
Malignant neoplasm of maxilla (superior)
Malignant neoplasm of orbital bone

Excludes 2: carcinoma, any type except intraosseous or odontogenic of:
maxillary sinus (C31.0)
upper jaw (C03.0)
malignant neoplasm of jaw bone (lower) (C41.1)

C41.1 Malignant neoplasm of mandible
Malignant neoplasm of inferior maxilla
Malignant neoplasm of lower jaw bone

Excludes 2: carcinoma, any type except intraosseous or odontogenic of:
jaw NOS (C03.9)
lower (C03.1)
malignant neoplasm of upper jaw bone (C41.0)

C41.2 Malignant neoplasm of vertebral column

Excludes 1: malignant neoplasm of sacrum and coccyx (C41.4)

C41.3 Malignant neoplasm of ribs, sternum and clavicle

FORWARD MAPPING SAMPLE (ICD-9-CM ➡ ICD-10-CM)

ICD-9-CM CODE & DESCRIPTION		ICD-10-CM CODE & DESCRIPTION	
150.0	Malignant neoplasm of cervical esophagus	C15.3	Malignant neoplasm of upper third of esophagus
150.1	Malignant neoplasm of thoracic esophagus	C15.4	Malignant neoplasm of middle third of esophagus
150.2	Malignant neoplasm of abdominal esophagus	C15.5	Malignant neoplasm of lower third of esophagus
150.3	Malignant neoplasm of upper third of esophagus	C15.3	Malignant neoplasm of upper third of esophagus
150.4	Malignant neoplasm of middle third of esophagus	C15.4	Malignant neoplasm of middle third of esophagus
150.5	Malignant neoplasm of lower third of esophagus	C15.5	Malignant neoplasm of lower third of esophagus
150.8	Malignant neoplasm of other specified part of esophagus	C15.8	Malignant neoplasm of overlapping sites of esophagus
150.9	Malignant neoplasm of esophagus unspecified site	C15.9	Malignant neoplasm of esophagus unspecified
151.0	Malignant neoplasm of cardia	C16.0	Malignant neoplasm of cardia
151.1	Malignant neoplasm of pylorus	C16.4	Malignant neoplasm of pylorus
151.2	Malignant neoplasm of pyloric antrum	C16.3	Malignant neoplasm of pyloric antrum
151.3	Malignant neoplasm of fundus of stomach	C16.1	Malignant neoplasm of fundus of stomach
151.4	Malignant neoplasm of body of stomach	C16.2	Malignant neoplasm of body of stomach
151.5	Malignant neoplasm of lesser curvature of stomach unspecified	C16.5	Malignant neoplasm of lesser curvature of stomach unspecified
151.6	Malignant neoplasm of greater curvature of stomach unspecified	C16.6	Malignant neoplasm of greater curvature of stomach unspecified
151.8	Malignant neoplasm of other specified sites of stomach	C16.8	Malignant neoplasm of overlapping sites of stomach
151.9	Malignant neoplasm of stomach unspecified site	C16.9	Malignant neoplasm of stomach unspecified
152.0	Malignant neoplasm of duodenum	C17.0	Malignant neoplasm of duodenum
152.1	Malignant neoplasm of jejunum	C17.1	Malignant neoplasm of jejunum
152.2	Malignant neoplasm of ileum	C17.2	Malignant neoplasm of ileum
152.3	Malignant neoplasm of Meckel's diverticulum	C17.3	Meckel's diverticulum malignant
152.8	Malignant neoplasm of other specified sites of small intestine	C17.8	Malignant neoplasm of overlapping sites of small intestine
152.9	Malignant neoplasm of small intestine unspecified site	C17.9	Malignant neoplasm of small intestine unspecified

153.0	Malignant neoplasm of hepatic flexure	C18.3	Malignant neoplasm of hepatic flexure
153.1	Malignant neoplasm of transverse colon	C18.4	Malignant neoplasm of transverse colon
153.2	Malignant neoplasm of descending colon	C18.6	Malignant neoplasm of descending colon
153.3	Malignant neoplasm of sigmoid colon	C18.7	Malignant neoplasm of sigmoid colon
153.4	Malignant neoplasm of cecum	C18.0	Malignant neoplasm of cecum
153.5	Malignant neoplasm of appendix vermiformis	C18.1	Malignant neoplasm of appendix
153.6	Malignant neoplasm of ascending colon	C18.2	Malignant neoplasm of ascending colon
153.7	Malignant neoplasm of splenic flexure	C18.5	Malignant neoplasm of splenic flexure
153.8	Malignant neoplasm of other specified sites of large intestine	C18.8	Malignant neoplasm of overlapping sites of colon
153.9	Malignant neoplasm of colon unspecified site	C18.9	Malignant neoplasm of colon unspecified
154.0	Malignant neoplasm of rectosigmoid junction	C19	Malignant neoplasm of rectosigmoid junction
154.1	Malignant neoplasm of rectum	C20	Malignant neoplasm of rectum
154.2	Malignant neoplasm of anal canal	C21.1	Malignant neoplasm of anal canal
154.3	Malignant neoplasm of anus unspecified site	C21.0	Malignant neoplasm of anus unspecified
154.8	Malignant neoplasm of other sites of rectum rectosigmoid junction and anus	C21.8	Malignant neoplasm of overlapping sites of rectum anus and anal canal
155.0	Malignant neoplasm of liver primary	C22.0	Liver cell carcinoma
155.0	Malignant neoplasm of liver primary	C22.2	Hepatoblastoma

BACKWARD MAPPING SAMPLE (ICD-10-CM ➡ ICD-9-CM)			
ICD-10-CM CODE & DESCRIPTION		ICD-9-CM CODE & DESCRIPTION	
C00.0	Malignant neoplasm of external upper lip	140.0	Malignant neoplasm of upper lip vermilion border
C00.1	Malignant neoplasm of external lower lip	140.1	Malignant neoplasm of lower lip vermilion border
C00.2	Malignant neoplasm of external lip unspecified	140.9	Malignant neoplasm of lip unspecified vermilion border
C00.3	Malignant neoplasm of upper lip inner aspect	140.3	Malignant neoplasm of upper lip inner aspect
C00.4	Malignant neoplasm of lower lip inner aspect	140.4	Malignant neoplasm of lower lip inner aspect

C00.5	Malignant neoplasm of lip unspecified inner aspect	140.5	Malignant neoplasm of lip unspecified inner aspect
C00.6	Malignant neoplasm of commissure of lip unspecified	140.6	Malignant neoplasm of commissure of lip
C00.8	Malignant neoplasm of overlapping sites of lip	140.8	Malignant neoplasm of other sites of lip
C00.9	Malignant neoplasm of lip unspecified	140.9	Malignant neoplasm of lip unspecified vermilion border
C01	Malignant neoplasm of base of tongue	141.0	Malignant neoplasm of base of tongue
C02.0	Malignant neoplasm of dorsal surface of tongue	141.1	Malignant neoplasm of dorsal surface of tongue
C02.1	Malignant neoplasm of border of tongue	141.2	Malignant neoplasm of tip and lateral border of tongue
C02.2	Malignant neoplasm of ventral surface of tongue	141.3	Malignant neoplasm of ventral surface of tongue
C02.3	Malignant neoplasm of anterior two-thirds of tongue part unspecified	141.4	Malignant neoplasm of anterior two-thirds of tongue part unspecified
C02.4	Malignant neoplasm of lingual tonsil	141.6	Malignant neoplasm of lingual tonsil
C02.8	Malignant neoplasm of overlapping sites of tongue	141.8	Malignant neoplasm of other sites of tongue
C02.9	Malignant neoplasm of tongue unspecified	141.9	Malignant neoplasm of tongue unspecified
C03.0	Malignant neoplasm of upper gum	143.0	Malignant neoplasm of upper gum
C03.1	Malignant neoplasm of lower gum	143.1	Malignant neoplasm of lower gum
C03.9	Malignant neoplasm of gum unspecified	143.8	Malignant neoplasm of other sites of gum
D00.00	Carcinoma in situ of oral cavity unspecified site	230.0	Carcinoma in situ of lip oral cavity and pharynx
D00.01	Carcinoma in situ of labial mucosa and vermilion border	230.0	Carcinoma in situ of lip oral cavity and pharynx
D00.02	Carcinoma in situ of buccal mucosa	230.0	Carcinoma in situ of lip oral cavity and pharynx
D00.03	Carcinoma in situ of gingiva and edentulous alveolar ridge	230.0	Carcinoma in situ of lip oral cavity and pharynx
D00.04	Carcinoma in situ of soft palate	230.0	Carcinoma in situ of lip oral cavity and pharynx
D00.05	Carcinoma in situ of hard palate	230.0	Carcinoma in situ of lip oral cavity and pharynx
D00.06	Carcinoma in situ of floor of mouth	230.0	Carcinoma in situ of lip oral cavity and pharynx
D00.07	Carcinoma in situ of tongue	230.0	Carcinoma in situ of lip oral cavity and pharynx

D00.08	Carcinoma in situ of pharynx	230.0	Carcinoma in situ of lip oral cavity and pharynx
D00.1	Carcinoma in situ of esophagus	230.1	Carcinoma in situ of esophagus
D00.2	Carcinoma in situ of stomach	230.2	Carcinoma in situ of stomach
D01.0	Carcinoma in situ of colon	230.3	Carcinoma in situ of colon
D01.1	Carcinoma in situ of rectosigmoid junction	230.4	Carcinoma in situ of rectum
D01.2	Carcinoma in situ of rectum	230.4	Carcinoma in situ of rectum
D01.3	Carcinoma in situ of anus and anal canal	230.5	Carcinoma in situ of anal canal
D01.3	Carcinoma in situ of anus and anal canal	230.6	Carcinoma in situ of anus unspecified
D01.40	Carcinoma in situ of unspecified part of intestine	230.7	Carcinoma in situ of other and unspecified parts of intestine
D01.49	Carcinoma in situ of other parts of intestine	230.7	Carcinoma in situ of other and unspecified parts of intestine
D01.5	Carcinoma in situ of liver gallbladder and bile ducts	230.8	Carcinoma in situ of liver and biliary system
D01.7	Carcinoma in situ of other specified digestive organs	230.9	Carcinoma in situ of other and unspecified digestive organs

ICD-10-CM TABLE OF NEOPLASMS

The list below gives the code numbers for neoplasms by anatomical site. For each site there are six possible code numbers according to whether the neoplasm in question is malignant, benign, in situ, of uncertain behavior, or of unspecified nature. The description of the neoplasm will often indicate which of the six columns is appropriate; e.g., malignant melanoma of skin, benign fibroadenoma of breast, carcinoma in situ of cervix uteri.

	Malignant Primary	Malignant Secondary	Ca in Situ	Benign	Uncertain Behavior	Unspecified Behavior
Neoplasm, neoplastic	C80.1	C79.9	D09.9	D36.9	D48.9	D49.9
abdomen, abdominal	C76.2	C79.8-	D09.8	D36.7	D48.7	D49.89
- cavity	C76.2	C79.8-	D09.8	D36.7	D48.7	D49.89
- organ	C76.2	C79.8-	D09.8	D36.7	D48.7	D49.89
- viscera	C76.2	C79.8-	D09.8	D36.7	D48.7	D49.89
- wall	C44.59	C79.2-	D04.5	D23.5	D48.5	D49.2
- - connective tissue	C49.4	C79.8-	-	D21.4	D48.1	D49.2
abdominopelvic	C76.8	C79.8-	-	D36.7	D48.7	D49.89
accessory sinus-see Neoplasm, sinus						
acoustic nerve	C72.4-	C79.49	-	D33.3	D43.3	D49.7
adenoid (pharynx) (tissue)	C11.1	C79.89	D00.08	D10.6	D37.05	D49.0
adipose tissue—see also Neoplasm, connective tissue	C49.4	C79.89	-	D21.9	D48.1	D49.2
adnexa (uterine)	C57.4	C79.89	D07.39	D28.7	D39.8	D49.5
adrenal	C74.9-	C79.7-	D09.3	D35.0-	D44.1-	D49.7
- capsule	C74.9-	C79.7-	D09.3	D35.0-	D44.1-	D49.7

- cortex	C74.0-	C79.7-	D09.3	D35.0-	D44.1-	D49.7
- gland	C74.9-	C79.7-	D09.3	D35.0-	D44.1-	D49.7
- medulla	C74.1-	C79.7-	D09.3	D35.0-	D44.1-	D49.7
ala nasi (external)	C44.31	C79.2	D04.39	D23.39	D48.5	D49.2
alimentary canal or tract NEC	C26.9	C78.80	D01.9	D13.9	D37.9	D49.0

Codes listed with a dash -, following the code have a required 5th character for laterality. The tabular list must be reviewed for the complete code.

CHAPTER 3: DISEASE OF THE BLOOD AND BLOOD-FORMING ORGANS AND CERTAIN DISORDERS INVOLVING THE IMMUNE MECHANISM (D50-D89)

GENERAL GUIDELINES

Excludes2: autoimmune disease (systemic) NOS (M35.9)
certain conditions originating in the perinatal period (P00-P96)
complications of pregnancy, childbirth and the puerperium (O00-O99)
congenital malformations, deformations and chromosomal abnormalities (Q00-Q99)
endocrine, nutritional and metabolic diseases (E00-E88)
human immunodeficiency virus [HIV] disease (B20)
injury, poisoning and certain other consequences of external causes (S00-T88)
neoplasms (C00-D49)
symptoms, signs and abnormal clinical and laboratory findings, not elsewhere classified (R00-R94)

This chapter contains the following blocks:	
D50-D53	Nutritional anemias
D55-D59	Hemolytic anemias
D60-D64	Aplastic and other anemias and other bone marrow failure syndromes
D65-D69	Coagulation defects, purpura and other hemorrhagic conditions
D70-D77	Other disorders of blood and blood-forming organs
D78	Intraoperative and postprocedural complications of the spleen
D80-D89	Certain disorders involving the immune mechanism

SAMPLE ICD-10-CM CODES FROM THIS CHAPTER

NUTRITIONAL ANEMIAS (D50-D53)

D50   Iron deficiency anemia

> *Includes:*   asiderotic anemia
> hypochromic anemia

> **D50.0   Iron deficiency anemia secondary to blood loss (chronic)**
> Posthemorrhagic anemia (chronic)

Excludes 1: acute posthemorrhagic anemia (D62)
  congenital anemia from fetal blood loss (P61.3)

D50.1 Sideropenic dysphagia
Kelly-Paterson syndrome
Plummer-Vinson syndrome

D50.8 Other iron deficiency anemias
Iron deficiency anemia due to inadequate dietary iron intake

D50.9 Iron deficiency anemia, unspecified

D51 Vitamin B12 deficiency anemia

Excludes 1: vitamin B12   deficiency (E53.8)

D51.0 Vitamin B12 deficiency anemia due to intrinsic factor deficiency
Addison anemia
Biermer anemia
Pernicious (congenital) anemia
Congenital intrinsic factor deficiency

D51.1 Vitamin B12 deficiency anemia due to selective vitamin B12 malabsorption with proteinuria
Imerslund (Gräsbeck) syndrome
Megaloblastic hereditary anemia

D51.2 Transcobalamin II deficiency

D51.3 Other dietary vitamin B12 deficiency anemia
Vegan anemia

D51.8 Other vitamin B12 deficiency anemias

D51.9 Vitamin B12 deficiency anemia, unspecified

D52 Folate deficiency anemia

Excludes 1: folate deficiency without anemia (E53.8)

D52.0 Dietary folate deficiency anemia
Nutritional megaloblastic anemia

D52.1 Drug-induced folate deficiency anemia
Code first (T36-T50) to identify drug

D52.8 Other folate deficiency anemias

D52.9 Folate deficiency anemia, unspecified
Folic acid deficiency anemia NOS

D53   Other nutritional anemias

Includes: megaloblastic anemia unresponsive to vitamin B12 or folate therapy

D53.0   Protein deficiency anemia
Amino-acid deficiency anemia
Orotaciduric anemia
Excludes 1: Lesch-Nyhan syndrome (E79.1)

D53.1   Other megaloblastic anemias, not elsewhere classified
Megaloblastic anemia NOS

Excludes 1: Di Guglielmo's disease (C94.0)

D53.2   Scorbutic anemia

Excludes 1: scurvy (E54)

D53.8   Other specified nutritional anemias
Anemia associated with deficiency of copper
Anemia associated with deficiency of molybdenum
Anemia associated with deficiency of zinc

Excludes 1:   nutritional deficiencies without anemia, such as:
copper deficiency NOS (E61.0)
molybdenum deficiency NOS (E61.5)
zinc deficiency NOS (E60)

D53.9   Nutritional anemia, unspecified
Simple chronic anemia

Excludes 1: anemia NOS (D64.9)

HEMOLYTIC ANEMIAS (D55-D59)

D55   Anemia due to enzyme disorders

Excludes 1: drug-induced enzyme deficiency anemia (D59.2)

D55.0   Anemia due to glucose-6-phosphate dehydrogenase [G6PD] deficiency
Favism
G6PD deficiency anemia

D55.1   Anemia due to other disorders of glutathione metabolism
Anemia (due to) enzyme deficiencies, except G6PD, related to the hexose
monophosphate [HMP] shunt pathway
Anemia (due to) hemolytic nonspherocytic (hereditary), type I

D55.2   Anemia due to disorders of glycolytic enzymes
Hemolytic nonspherocytic (hereditary) anemia, type II
Hexokinase deficiency anemia

Pyruvate kinase [PK] deficiency anemia
Triose-phosphate isomerase deficiency anemia

Excludes 1: disorders of glycolysis not associated with anemia (E74.8)

D55.3 Anemia due to disorders of nucleotide metabolism

D55.8 Other anemias due to enzyme disorders

D55.9 Anemia due to enzyme disorder, unspecified

FORWARD MAPPING SAMPLE (ICD-9-CM ➡ ICD-10-CM)			
ICD-9-CM CODE & DESCRIPTION		**ICD-10-CM CODE & DESCRIPTION**	
280.0	Iron deficiency anemia secondary to blood loss (chronic)	D50.0	Iron deficiency anemia secondary to blood loss (chronic)
280.1	Iron deficiency anemia secondary to inadequate dietary iron intake	D50.8	Other iron deficiency anemias
280.8	Other specified iron deficiency anemias	D50.1	Sideropenic dysphagia
280.8	Other specified iron deficiency anemias	D50.8	Other iron deficiency anemias
280.9	Iron deficiency anemia unspecified	D50.9	Iron deficiency anemia unspecified
281.0	Pernicious anemia	D51.0	Vitamin B12 deficiency anemia due to intrinsic factor deficiency
281.1	Other vitamin B12 deficiency anemia	D51.1	Vitamin B12 deficiency anemia due to selective vitamin B12 malabsorption with proteinuria
281.1	Other vitamin B12 deficiency anemia	D51.3	Other dietary vitamin B12 deficiency anemia
281.1	Other vitamin B12 deficiency anemia	D51.8	Other vitamin B12 deficiency anemias
281.2	Folate-deficiency anemia	D52.1	Drug-induced folate deficiency anemia
281.2	Folate-deficiency anemia	D52.8	Other folate deficiency anemias
281.2	Folate-deficiency anemia	D52.0	Dietary folate deficiency anemia
281.2	Folate-deficiency anemia	D52.9	Folate deficiency anemia unspecified
281.3	Other specified megaloblastic anemias not elsewhere classified	D53.1	Other megaloblastic anemias not elsewhere classified
281.4	Protein-deficiency anemia	D53.0	Protein deficiency anemia
281.8	Anemia associated with other specified nutritional deficiency	D53.2	Scorbutic anemia
281.9	Unspecified deficiency anemia	D53.9	Nutritional anemia unspecified
282.0	Hereditary spherocytosis	D58.0	Hereditary spherocytosis
282.1	Hereditary elliptocytosis	D58.1	Hereditary elliptocytosis

282.2	Anemias due to disorders of glutathione metabolism	D55.0	Anemia due to glucose-6-phosphate dehydrogenase [G6PD] deficiency
282.2	Anemias due to disorders of glutathione metabolism	D55.1	Anemia due to other disorders of glutathione metabolism
282.3	Other hemolytic anemias due to enzyme deficiency	D55.8	Other anemias due to enzyme disorders
282.41	Sickle-cell thalassemia without crisis	D57.40	Sickle-cell thalassemia without crisis
282.42	Sickle-cell thalassemia with crisis	D57.419	Sickle-cell thalassemia with crisis unspecified
282.49	Other thalassemia	D56.3	Thalassemia minor
282.49	Other thalassemia	D56.8	Other thalassemias
282.49	Other thalassemia	D56.2	Delta-beta thalassemia
282.49	Other thalassemia	D56.1	Beta thalassemia
282.49	Other thalassemia	D56.0	Alpha thalassemia
282.5	Sickle-cell trait	D57.3	Sickle-cell trait
282.60	Sickle-cell disease, unspecified	D57.1	Sickle-cell disease without crisis
282.61	Hb-ss disease without crisis	D57.1	Sickle-cell disease without crisis
282.62	Hb-ss disease with crisis	D57.00	Hb-SS disease with crisis unspecified
282.63	Sickle-cell/hb-c disease without crisis	D57.20	Sickle-cell/Hb-C disease without crisis
282.64	Sickle-cell/hb c disease with crisis	D57.219	Sickle-cell/Hb-C disease with crisis unspecified
282.68	Other sickle-cell disease without crisis	D57.80	Other sickle-cell disorders without crisis
282.69	Other sickle-cell disease with crisis	D57.819	Other sickle-cell disorders with crisis unspecified
282.7	Other hemoglobinopathies	D58.2	Other hemoglobinopathies
282.7	Other hemoglobinopathies	D56.4	Hereditary persistence of fetal hemoglobin [HPFH]
282.8	Other specified hereditary hemolytic anemias	D58.8	Other specified hereditary hemolytic anemias

BACKWARD MAPPING SAMPLE (ICD-10-CM ➡ ICD-9-CM)

ICD-10-CM CODE & DESCRIPTION		ICD-9-CM CODE & DESCRIPTION	
D50.0	Iron deficiency anemia secondary to blood loss (chronic)	280.0	Iron deficiency anemia secondary to blood loss (chronic)
D50.1	Sideropenic dysphagia	280.8	Other specified iron deficiency anemias
D50.8	Other iron deficiency anemias	280.1	Iron deficiency anemia secondary to inadequate dietary iron intake

D50.8	Other iron deficiency anemias	280.8	Other specified iron deficiency anemias
D50.9	Iron deficiency anemia unspecified	280.9	Iron deficiency anemia unspecified
D51.0	Vitamin B12 deficiency anemia due to intrinsic factor deficiency	281.0	Pernicious anemia
D51.1	Vitamin B12 deficiency anemia due to selective vitamin B12 malabsorption with proteinuria	281.1	Other vitamin B12 deficiency anemia
D51.2	Transcobalamin II deficiency	281.1	Other vitamin B12 deficiency anemia
D51.3	Other dietary vitamin B12 deficiency anemia	281.1	Other vitamin B12 deficiency anemia
D51.8	Other vitamin B12 deficiency anemias	281.1	Other vitamin B12 deficiency anemia
D51.9	Vitamin B12 deficiency anemia unspecified	281.1	Other vitamin B12 deficiency anemia
D52.0	Dietary folate deficiency anemia	281.2	Folate-deficiency anemia
D52.1	Drug-induced folate deficiency anemia	281.2	Folate-deficiency anemia
D52.8	Other folate deficiency anemias	281.2	Folate-deficiency anemia
D52.9	Folate deficiency anemia unspecified	281.2	Folate-deficiency anemia
D53.0	Protein deficiency anemia	281.4	Protein-deficiency anemia
D53.1	Other megaloblastic anemias not elsewhere classified	281.3	Other specified megaloblastic anemias not elsewhere classified
D53.2	Scorbutic anemia	281.8	Anemia associated with other specified nutritional deficiency
D53.8	Other specified nutritional anemias	281.8	Anemia associated with other specified nutritional deficiency
D53.9	Nutritional anemia unspecified	281.9	Unspecified deficiency anemia
D55.0	Anemia due to glucose-6-phosphate dehydrogenase [G6PD] deficiency	282.2	Anemias due to disorders of glutathione metabolism
D55.1	Anemia due to other disorders of glutathione metabolism	282.2	Anemias due to disorders of glutathione metabolism
D55.2	Anemia due to disorders of glycolytic enzymes	282.3	Other hemolytic anemias due to enzyme deficiency
D55.3	Anemia due to disorders of nucleotide metabolism	282.3	Other hemolytic anemias due to enzyme deficiency
D55.8	Other anemias due to enzyme disorders	282.3	Other hemolytic anemias due to enzyme deficiency
D55.9	Anemia due to enzyme disorder unspecified	282.3	Other hemolytic anemias due to enzyme deficiency
D56.0	Alpha thalassemia	282.49	Other thalassemia

D56.1	Beta thalassemia	282.49	Other thalassemia
D56.2	Delta-beta thalassemia	282.49	Other thalassemia
D56.3	Thalassemia minor	282.49	Other thalassemia
D56.4	Hereditary persistence of fetal hemoglobin [HPFH]	282.7	Other hemoglobinopathies
D56.8	Other thalassemias	282.49	Other thalassemia
D56.9	Thalassemia unspecified	282.49	Other thalassemia
D57.00	Hb-SS disease with crisis unspecified	282.62	Hb-ss disease with crisis
D57.01	Hb-SS disease with acute chest syndrome	282.62	Hb-ss disease with crisis
D57.01	Hb-SS disease with acute chest syndrome	517.3	Acute chest syndrome
D57.02	Hb-SS disease with splenic sequestration	282.62	Hb-ss disease with crisis
D57.02	Hb-SS disease with splenic sequestration	289.52	Splenic sequestration
D57.1	Sickle-cell disease without crisis	282.60	Sickle-cell disease, unspecified
D57.1	Sickle-cell disease without crisis	282.61	Hb-ss disease without crisis

CHAPTER 4: ENDOCRINE, NUTRITIONAL, AND METABOLIC DISEASES (E00-E89)

GENERAL GUIDELINES

DIABETES MELLITUS

The diabetes mellitus codes are combination codes that include the type of diabetes mellitus, the body system affected, and the complications affecting that body system. As many codes within a particular category as are necessary to describe all of the complications of the disease may be used. They should be sequenced based on the reason for a particular encounter. Assign as many codes from categories E08 - E13 as needed to identify all of the associated conditions that the patient has.

1) **Type of diabetes**

   The age of a patient is not the sole determining factor, though most type 1 diabetics develop the condition before reaching puberty. For this reason type 1 diabetes mellitus is also referred to as juvenile diabetes.

2) **Type of diabetes mellitus not documented**

   If the type of diabetes mellitus is not documented in the medical record the default is E11.-, Type 2 diabetes mellitus.

3) Diabetes mellitus and the use of insulin

If the documentation in a medical record does not indicate the type of diabetes but does indicate that the patient uses insulin, code E11, Type 2 diabetes mellitus, should be assigned. Code Z79.4, Long-term (current) use of insulin, should also be assigned to indicate that the patient uses insulin. Code Z79.4 should not be assigned if insulin is given temporarily to bring a type 2 patient's blood sugar under control during an encounter.

4) Complications due to insulin pump malfunction

(a) Underdose of insulin due *to* insulin pump failure

An underdose of insulin due to an insulin pump failure should be assigned to a code from subcategory T85.6, Mechanical complication of other specified internal and external prosthetic devices, implants and grafts, that specifies the type of pump malfunction, as the principal or first-listed code, followed by code T38.3x6-, Underdosing of insulin and oral hypoglycemic [antidiabetic] drugs. Additional codes for the type of diabetes mellitus and any associated complications due to the underdosing should also be assigned.

(b) Overdose of insulin due to insulin pump failure

The principal or first-listed code for an encounter due to an insulin pump malfunction resulting in an overdose of insulin, should also be T85.6-, Mechanical complication of other specified internal and external prosthetic devices, implants and grafts, followed by code T38.3x1-, Poisoning by insulin and oral hypoglycemic [antidiabetic] drugs, accidental (unintentional).

5) Secondary Diabetes Mellitus

Codes under categories E08, Diabetes mellitus due to underlying condition, and E09, Drug or chemical induced diabetes mellitus, identify complications/manifestations associated with secondary diabetes mellitus. Secondary diabetes is always caused by another condition or event (e.g., cystic fibrosis, malignant neoplasm of pancreas, pancreatectomy, adverse effect of drug, or poisoning).

(a) Secondary diabetes mellitus and the use of insulin

For patients who routinely use insulin, code Z79.4, Long-term (current) use of insulin, should also be assigned. Code Z79.4 should not be assigned if insulin is given temporarily to bring a patient's blood sugar under control during an encounter.

(b) Assigning and sequencing secondary diabetes codes and its causes

The sequencing of the secondary diabetes codes in relationship to codes for the cause of the diabetes is based on the Tabular List instructions for categories E08 and E09. For example, for category E08, Diabetes mellitus due to underlying condition, code first the underlying condition; for category E09, Drug or chemical induced diabetes mellitus, code first the drug or chemical (T36-T65).

(i) Secondary diabetes mellitus due to pancreatectomy

For post-pancreatectomy diabetes mellitus (lack of insulin due to the surgical removal of all or part of the pancreas), assign code E89.1, Postprocedural hypoinsulinemia. Assign a code from category E13 and a code from subcategory Z90.41-, Acquired absence of pancreas, as additional codes.

(ii) Secondary diabetes due to drugs

Secondary diabetes may be caused by an adverse effect of correctly administered medications, poisoning or late effect of poisoning. See section I.C.19.e for coding of adverse effects and poisoning, and section I.C.20 for external cause code reporting.

SAMPLE ICD-10-CM CODES FROM THIS CHAPTER

Note: All neoplasms, whether functionally active or not, are classified in Chapter 2. Appropriate codes in this chapter (i.e. E05.8, E07.0, E16-E31, E34.-) may be used as additional codes to indicate either functional activity by neoplasms and ectopic endocrine tissue or hyperfunction and hypofunction of endocrine glands associated with neoplasms and other conditions classified elsewhere.

Excludes 1: transitory endocrine and metabolic disorders specific to newborn (P70-P74)

This chapter contains the following blocks:	
E00-E07	Disorders of thyroid gland
E08-E13	Diabetes mellitus
E15-E16	Other disorders of glucose regulation and pancreatic internal secretion
E20-E35	Disorders of other endocrine glands
E36	Intraoperative complications of endocrine system
E40-E46	Malnutrition
E50-E64	Other nutritional deficiencies
E65-E68	Overweight, obesity and other hyperalimentation
E70-E88	Metabolic disorders
E89	Postprocedural endocrine and metabolic complications and disorders, not elsewhere classified

DISORDERS OF THYROID GLAND (E00-E07)

E00 Congenital iodine-deficiency syndrome

Use additional code (F70-F79) to identify associated mental retardation.

Excludes 1: subclinical iodine-deficiency hypothyroidism (E02)

E00.0 Congenital iodine-deficiency syndrome, neurological type
Endemic cretinism, neurological type

E00.1 Congenital iodine-deficiency syndrome, myxedematous type
Endemic hypothyroid cretinism

Endemic cretinism, myxedematous type

E00.2 **Congenital iodine-deficiency syndrome, mixed type**
Endemic cretinism, mixed type

E00.9 **Congenital iodine-deficiency syndrome, unspecified**
Congenital iodine-deficiency hypothyroidism NOS
Endemic cretinism NOS

E01 **Iodine-deficiency related thyroid disorders and allied conditions**

Excludes 1: congenital iodine-deficiency syndrome (E00.-)
subclinical iodine-deficiency hypothyroidism (E02)

E01.0 **Iodine-deficiency related diffuse (endemic) goiter**

E01.1 **Iodine-deficiency related multinodular (endemic) goiter**
Iodine-deficiency related nodular goiter

E01.2 **Iodine-deficiency related (endemic) goiter, unspecified**
Endemic goiter NOS

E01.8 **Other iodine-deficiency related thyroid disorders and allied conditions**
Acquired iodine-deficiency hypothyroidism NOS

E02 **Subclinical iodine-deficiency hypothyroidism**

E03 **Other hypothyroidism**

Excludes 1: iodine-deficiency related hypothyroidism (E00-E02)
postprocedural hypothyroidism (E89.0)

E03.0 **Congenital hypothyroidism with diffuse goiter**
Congenital parenchymatous goiter (nontoxic)
Congenital goiter (nontoxic) NOS

Excludes 1: transitory congenital goiter with normal function (P72.0)

E03.1 **Congenital hypothyroidism without goiter**
Aplasia of thyroid (with myxedema)
Congenital atrophy of thyroid
Congenital hypothyroidism NOS

E03.2 **Hypothyroidism due to medicaments and other exogenous substances**
Code first (T36-T65) to identify drug or substance

E03.3 **Postinfectious hypothyroidism**

E03.4 **Atrophy of thyroid (acquired)**

Excludes 1: congenital atrophy of thyroid (E03.1)

E03.5 Myxedema coma

E03.8 Other specified hypothyroidism

E03.9 Hypothyroidism, unspecified
Myxedema NOS

E04 Other nontoxic goiter

Excludes 1: congenital goiter (NOS) (diffuse) (parenchymatous) (E03.0)
iodine-deficiency related goiter (E00-E02)

E04.0 Nontoxic diffuse goiter
Diffuse (colloid) nontoxic goiter
Simple nontoxic goiter

E04.1 Nontoxic single thyroid nodule
Colloid nodule (cystic) (thyroid)
Nontoxic uninodular goiter
Thyroid (cystic) nodule NOS

E04.2 Nontoxic multinodular goiter
Cystic goiter NOS
Multinodular (cystic) goiter NOS

E04.8 Other specified nontoxic goiter

E04.9 Nontoxic goiter, unspecified
Goiter NOS
Nodular goiter (nontoxic) NOS

E05 Thyrotoxicosis [hyperthyroidism]

Excludes 1: chronic thyroiditis with transient thyrotoxicosis (E06.2)
neonatal thyrotoxicosis (P72.1)

E05.0 Thyrotoxicosis with diffuse goiter
Exophthalmic or toxic goiter NOS
Graves' disease
Toxic diffuse goiter

    E05.00 Thyrotoxicosis with diffuse goiter without thyrotoxic crisis or storm

    E05.01 Thyrotoxicosis with diffuse goiter with thyrotoxic crisis or storm

E05.1 Thyrotoxicosis with toxic single thyroid nodule
Thyrotoxicosis with toxic uninodular goiter

    E05.10 Thyrotoxicosis with toxic single thyroid nodule without thyrotoxic crisis or storm

E05.11   **Thyrotoxicosis with toxic single thyroid nodule with thyrotoxic crisis or storm**

E05.2   **Thyrotoxicosis with toxic multinodular goiter**
Toxic nodular goiter NOS

E05.20   **Thyrotoxicosis with toxic multinodular goiter without thyrotoxic crisis or storm**

E05.21   **Thyrotoxicosis with toxic multinodular goiter with thyrotoxic crisis or storm**

E05.3   **Thyrotoxicosis from ectopic thyroid tissue**

FORWARD MAPPING SAMPLE (ICD-9-CM ➡ ICD-10-CM)

ICD-9-CM CODE & DESCRIPTION		ICD-9-CM CODE & DESCRIPTION	
245.0	Acute thyroiditis	E06.0	Acute thyroiditis
245.1	Subacute thyroiditis	E06.1	Subacute thyroiditis
245.2	Chronic lymphocytic thyroiditis	E06.3	Autoimmune thyroiditis
245.3	Chronic fibrous thyroiditis	E06.5	Other chronic thyroiditis
245.4	Iatrogenic thyroiditis	E06.4	Drug-induced thyroiditis
245.8	Other and unspecified chronic thyroiditis	E06.5	Other chronic thyroiditis
245.9	Thyroiditis unspecified	E06.9	Thyroiditis unspecified
246.0	Disorders of thyrocalcitonin secretion	E07.0	Hypersecretion of calcitonin
246.1	Dyshormonogenic goiter	E07.1	Dyshormogenetic goiter
246.2	Cyst of thyroid	E04.1	Nontoxic single thyroid nodule
246.3	Hemorrhage and infarction of thyroid	E07.89	Other specified disorders of thyroid
246.8	Other specified disorders of thyroid	E03.4	Atrophy of thyroid (acquired)
246.8	Other specified disorders of thyroid	E07.89	Other specified disorders of thyroid
246.9	Unspecified disorder of thyroid	E07.9	Disorder of thyroid unspecified
249.00	Secondary diabetes mellitus without mention of complication, not stated as uncontrolled, or unspecified	E09.9	Drug or chemical induced diabetes mellitus without complications
249.01	Secondary diabetes mellitus without mention of complication, uncontrolled	E09.9	Drug or chemical induced diabetes mellitus without complications
249.10	Secondary diabetes mellitus with ketoacidosis, not stated as uncontrolled, or unspecified	E09.10	Drug or chemical induced diabetes mellitus with ketoacidosis without coma

249.11	Secondary diabetes mellitus with ketoacidosis, uncontrolled	E09.10	Drug or chemical induced diabetes mellitus with ketoacidosis without coma
249.20	Secondary diabetes mellitus with hyperosmolarity, not stated as uncontrolled, or unspecified	E09.01	Drug or chemical induced diabetes mellitus with hyperosmolarity with coma
249.21	Secondary diabetes mellitus with hyperosmolarity, uncontrolled	E09.01	Drug or chemical induced diabetes mellitus with hyperosmolarity with coma
249.30	Secondary diabetes mellitus with other coma, not stated as uncontrolled, or unspecified	E09.11	Drug or chemical induced diabetes mellitus with ketoacidosis with coma
249.30	Secondary diabetes mellitus with other coma, not stated as uncontrolled, or unspecified	E09.641	Drug or chemical induced diabetes mellitus with hypoglycemia with coma
249.31	Secondary diabetes mellitus with other coma, uncontrolled	E09.11	Drug or chemical induced diabetes mellitus with ketoacidosis with coma
249.31	Secondary diabetes mellitus with other coma, uncontrolled	E09.641	Drug or chemical induced diabetes mellitus with hypoglycemia with coma
249.40	Secondary diabetes mellitus with renal manifestations, not stated as uncontrolled, or unspecified	E09.22	Drug or chemical induced diabetes mellitus with diabetic chronic kidney disease
249.40	Secondary diabetes mellitus with renal manifestations, not stated as uncontrolled, or unspecified	E09.29	Drug or chemical induced diabetes mellitus with other diabetic kidney complication
249.40	Secondary diabetes mellitus with renal manifestations, not stated as uncontrolled, or unspecified	E09.21	Drug or chemical induced diabetes mellitus with diabetic nephropathy
249.41	Secondary diabetes mellitus with renal manifestations, uncontrolled	E09.22	Drug or chemical induced diabetes mellitus with diabetic chronic kidney disease
249.41	Secondary diabetes mellitus with renal manifestations, uncontrolled	E09.29	Drug or chemical induced diabetes mellitus with other diabetic kidney complication
249.41	Secondary diabetes mellitus with renal manifestations, uncontrolled	E09.21	Drug or chemical induced diabetes mellitus with diabetic nephropathy
249.50	Secondary diabetes mellitus with ophthalmic manifestations, not stated as uncontrolled, or unspecified	E09.311	Drug or chemical induced diabetes mellitus with unspecified diabetic retinopathy with macular edema
249.50	Secondary diabetes mellitus with ophthalmic manifestations, not stated as uncontrolled, or unspecified	E09.349	Drug or chemical induced diabetes mellitus with severe nonproliferative diabetic retinopathy without macular edema

249.50	Secondary diabetes mellitus with ophthalmic manifestations, not stated as uncontrolled, or unspecified	E09.39	Drug or chemical induced diabetes mellitus with other diabetic ophthalmic complication
249.50	Secondary diabetes mellitus with ophthalmic manifestations, not stated as uncontrolled, or unspecified	E09.36	Drug or chemical induced diabetes mellitus with diabetic cataract
249.50	Secondary diabetes mellitus with ophthalmic manifestations, not stated as uncontrolled, or unspecified	E09.359	Drug or chemical induced diabetes mellitus with proliferative diabetic retinopathy without macular edema
249.50	Secondary diabetes mellitus with ophthalmic manifestations, not stated as uncontrolled, or unspecified	E09.351	Drug or chemical induced diabetes mellitus with proliferative diabetic retinopathy with macular edema
249.50	Secondary diabetes mellitus with ophthalmic manifestations, not stated as uncontrolled, or unspecified	E09.341	Drug or chemical induced diabetes mellitus with severe nonproliferative diabetic retinopathy with macular edema
249.50	Secondary diabetes mellitus with ophthalmic manifestations, not stated as uncontrolled, or unspecified	E09.339	Drug or chemical induced diabetes mellitus with moderate nonproliferative diabetic retinopathy without macular edema
249.50	Secondary diabetes mellitus with ophthalmic manifestations, not stated as uncontrolled, or unspecified	E09.331	Drug or chemical induced diabetes mellitus with moderate nonproliferative diabetic retinopathy with macular edema
249.50	Secondary diabetes mellitus with ophthalmic manifestations, not stated as uncontrolled, or unspecified	E09.329	Drug or chemical induced diabetes mellitus with mild nonproliferative diabetic retinopathy without macular edema

BACKWARD MAPPING SAMPLE (ICD-10-CM ➡ ICD-9-CM)			
ICD-9-CM CODE & DESCRIPTION		**ICD-9-CM CODE & DESCRIPTION**	
E06.0	Acute thyroiditis	245.0	Acute thyroiditis
E06.1	Subacute thyroiditis	245.1	Subacute thyroiditis
E06.2	Chronic thyroiditis with transient thyrotoxicosis	245.8	Other and unspecified chronic thyroiditis
E06.3	Autoimmune thyroiditis	245.2	Chronic lymphocytic thyroiditis
E06.4	Drug-induced thyroiditis	245.4	Iatrogenic thyroiditis
E06.5	Other chronic thyroiditis	245.3	Chronic fibrous thyroiditis
E06.5	Other chronic thyroiditis	245.8	Other and unspecified chronic thyroiditis

E06.9	Thyroiditis unspecified	245.9	Thyroiditis unspecified
E07.0	Hypersecretion of calcitonin	246.0	Disorders of thyrocalcitonin secretion
E07.1	Dyshormogenetic goiter	246.1	Dyshormonogenic goiter
E07.81	Sick-euthyroid syndrome	790.94	Euthyroid sick syndrome
E07.89	Other specified disorders of thyroid	246.3	Hemorrhage and infarction of thyroid
E07.89	Other specified disorders of thyroid	246.8	Other specified disorders of thyroid
E07.9	Disorder of thyroid unspecified	246.9	Unspecified disorder of thyroid
E08.00	Diabetes mellitus due to underlying condition with hyperosmolarity without nonketotic hyperglycemic-hyperosmolar coma (NKHHC)	251.8	Other specified disorders of pancreatic internal secretion
E08.00	Diabetes mellitus due to underlying condition with hyperosmolarity without nonketotic hyperglycemic-hyperosmolar coma (NKHHC)	276.0	Hyperosmolality and/or hypernatremia
E08.01	Diabetes mellitus due to underlying condition with hyperosmolarity with coma	251.8	Other specified disorders of pancreatic internal secretion
E08.01	Diabetes mellitus due to underlying condition with hyperosmolarity with coma	276.0	Hyperosmolality and/or hypernatremia
E08.01	Diabetes mellitus due to underlying condition with hyperosmolarity with coma	780.01	Coma
E08.10	Diabetes mellitus due to underlying condition with ketoacidosis without coma	251.8	Other specified disorders of pancreatic internal secretion
E08.10	Diabetes mellitus due to underlying condition with ketoacidosis without coma	276.2	Acidosis
E08.11	Diabetes mellitus due to underlying condition with ketoacidosis with coma	251.8	Other specified disorders of pancreatic internal secretion
E08.11	Diabetes mellitus due to underlying condition with ketoacidosis with coma	276.2	Acidosis
E08.11	Diabetes mellitus due to underlying condition with ketoacidosis with coma	780.01	Coma
E08.21	Diabetes mellitus due to underlying condition with diabetic nephropathy	251.8	Other specified disorders of pancreatic internal secretion

E08.21	Diabetes mellitus due to underlying condition with diabetic nephropathy	581.81	Nephrotic syndrome in diseases classified elsewhere
E08.22	Diabetes mellitus due to underlying condition with diabetic chronic kidney disease	251.8	Other specified disorders of pancreatic internal secretion
E08.22	Diabetes mellitus due to underlying condition with diabetic chronic kidney disease	581.81	Nephrotic syndrome in diseases classified elsewhere
E08.29	Diabetes mellitus due to underlying condition with other diabetic kidney complication	251.8	Other specified disorders of pancreatic internal secretion
E08.29	Diabetes mellitus due to underlying condition with other diabetic kidney complication	581.81	Nephrotic syndrome in diseases classified elsewhere
E08.311	Diabetes mellitus due to underlying condition with unspecified diabetic retinopathy with macular edema	251.8	Other specified disorders of pancreatic internal secretion
E08.311	Diabetes mellitus due to underlying condition with unspecified diabetic retinopathy with macular edema	362.10	Background retinopathy unspecified
E08.311	Diabetes mellitus due to underlying condition with unspecified diabetic retinopathy with macular edema	362.83	Retinal edema
E08.319	Diabetes mellitus due to underlying condition with unspecified diabetic retinopathy without macular edema	251.8	Other specified disorders of pancreatic internal secretion
E08.319	Diabetes mellitus due to underlying condition with unspecified diabetic retinopathy without macular edema	362.10	Background retinopathy unspecified
E08.321	Diabetes mellitus due to underlying condition with mild nonproliferative diabetic retinopathy with macular edema	251.8	Other specified disorders of pancreatic internal secretion
E08.321	Diabetes mellitus due to underlying condition with mild nonproliferative diabetic retinopathy with macular edema	362.10	Background retinopathy unspecified
E08.321	Diabetes mellitus due to underlying condition with mild nonproliferative diabetic retinopathy with macular edema	362.83	Retinal edema
E08.329	Diabetes mellitus due to underlying condition with mild nonproliferative diabetic retinopathy without macular edema	251.8	Other specified disorders of pancreatic internal secretion

E08.329	Diabetes mellitus due to underlying condition with mild nonproliferative diabetic retinopathy without macular edema	362.10	Background retinopathy unspecified

CHAPTER 5: MENTAL AND BEHAVIORAL DISORDERS (F01 - F99)

GENERAL GUIDELINES

PAIN DISORDERS RELATED TO PSYCHOLOGICAL FACTORS

Assign code F45.41, for pain that is exclusively psychological. Code F45.41, Pain disorder exclusively related to psychological factors, should be used following the appropriate code from category G89, Pain, not elsewhere classified, if there is documentation of a psychological component for a patient with acute or chronic pain.

MENTAL AND BEHAVIORAL DISORDERS DUE TO PSYCHOACTIVE SUBSTANCE USE

1) **In Remission**

    Selection of codes for "in remission" for categories F10- F19, Mental and behavioral disorders due to psychoactive substance use (categories F10-F19 with -.21) requires the provider's clinical judgment. The appropriate codes for "in remission" are assigned only on the basis of provider documentation (as defined in the Official Guidelines for Coding and Reporting).

2) **Psychoactive Substance Use, Abuse And Dependence**

    When the provider documentation refers to use, abuse and dependence of the same substance (e.g. alcohol, opioid, cannabis, etc.), only one code should be assigned to identify the pattern of use based on the following hierarchy:

    - If both use and abuse are documented, assign only the code for abuse
    - If both abuse and dependence are documented, assign only the code for dependence
    - If use, abuse and dependence are all documented, assign only the code for dependence
    - If both use and dependence are documented, assign only the code for dependence.

3) **Psychoactive Substance Use**

    As with all other diagnoses, the codes for psychoactive substance use (F10.9-, F11.9-, F12.9-, F13.9-, F14.9-, F15.9-, F16.9-) should only be assigned based on provider documentation and when they meet the definition of a reportable diagnosis (see Section III, Reporting Additional Diagnoses). The codes are to be used only when the psychoactive substance use is associated with a mental or behavioral disorder, and such a relationship is documented by the provider.

SAMPLE ICD-10-CM CODES FROM THIS CHAPTER

Includes: disorders of psychological development

Excludes 2: symptoms, signs and abnormal clinical laboratory findings, not elsewhere classified (R00-R99)

This chapter contains the following blocks:	
F01-F09	Mental disorders due to known physiological conditions
F10-F19	Mental and behavioral disorders due to psychoactive substance use
F20-F29	Schizophrenia, schizotypal, delusional, and other non-mood psychotic disorders
F30-F39	Mood [affective] disorders
F40-F48	Anxiety, dissociative, stress-related, somatoform and other nonpsychotic mental disorders
F50-F59	Behavioral syndromes associated with physiological disturbances and physical factors
F60-F69	Disorders of adult personality and behavior
F70-F79	Mental retardation
F80-F89	Pervasive and specific developmental disorders
F90-F98	Behavioral and emotional disorders with onset usually occurring in childhood and adolescence
F99	Unspecified mental disorder

MENTAL DISORDERS DUE TO KNOWN PHYSIOLOGICAL CONDITIONS (F01-F09)

Note: This block comprises a range of mental disorders grouped together on the basis of their having in common a demonstrable etiology in cerebral disease, brain injury, or other insult leading to cerebral dysfunction. The dysfunction may be primary, as in diseases, injuries, and insults that affect the brain directly and selectively; or secondary, as in systemic diseases and disorders that attack the brain only as one of the multiple organs or systems of the body that are involved.

F01 Vascular Dementia

Vascular dementia as a result of infarction of the brain due to vascular disease, including hypertensive cerebrovascular disease.

Includes: arteriosclerotic dementia

Code first the underlying physiological condition or sequelae of cerebrovascular disease.

F01.5 Vascular dementia

F01.50 Vascular dementia without behavioral disturbance

F01.51 Vascular dementia with behavioral disturbance
Vascular dementia with aggressive behavior
Vascular dementia with combative behavior
Vascular dementia with violent behavior

Vascular dementia with wandering off

F02   Dementia in other diseases classified elsewhere

Code first the underlying physiological condition, such as:

Alzheimer's (G30.-)
cerebral lipidosis (E75.4)
Creutzfeldt-Jakob disease (A81.0-)
dementia with Lewy bodies (G31.83)
epilepsy and recurrent seizures (G40.-)
frontotemporal dementia (G31.09)
hepatolenticular degeneration (E83.0)
human immunodeficiency virus [HIV] disease (B20)
hypercalcemia (E83.52)
hypothyroidism, acquired (E00-E03.-)
intoxications (T36-T65)
Jakob-Creutzfeldt disease (A81.0-)
multiple sclerosis (G35)
neurosyphilis (A52.17)
niacin deficiency [pellagra] (E52)
Parkinson's disease (G20)
Pick's disease (G31.01)
polyarteritis nodosa (M30.0)
systemic lupus erythematosus (M32.-)
trypanosomiasis (B56.-, B57.-)
vitamin B deficiency (E53.8)

Excludes 1: dementia with Parkinsonism (G31.83)

Excludes 2: dementia in alcohol and psychoactive substance disorders (F10-F19,
           with .17, .27, .97)
           vascular dementia (F01.5-)

F02.8   Dementia in other diseases classified elsewhere

**F02.80   Dementia in other diseases classified elsewhere, without behavioral
           disturbance**
           Dementia in other diseases classified elsewhere NOS

**F02.81   Dementia in other diseases classified elsewhere, with behavioral
           disturbance**
           Dementia in other diseases classified elsewhere with aggressive behavior
           Dementia in other diseases classified elsewhere with combative behavior
           Dementia in other diseases classified elsewhere with violent behavior
           Dementia in other diseases classified elsewhere with wandering off

F03   Unspecified dementia
Presenile dementia NOS
Presenile psychosis NOS
Primary degenerative dementia NOS

Senile dementia NOS
Senile dementia depressed or paranoid type
Senile psychosis NOS

Excludes 1: senility NOS (R41.81)

Excludes 2: senile dementia with delirium or acute confusional state (F05)

F04   Amnestic disorder due to known physiological condition

Korsakov's psychosis or syndrome, nonalcoholic
Code first the underlying physiological condition

Excludes 1: amnesia NOS (R41.3)
            anterograde amnesia (R41.1)
            dissociative amnesia (F44.0)
            retrograde amnesia (R41.2)

Excludes 2: alcohol-induced or unspecified Korsakov's syndrome (F10.26, F10.96)
            Korsakov's syndrome induced by other psychoactive substances (F13.26,
            F13.96, F19.16, F19.26, F19.96)

F05   Delirium due to known physiological condition

Acute or subacute brain syndrome
Acute or subacute confusional state (nonalcoholic)
Acute or subacute infective psychosis
Acute or subacute organic reaction
Acute or subacute psycho-organic syndrome
Delirium of mixed etiology
Delirium superimposed on dementia
Sundowning

Code first the underlying physiological condition

Excludes 1: delirium NOS (R41.0)

Excludes 2: delirium tremens alcohol-induced or unspecified (F10.231, F10.921)

FORWARD MAPPING SAMPLE (ICD-9-CM ➡ ICD-10-CM)			
ICD-9-CM CODE & DESCRIPTION		**ICD-10-CM CODE & DESCRIPTION**	
292.0	Drug withdrawal	**F19.939**	Other psychoactive substance use unspecified with withdrawal unspecified
292.11	Drug-induced psychotic disorder with delusions	**F19.950**	Other psychoactive substance use unspecified with psychoactive substance-induced psychotic disorder with delusions

292.12	Drug-induced psychotic disorder with hallucinations	F19.951	Other psychoactive substance use unspecified with psychoactive substance-induced psychotic disorder with hallucinations
292.2	Pathological drug intoxication	F15.920	Other stimulant use unspecified with intoxication uncomplicated
292.81	Drug-induced persisting delirium	F19.921	Other psychoactive substance use unspecified with intoxication with delirium
292.82	Drug-induced persisting dementia	F19.97	Other psychoactive substance use unspecified with psychoactive substance-induced persisting dementia
292.83	Drug-induced persisting amnestic disorder	F19.96	Other psychoactive substance use unspecified with psychoactive substance-induced persisting amnestic disorder
292.84	Drug-induced mood disorder	F19.94	Other psychoactive substance use unspecified with psychoactive substance-induced mood disorder
292.85	Drug-induced sleep disorders	F19.982	Other psychoactive substance use unspecified with psychoactive substance-induced sleep disorder
292.89	Other specified drug-induced mental disorders	F19.988	Other psychoactive substance use unspecified with other psychoactive substance-induced disorder
292.9	Unspecified drug-induced mental disorder	F19.99	Other psychoactive substance use unspecified with unspecified psychoactive substance-induced disorder
293.0	Delirium due to conditions classified elsewhere	F05	Delirium due to known physiological condition
293.1	Subacute delirium	F05	Delirium due to known physiological condition
293.81	Psychotic disorder with delusions in conditions classified elsewhere	F06.2	Psychotic disorder with delusions due to known physiological condition
293.82	Psychotic disorder with hallucinations in conditions classified elsewhere	F06.0	Psychotic disorder with hallucinations due to known physiological condition
293.83	Mood disorder in conditions classified elsewhere	F06.30	Mood disorder due to known physiological condition unspecified
293.84	Anxiety disorder in conditions classified elsewhere	F06.4	Anxiety disorder due to known physiological condition

293.89	Other catatonic disorder in conditions classified elsewhere	F06.1	Catatonic disorder due to known physiological condition
294.0	Amnestic disorder in conditions classified elsewhere	F04	Amnestic disorder due to known physiological condition
294.10	Dementia in conditions classified elsewhere without behavioral disturbance	F02.80	Dementia in other diseases classified elsewhere without behavioral disturbance
294.11	Dementia in conditions classified elsewhere with behavioral disturbance	F02.81	Dementia in other diseases classified elsewhere with behavioral disturbance
294.8	Other persistent mental disorders due to conditions classified elsewhere	F06.0	Psychotic disorder with hallucinations due to known physiological condition
294.8	Other persistent mental disorders due to conditions classified elsewhere	F06.8	Other specified mental disorders due to known physiological condition
295.00	Simple type schizophrenia unspecified state	F20.89	Other schizophrenia
295.01	Simple type schizophrenia subchronic state	F20.89	Other schizophrenia
295.02	Simple type schizophrenia chronic state	F20.89	Other schizophrenia
295.03	Simple type schizophrenia subchronic state with acute exacerbation	F20.89	Other schizophrenia
295.04	Simple type schizophrenia chronic state with acute exacerbation	F20.89	Other schizophrenia
295.05	Simple type schizophrenia in remission	F20.89	Other schizophrenia
295.10	Disorganized type schizophrenia unspecified state	F20.1	Disorganized schizophrenia
295.11	Disorganized type schizophrenia subchronic state	F20.1	Disorganized schizophrenia
295.12	Disorganized type schizophrenia chronic state	F20.1	Disorganized schizophrenia
295.13	Disorganized type schizophrenia subchronic state with acute exacerbation	F20.1	Disorganized schizophrenia
295.14	Disorganized type schizophrenia chronic state with acute exacerbation	F20.1	Disorganized schizophrenia
295.15	Disorganized type schizophrenia in remission	F20.1	Disorganized schizophrenia
295.20	Catatonic type schizophrenia unspecified state	F20.2	Catatonic schizophrenia

295.21	Catatonic type schizophrenia subchronic state	F20.2	Catatonic schizophrenia
295.22	Catatonic type schizophrenia chronic state	F20.2	Catatonic schizophrenia

BACKWARD MAPPING SAMPLE (ICD-10-CM ➡ ICD-9-CM)

ICD-10-CM CODE & DESCRIPTION		ICD-9-CM CODE & DESCRIPTION	
F32.0	Major depressive disorder single episode mild	296.21	Major depressive affective disorder single episode mild degree
F32.1	Major depressive disorder single episode moderate	296.22	Major depressive affective disorder single episode moderate degree
F32.2	Major depressive disorder single episode severe without psychotic features	296.23	Major depressive affective disorder single episode severe degree without psychotic behavior
F32.3	Major depressive disorder single episode severe with psychotic features	296.24	Major depressive affective disorder single episode severe degree specified as with psychotic behavior
F32.3	Major depressive disorder single episode severe with psychotic features	298.0	Depressive type psychosis
F32.4	Major depressive disorder single episode in partial remission	296.25	Major depressive affective disorder single episode in partial or unspecified remission
F32.5	Major depressive disorder single episode in full remission	296.26	Major depressive affective disorder single episode in full remission
F32.8	Other depressive episodes	296.82	Atypical depressive disorder
F32.9	Major depressive disorder single episode unspecified	296.20	Major depressive affective disorder single episode unspecified degree
F33.0	Major depressive disorder recurrent mild	296.31	Major depressive affective disorder recurrent episode mild degree
F33.1	Major depressive disorder recurrent moderate	296.32	Major depressive affective disorder recurrent episode moderate degree
F33.2	Major depressive disorder recurrent severe without psychotic features	296.33	Major depressive affective disorder recurrent episode severe degree without psychotic behavior
F33.3	Major depressive disorder recurrent severe with psychotic symptoms	296.34	Major depressive affective disorder recurrent episode severe degree specified as with psychotic behavior
F33.3	Major depressive disorder recurrent severe with psychotic symptoms	298.0	Depressive type psychosis
F33.40	Major depressive disorder recurrent in remission	296.30	Major depressive affective disorder recurrent episode unspecified degree
F33.41	Major depressive disorder recurrent in partial remission	296.35	Major depressive affective disorder recurrent episode in partial or unspecified remission

F33.42	Major depressive disorder recurrent in full remission	296.36	Major depressive affective disorder recurrent episode in full remission
F33.8	Other recurrent depressive disorders	296.99	Other specified episodic mood disorder
F33.9	Major depressive disorder recurrent unspecified	296.30	Major depressive affective disorder recurrent episode unspecified degree
F34.0	Cyclothymic disorder	301.10	Affective personality disorder unspecified
F34.0	Cyclothymic disorder	301.13	Cyclothymic disorder
F34.1	Dysthymic disorder	300.4	Dysthymic disorder
F34.1	Dysthymic disorder	301.12	Chronic depressive personality disorder
F34.8	Other persistent mood [affective] disorders	296.99	Other specified episodic mood disorder
F34.9	Persistent mood [affective] disorder unspecified	296.99	Other specified episodic mood disorder
F39	Unspecified mood [affective] disorder	296.90	Unspecified episodic mood disorder
F40.00	Agoraphobia unspecified	300.22	Agoraphobia without panic attacks
F40.01	Agoraphobia with panic disorder	300.21	Agoraphobia with panic attacks
F40.02	Agoraphobia without panic disorder	300.22	Agoraphobia without panic attacks
F40.10	Social phobia unspecified	300.23	Social phobia
F40.11	Social phobia generalized	300.23	Social phobia
F40.210	Arachnophobia	300.29	Other isolated or specific phobias
F40.218	Other animal type phobia	300.29	Other isolated or specific phobias
F40.220	Fear of thunderstorms	300.29	Other isolated or specific phobias
F40.228	Other natural environment type phobia	300.29	Other isolated or specific phobias
F40.230	Fear of blood	300.29	Other isolated or specific phobias
F40.231	Fear of injections and transfusions	300.29	Other isolated or specific phobias
F40.232	Fear of other medical care	300.29	Other isolated or specific phobias
F40.233	Fear of injury	300.29	Other isolated or specific phobias
F40.240	Claustrophobia	300.29	Other isolated or specific phobias

CHAPTER 6: DISEASES OF NERVOUS SYSTEM AND SENSE ORGANS (G00-G99)

GENERAL GUIDELINES

DOMINANT/NONDOMINANT SIDE

Codes from category G81, Hemiplegia and hemiparesis, and subcategories, G83.1, Monoplegia of lower limb, G83.2, Monoplegia of upper limb, and G83.3, Monoplegia, unspecified, identify whether the dominant or nondominant side is affected. Should the affected side be documented, but not specified as dominant or nondominant, and the classification system does not indicate a default, code selection is as follows:

- For ambidextrous patients, the default should be dominant.
- If the left side is affected, the default is non-dominant.
- If the right side is affected, the default is dominant.

PAIN - CATEGORY G89

1) General coding information

Codes in category G89, Pain, not elsewhere classified, may be used in conjunction with codes from other categories and chapters to provide more detail about acute or chronic pain and neoplasm-related pain, unless otherwise indicated below.

If the pain is not specified as acute or chronic, post- thoracotomy, postprocedural, or neoplasm-related, do not assign codes from category G89.

A code from category G89 should not be assigned if the underlying (definitive) diagnosis is known, unless the reason for the encounter is pain control/ management and not management of the underlying condition.

(a) When an admission or encounter is for a procedure aimed at treating the underlying condition (e.g., spinal fusion, kyphoplasty), a code for the underlying condition (e.g., vertebral fracture, spinal stenosis) should be assigned as the principal diagnosis. No code from category G89 should be assigned. Category G89 Codes as Principal or First-Listed Diagnosis
Category G89 codes are acceptable as principal diagnosis or the first-listed code:

- When pain control or pain management is the reason for the admission/encounter (e.g., a patient with displaced intervertebral disc, nerve impingement and severe back pain presents for injection of steroid into the spinal canal). The underlying cause of the pain should be reported as an additional diagnosis, if known.

- When a patient is admitted for the insertion of a neurostimulator for pain control, assign the appropriate pain code as the principal or first-listed diagnosis. When an admission or encounter is for a procedure aimed at treating the underlying condition and a neurostimulator is inserted for pain control during the same admission/ encounter, a code for the underlying condition should be assigned as the principal diagnosis and the appropriate pain code should be assigned as a secondary diagnosis.

(b) Use of Category G89 Codes in Conjunction with Site Specific Pain Codes

(i) Assigning Category G89 and Site-Specific Pain Codes

Codes from category G89 may be used in conjunction with codes that identify the site of pain (including codes from chapter 18) if the category G89 code provides additional information. For example, if the code describes the site of the pain, but does not fully describe whether the pain is acute or chronic, then both codes should be assigned.

(ii) Sequencing of Category G89 Codes with Site- Specific Pain Codes

- The sequencing of category G89 codes with site-specific pain codes (including chapter 18 codes), is dependent on the circumstances of the encounter/admission as follows: If the encounter is for pain control or pain management, assign the code from category G89 followed by the code identifying the specific site of pain (e.g., encounter for pain management for acute neck pain from trauma is assigned code G89.11, Acute pain due to trauma, followed by code M54.2, Cervicalgia, to identify the site of pain).

- If the encounter is for any other reason except pain control or pain management, and a related definitive diagnosis has not been established (confirmed) by the provider, assign the code for the specific site of pain first, followed by the appropriate code from category G89.

2) **Pain due to devices, implants and grafts**

See Section I.C.19. Pain due to medical devices

3) **Postoperative Pain**

The provider's documentation should be used to guide the coding of postoperative pain, as well as Section III. Reporting Additional Diagnoses *and* Section IV. Diagnostic Coding and Reporting in the Outpatient Setting.

The default for post-thoracotomy and other postoperative pain not specified as acute or chronic is the code for the acute form.

Routine or expected postoperative pain immediately after surgery should not be coded.

(a) Postoperative pain not associated with specific postoperative complication

Postoperative pain not associated with a specific postoperative complication is assigned to the appropriate postoperative pain code in category G89.

(b) Postoperative pain associated with specific postoperative complication

Postoperative pain associated with a specific postoperative complication (such as painful wire sutures) is assigned to the appropriate code(s) found in Chapter 19, Injury, poisoning, and certain other consequences of external causes. If appropriate, use additional code(s) from category G89 to identify acute or chronic pain (G89.18 or G89.28).

4) **Chronic pain**

Chronic pain is classified to subcategory G89.2. There is no time frame defining when pain becomes chronic pain. The provider's documentation should be used to guide use of these codes.

5) Neoplasm Related Pain

Code G89.3 is assigned to pain documented as being related, associated or due to cancer, primary or secondary malignancy, or tumor. This code is assigned regardless of whether the pain is acute or chronic.

This code may be assigned as the principal or first- listed code when the stated reason for the admission/encounter is documented as pain control/pain management. The underlying neoplasm should be reported as an additional diagnosis.

When the reason for the admission/encounter is management of the neoplasm and the pain associated with the neoplasm is also documented, code G89.3 may be assigned as an additional diagnosis. It is not necessary to assign an additional code for the site of the pain.

6) Chronic pain syndrome

Central pain syndrome (G89.0) and chronic pain syndrome (G89.4) are different than the term "chronic pain," and therefore codes should only be used when the provider has specifically documented this condition.

SAMPLE ICD-10-CM CODES FROM THIS CHAPTER

Excludes 2: certain conditions originating in the perinatal period (P04-P96)
certain infectious and parasitic diseases (A00-B99)
complications of pregnancy, childbirth and the puerperium (O00-O99)
congenital malformations, deformations, and chromosomal abnormalities (Q00-Q99)
endocrine, nutritional and metabolic diseases (E00-E88)
injury, poisoning and certain other consequences of external causes (S00-T88)
neoplasms (C00-D49)
symptoms, signs and abnormal clinical and laboratory findings, not elsewhere classified (R00-R94)

This chapter contains the following blocks:	
G00-G09	Inflammatory diseases of the central nervous system
G10-G14	Systemic atrophies primarily affecting the central nervous system
G20-G26	Extrapyramidal and movement disorders
G30-G32	Other degenerative diseases of the nervous system
G35-G37	Demyelinating diseases of the central nervous system
G40-G47	Episodic and paroxysmal disorders
G50-G59	Nerve, nerve root and plexus disorders
G60-G65	Polyneuropathies and other disorders of the peripheral nervous system
G70-G73	Diseases of myoneural junction and muscle
G80-G83	Cerebral palsy and other paralytic syndromes

| **G89-G99** | Other disorders of the nervous system |

INFLAMMATORY DISEASES OF THE CENTRAL NERVOUS SYSTEM (G00-G09)

G00   Bacterial meningitis, not elsewhere classified

> ***Includes:***   bacterial arachnoiditis
> bacterial leptomeningitis
> bacterial meningitis
> bacterial pachymeningitis

> ***Excludes 1***: bacterial:
> meningoencephalitis (G04.2)
> meningomyelitis (G04.2)

G00.0 Hemophilus meningitis
Meningitis due to Hemophilus influenzae

G00.1 Pneumococcal meningitis

G00.2 Streptococcal meningitis
Use additional code to further identify organism (B95.0-B95.5)

G00.3 Staphylococcal meningitis
Use additional code to further identify organism (B95.6-B95.8)

G00.8 Other bacterial meningitis
Meningitis due to Escherichia coli
Meningitis due to Friedländer's bacillus
Meningitis due to Klebsiella
Use additional code to further identify organism (B96.-)

G00.9 Bacterial meningitis, unspecified
Meningitis due to gram-negative bacteria, unspecified
Purulent meningitis NOS
Pyogenic meningitis NOS
Suppurative meningitis NOS

G01   Meningitis in bacterial diseases classified elsewhere

Code first underlying disease

> ***Excludes 1***: meningitis (in):
> gonococcal (A54.81)
> leptospirosis (A27.81)
> listeriosis (A32.11)
> Lyme disease (A69.21)
> meningococcal (A39.0)
> neurosyphilis (A52.13)
> tuberculosis (A17.0)

meningoencephalitis and meningomyelitis in bacterial diseases classified elsewhere (G05)

G02 Meningitis in other infectious and parasitic diseases classified elsewhere

Code first underlying disease, such as:
  poliovirus infection (A80.-)
Excludes 1: meningitis (due to):
  candidal (B37.5)
  coccidioidomycosis (B38.4)
  cryptococcal meningitis (B45.1)
  herpesviral [herpes simplex] (B00.3)
  infectious mononucleosis (B27.-2)
  measles (B05.1)
  mumps (B26.1)
  rubella (B06.02)
  varicella [chickenpox] (B01.0)
  zoster (B02.1)
  meningoencephalitis and meningomyelitis in other infectious and parasitic diseases classified elsewhere (G05)

G03 Meningitis due to other and unspecified causes

Includes: arachnoiditis NOS
    leptomeningitis NOS
    meningitis NOS
    pachymeningitis NOS

Excludes 1: meningoencephalitis (G04.-)
     meningomyelitis (G04.-)

G03.0 Nonpyogenic meningitis
Aseptic meningitis
Nonbacterial meningitis

G03.1 Chronic meningitis

G03.2 Benign recurrent meningitis [Mollaret]

G03.8 Meningitis due to other specified causes

G03.9 Meningitis, unspecified
Arachnoiditis (spinal) NOS

G04 Encephalitis, myelitis and encephalomyelitis

Includes: acute ascending myelitis
    meningoencephalitis
    meningomyelitis

Excludes 1: encephalopathy NOS (G93.40)

Excludes 2: acute transverse myelitis (G37.3-)
   alcoholic encephalopathy (G31.2)
   benign myalgic encephalomyelitis (G93.3)
   multiple sclerosis (G35)
   subacute necrotizing myelitis (G37.4)
   toxic encephalitis (G92)
   toxic encephalopathy (G92)

G04.0   Acute disseminated encephalitis and encephalomyelitis (ADEM)

Excludes 1: acute necrotizing hemorrhagic encephalopathy (G04.3-)

FORWARD MAPPING SAMPLE (ICD-9-CM ➡ ICD-10-CM)			
ICD-9-CM CODE & DESCRIPTION		**ICD-10-CM CODE & DESCRIPTION**	
320.0	Hemophilus meningitis	G00.0	Hemophilus meningitis
320.1	Pneumococcal meningitis	G00.1	Pneumococcal meningitis
320.2	Streptococcal meningitis	G00.2	Streptococcal meningitis
320.3	Staphylococcal meningitis	G00.3	Staphylococcal meningitis
320.7	Meningitis in other bacterial diseases classified elsewhere	G01	Meningitis in bacterial diseases classified elsewhere
320.81	Anaerobic meningitis	G00.8	Other bacterial meningitis
320.82	Meningitis due to gram-negative bacteria not elsewhere classified	G00.9	Bacterial meningitis unspecified
320.89	Meningitis due to other specified bacteria	G00.8	Other bacterial meningitis
320.9	Meningitis due to unspecified bacterium	G00.9	Bacterial meningitis unspecified
320.9	Meningitis due to unspecified bacterium	G04.2	Bacterial meningoencephalitis and meningomyelitis not elsewhere classified
321.0	Cryptococcal meningitis	B45.1	Cerebral cryptococcosis
321.1	Meningitis in other fungal diseases	G02	Meningitis in other infectious and parasitic diseases classified elsewhere
321.2	Meningitis due to viruses not elsewhere classified	G02	Meningitis in other infectious and parasitic diseases classified elsewhere
321.3	Meningitis due to trypanosomiasis	G02	Meningitis in other infectious and parasitic diseases classified elsewhere
321.4	Meningitis in sarcoidosis	G02	Meningitis in other infectious and parasitic diseases classified elsewhere
321.8	Meningitis due to other nonbacterial organisms classified elsewhere	G02	Meningitis in other infectious and parasitic diseases classified elsewhere

322.0	Nonpyogenic meningitis	G03.0	Nonpyogenic meningitis
322.1	Eosinophilic meningitis	G03.8	Meningitis due to other specified causes
322.2	Chronic meningitis	G03.1	Chronic meningitis
322.9	Meningitis unspecified	G03.9	Meningitis unspecified
323.01	Encephalitis and encephalomyelitis in viral diseases classified elsewhere	G05.3	Encephalitis and encephalomyelitis in diseases classified elsewhere
323.02	Myelitis in viral diseases classified elsewhere	G05.4	Myelitis in diseases classified elsewhere
323.1	Encephalitis in rickettsial diseases classified elsewhere	G05.3	Encephalitis and encephalomyelitis in diseases classified elsewhere
323.2	Encephalitis in protozoal diseases classified elsewhere	G05.3	Encephalitis and encephalomyelitis in diseases classified elsewhere
323.41	Other encephalitis and encephalomyelitis due to infection classified elsewhere	G05.3	Encephalitis and encephalomyelitis in diseases classified elsewhere
323.42	Other myelitis due to infection classified elsewhere	G05.4	Myelitis in diseases classified elsewhere
323.51	Encephalitis and encephalomyelitis following immunization procedures	G04.31	Postimmunization acute necrotizing hemorrhagic encephalopathy
323.52	Myelitis following immunization procedures	G04.01	Postimmunization acute disseminated encephalitis myelitis and encephalomyelitis
323.61	Infectious acute disseminated encephalomyelitis (adem)	G04.00	Postinfectious acute disseminated encephalitis and encephalomyelitis (postinfectious ADEM)
323.62	Other postinfectious encephalitis and encephalomyelitis	G04.30	Postinfectious acute necrotizing hemorrhagic encephalopathy
323.63	Postinfectious myelitis	G05.4	Myelitis in diseases classified elsewhere
323.71	Toxic encephalitis and encephalomyelitis	G92	Toxic encephalopathy
323.72	Toxic myelitis	G92	Toxic encephalopathy
323.81	Other causes of encephalitis and encephalomyelitis	G04.81	Other encephalitis and encephalomyelitis
323.82	Other causes of myelitis	G04.89	Other myelitis
323.9	Unspecified cause of encephalitis	G04.90	Encephalitis and encephalomyelitis unspecified
323.9	Unspecified cause of encephalitis	G04.91	Myelitis unspecified
324.0	Intracranial abscess	G06.0	Intracranial abscess and granuloma
324.1	Intraspinal abscess	G06.1	Intraspinal abscess and granuloma
324.9	Intracranial and intraspinal abscess of unspecified site	G06.2	Extradural and subdural abscess unspecified

BACKWARD MAPPING SAMPLE (ICD-10-CM ➜ ICD-9-CM)

ICD-10-CM CODE & DESCRIPTION		ICD-9-CM CODE & DESCRIPTION	
G00.0	Hemophilus meningitis	320.0	Hemophilus meningitis
G00.1	Pneumococcal meningitis	320.1	Pneumococcal meningitis
G00.2	Streptococcal meningitis	320.2	Streptococcal meningitis
G00.3	Staphylococcal meningitis	320.3	Staphylococcal meningitis
G00.8	Other bacterial meningitis	320.89	Meningitis due to other specified bacteria
G00.9	Bacterial meningitis unspecified	320.82	Meningitis due to gram-negative bacteria not elsewhere classified
G00.9	Bacterial meningitis unspecified	320.9	Meningitis due to unspecified bacterium
G01	Meningitis in bacterial diseases classified elsewhere	320.7	Meningitis in other bacterial diseases classified elsewhere
G02	Meningitis in other infectious and parasitic diseases classified elsewhere	321.1	Meningitis in other fungal diseases
G02	Meningitis in other infectious and parasitic diseases classified elsewhere	321.2	Meningitis due to viruses not elsewhere classified
G02	Meningitis in other infectious and parasitic diseases classified elsewhere	321.8	Meningitis due to other nonbacterial organisms classified elsewhere
G03.0	Nonpyogenic meningitis	322.0	Nonpyogenic meningitis
G03.1	Chronic meningitis	322.2	Chronic meningitis
G03.2	Benign recurrent meningitis [Mollaret]	047.9	Unspecified viral meningitis
G03.8	Meningitis due to other specified causes	322.1	Eosinophilic meningitis
G03.9	Meningitis unspecified	322.9	Meningitis unspecified
G04.00	Postinfectious acute disseminated encephalitis and encephalomyelitis (postinfectious ADEM)	323.61	Infectious acute disseminated encephalomyelitis (adem)
G04.01	Postimmunization acute disseminated encephalitis myelitis and encephalomyelitis	323.52	Myelitis following immunization procedures
G04.1	Tropical spastic paraplegia	344.1	Paraplegia
G04.2	Bacterial meningoencephalitis and meningomyelitis not elsewhere classified	320.9	Meningitis due to unspecified bacterium
G04.30	Postinfectious acute necrotizing hemorrhagic encephalopathy	323.62	Other postinfectious encephalitis and encephalomyelitis
G04.31	Postimmunization acute necrotizing hemorrhagic encephalopathy	323.51	Encephalitis and encephalomyelitis following immunization procedures

G04.81	Other encephalitis and encephalomyelitis	323.81	Other causes of encephalitis and encephalomyelitis
G04.89	Other myelitis	323.82	Other causes of myelitis
G04.90	Encephalitis and encephalomyelitis unspecified	323.9	Unspecified cause of encephalitis
G04.91	Myelitis unspecified	323.9	Unspecified cause of encephalitis
G05.3	Encephalitis and encephalomyelitis in diseases classified elsewhere	323.41	Other encephalitis and encephalomyelitis due to infection classified elsewhere
G05.4	Myelitis in diseases classified elsewhere	323.42	Other myelitis due to infection classified elsewhere
G06.0	Intracranial abscess and granuloma	324.0	Intracranial abscess
G06.1	Intraspinal abscess and granuloma	324.1	Intraspinal abscess
G06.2	Extradural and subdural abscess unspecified	324.9	Intracranial and intraspinal abscess of unspecified site
G07	Intracranial and intraspinal abscess and granuloma in diseases classified elsewhere	324.9	Intracranial and intraspinal abscess of unspecified site
G08	Intracranial and intraspinal phlebitis and thrombophlebitis	325	Phlebitis and thrombophlebitis of intracranial venous sinuses
G09	Sequelae of inflammatory diseases of central nervous system	326	Late effects of intracranial abscess or pyogenic infection
G10	Huntington's disease	333.4	Huntington's chorea
G11.0	Congenital nonprogressive ataxia	334.1	Hereditary spastic paraplegia
G11.1	Early-onset cerebellar ataxia	334.0	Friedreich's ataxia
G11.1	Early-onset cerebellar ataxia	334.3	Other cerebellar ataxia
G11.2	Late-onset cerebellar ataxia	334.2	Primary cerebellar degeneration
G11.3	Cerebellar ataxia with defective DNA repair	334.8	Other spinocerebellar diseases

CHAPTER 7: DISEASES OF EYE AND ADNEXA (H00-H59)

GENERAL GUIDELINES

There are no published guidelines for this chapter.

SAMPLE ICD-10-CM CODES FROM THIS CHAPTER

Note: Use an external cause code following the code for the eye condition, if applicable, to identify the cause of the eye condition

Excludes 2: certain conditions originating in the perinatal period (P04-P96)
certain infectious and parasitic diseases (A00-B99)
complications of pregnancy, childbirth and the puerperium (O00-O99)

congenital malformations, deformations, and chromosomal abnormalities (Q00-Q99)
diabetes mellitus related eye conditions (E09.3-, E10.3-, E11.3-, E13.3-)
endocrine, nutritional and metabolic diseases (E00-E88)
injury (trauma) of eye and orbit (S05.-)
injury, poisoning and certain other consequences of external causes (S00-T88)
neoplasms (C00-D49)
symptoms, signs and abnormal clinical and laboratory findings, not elsewhere
classified (R00-R94)
syphilis related eye disorders (A50.01, A50.3-, A51.43, A52.71)

This chapter contains the following blocks:	
H00-H05	Disorders of eyelid, lacrimal system and orbit
H10-H11	Disorders of conjunctiva
H15-H22	Disorders of sclera, cornea, iris and ciliary body
H25-H28	Disorders of lens
H30-H36	Disorders of choroid and retina
H40-H42	Glaucoma
H43-H44	Disorders of vitreous body and globe
H46-H47	Disorders of optic nerve and visual pathways
H49-H52	Disorders of ocular muscles, binocular movement, accommodation and refraction
H53-H54	Visual disturbances and blindness
H55-H57	Other disorders of eye and adnexa
H59	Intraoperative and postprocedural complications and disorders of eye and adnexa, not elsewhere classified

DISORDERS OF EYELID, LACRIMAL SYSTEM AND ORBIT (H00-H05)

Excludes 2: open wound of eyelid (S01.1-)
        superficial injury of eyelid (S00.1-, S00.2-)

H00   Hordeolum and Chalazion

    H00.0 Hordeolum (externum) (internum) of eyelid

        H00.01   Hordeolum externum
        Hordeolum NOS
        Stye

           H00.011   Hordeolum externum right upper eyelid

           H00.012   Hordeolum externum right lower eyelid

           H00.013   Hordeolum externum right eye, unspecified eyelid

           H00.014   Hordeolum externum left upper eyelid

           H00.015   Hordeolum externum left lower eyelid

    H00.016   **Hordeolum externum left eye, unspecified eyelid**

    H00.019   **Hordeolum externum unspecified eye, unspecified eyelid**

H00.02   **Hordeolum internum**
Infection of meibomian gland

    H00.021   **Hordeolum internum right upper eyelid**

    H00.022   **Hordeolum internum right lower eyelid**

    H00.023   **Hordeolum internum right eye, unspecified eyelid**

    H00.024   **Hordeolum internum left upper eyelid**

    H00.025   **Hordeolum internum left lower eyelid**

    H00.026   **Hordeolum internum left eye, unspecified eyelid**

    H00.029   **Hordeolum internum unspecified eye, unspecified eyelid**

H00.03   **Abscess of eyelid**
Furuncle of eyelid

    H00.031   **Abscess of right upper eyelid**

    H00.032   **Abscess of right lower eyelid**

    H00.033   **Abscess of eyelid right eye, unspecified eyelid**

    H00.034   **Abscess of left upper eyelid**

    H00.035   **Abscess of left lower eyelid**

    H00.036   **Abscess of eyelid left eye, unspecified eyelid**

    H00.039   **Abscess of eyelid unspecified eye, unspecified eyelid**

H00.1 **Chalazion**
Meibomian (gland) cyst

Excludes 2: infected meibomian gland (H00.02-)

    H00.11   **Chalazion right upper eyelid**

    H00.12   **Chalazion right lower eyelid**

    H00.13   **Chalazion right eye, unspecified eyelid**

    H00.14   **Chalazion left upper eyelid**

 H00.15   Chalazion left lower eyelid

 H00.16   Chalazion left eye, unspecified eyelid

 H00.19   Chalazion unspecified eye, unspecified eyelid

H01   Other inflammation of eyelid

 H01.0 Blepharitis

 Excludes 1: blepharoconjunctivitis (H10.5-)

 H01.00   Unspecified blepharitis

  H01.001   Unspecified blepharitis right upper eyelid

  H01.002   Unspecified blepharitis right lower eyelid

  H01.003   Unspecified blepharitis right eye, unspecified eyelid

  H01.004   Unspecified blepharitis left upper eyelid

  H01.005   Unspecified blepharitis left lower eyelid

  H01.006   Unspecified blepharitis left eye, unspecified eyelid

  H01.009   Unspecified blepharitis unspecified eye, unspecified eyelid

 H01.01   Ulcerative blepharitis

  H01.011   Ulcerative blepharitis right upper eyelid

  H01.012   Ulcerative blepharitis right lower eyelid

  H01.013   Ulcerative blepharitis right eye, unspecified eyelid

  H01.014   Ulcerative blepharitis left upper eyelid

  H01.015   Ulcerative blepharitis left lower eyelid

  H01.016   Ulcerative blepharitis left eye, unspecified eyelid

  H01.019   Ulcerative blepharitis unspecified eye, unspecified eyelid

 H01.02   Squamous blepharitis

  H01.021   Squamous blepharitis right upper eyelid

  H01.022   Squamous blepharitis right lower eyelid

  H01.023   Squamous blepharitis right eye, unspecified eyelid

H01.024   **Squamous blepharitis left upper eyelid**

H01.025   **Squamous blepharitis left lower eyelid**

H01.026   **Squamous blepharitis left eye, unspecified eyelid**

H01.029   **Squamous blepharitis unspecified eye, unspecified eyelid**

H01.1   **Noninfectious dermatoses of eyelid**

   H01.11   **Allergic dermatitis of eyelid**
Contact dermatitis of eyelid

H01.111   **Allergic dermatitis of right upper eyelid**

H01.112   **Allergic dermatitis of right lower eyelid**

H01.113   **Allergic dermatitis of right eye, unspecified eyelid**

H01.114   **Allergic dermatitis of left upper eyelid**

H01.115   **Allergic dermatitis of left lower eyelid**

H01.116   **Allergic dermatitis of left eye, unspecified eyelid**

H01.119   **Allergic dermatitis of unspecified eye, unspecified eyelid**

   H01.12   **Discoid lupus erythematosus of eyelid**

FORWARD MAPPING SAMPLE (ICD-9-CM ➡ ICD-10-CM)

ICD-9-CM CODE & DESCRIPTION		ICD-10-CM CODE & DESCRIPTION	
379.00	Scleritis unspecified	H15.009	Unspecified scleritis unspecified eye
379.00	Scleritis unspecified	H15.109	Unspecified episcleritis unspecified eye
379.01	Episcleritis periodica fugax	H15.119	Episcleritis periodica fugax unspecified eye
379.02	Nodular episcleritis	H15.129	Nodular episcleritis unspecified eye
379.03	Anterior scleritis	H15.019	Anterior scleritis unspecified eye
379.04	Scleromalacia perforans	H15.059	Scleromalacia perforans unspecified eye
379.05	Scleritis with corneal involvement	H15.049	Scleritis with corneal involvement unspecified eye
379.06	Brawny scleritis	H15.029	Brawny scleritis unspecified eye
379.07	Posterior scleritis	H15.039	Posterior scleritis unspecified eye
379.09	Other scleritis	H15.099	Other scleritis unspecified eye
379.11	Scleral ectasia	H15.849	Scleral ectasia unspecified eye

379.12	Staphyloma posticum	H15.839	Staphyloma posticum unspecified eye
379.13	Equatorial staphyloma	H15.819	Equatorial staphyloma unspecified eye
379.14	Anterior staphyloma localized	H15.829	Localized anterior staphyloma unspecified eye
379.15	Ring staphyloma	H15.859	Ring staphyloma unspecified eye
379.16	Other degenerative disorders of sclera	H15.89	Other disorders of sclera
379.19	Other scleral disorders	H15.89	Other disorders of sclera
379.21	Vitreous degeneration	H43.819	Vitreous degeneration unspecified eye
379.22	Crystalline deposits in vitreous	H43.23	Crystalline deposits in vitreous body bilateral
379.23	Vitreous hemorrhage	H43.13	Vitreous hemorrhage bilateral
379.24	Other vitreous opacities	H43.399	Other vitreous opacities unspecified eye
379.25	Vitreous membranes and strands	H43.319	Vitreous membranes and strands unspecified eye
379.26	Vitreous prolapse	H43.03	Vitreous prolapse bilateral
379.29	Other disorders of vitreous	H43.89	Other disorders of vitreous body
379.31	Aphakia	H27.03	Aphakia bilateral
379.32	Subluxation of lens	H27.119	Subluxation of lens unspecified eye
379.33	Anterior dislocation of lens	H27.129	Anterior dislocation of lens unspecified eye
379.34	Posterior dislocation of lens	H27.139	Posterior dislocation of lens unspecified eye
379.39	Other disorders of lens	H27.8	Other specified disorders of lens
379.40	Abnormal pupillary function unspecified	H57.00	Unspecified anomaly of pupillary function
379.41	Anisocoria	H57.02	Anisocoria
379.42	Miosis (persistent) not due to miotics	H57.03	Miosis
379.43	Mydriasis (persistent) not due to mydriatics	H57.04	Mydriasis
379.45	Argyll Robertson pupil atypical	H57.01	Argyll Robertson pupil atypical
379.46	Tonic pupillary reaction	H57.059	Tonic pupil unspecified eye
379.49	Other anomalies of pupillary function	H57.09	Other anomalies of pupillary function
379.50	Nystagmus unspecified	H55.00	Unspecified nystagmus
379.51	Congenital nystagmus	H55.01	Congenital nystagmus
379.52	Latent nystagmus	H55.02	Latent nystagmus

| 379.53 | Visual deprivation nystagmus | H55.03 | Visual deprivation nystagmus |

BACKWARD MAPPING SAMPLE (ICD-10-CM ➡ ICD-9-CM)

ICD-10-CM CODE & DESCRIPTION		ICD-9-CM CODE AND DESCRIPTION	
H05.00	Unspecified acute inflammation of orbit	376.00	Acute inflammation of orbit unspecified
H05.011	Cellulitis of right orbit	376.01	Orbital cellulitis
H05.012	Cellulitis of left orbit	376.01	Orbital cellulitis
H05.013	Cellulitis of bilateral orbits	376.01	Orbital cellulitis
H05.019	Cellulitis of unspecified orbit	376.01	Orbital cellulitis
H05.021	Osteomyelitis of right orbit	376.03	Orbital osteomyelitis
H05.022	Osteomyelitis of left orbit	376.03	Orbital osteomyelitis
H05.023	Osteomyelitis of bilateral orbits	376.03	Orbital osteomyelitis
H05.029	Osteomyelitis of unspecified orbit	376.03	Orbital osteomyelitis
H05.031	Periostitis of right orbit	376.02	Orbital periostitis
H05.032	Periostitis of left orbit	376.02	Orbital periostitis
H05.033	Periostitis of bilateral orbits	376.02	Orbital periostitis
H05.039	Periostitis of unspecified orbit	376.02	Orbital periostitis
H05.041	Tenonitis of right orbit	376.04	Orbital tenonitis
H05.042	Tenonitis of left orbit	376.04	Orbital tenonitis
H05.043	Tenonitis of bilateral orbits	376.04	Orbital tenonitis
H05.049	Tenonitis of unspecified orbit	376.04	Orbital tenonitis
H05.10	Unspecified chronic inflammatory disorders of orbit	376.10	Chronic inflammation of orbit unspecified
H05.111	Granuloma of right orbit	376.11	Orbital granuloma
H05.112	Granuloma of left orbit	376.11	Orbital granuloma
H05.113	Granuloma of bilateral orbits	376.11	Orbital granuloma
H05.119	Granuloma of unspecified orbit	376.11	Orbital granuloma
H05.121	Orbital myositis right orbit	376.12	Orbital myositis
H05.122	Orbital myositis left orbit	376.12	Orbital myositis
H05.123	Orbital myositis bilateral	376.12	Orbital myositis
H05.129	Orbital myositis unspecified orbit	376.12	Orbital myositis
H05.20	Unspecified exophthalmos	376.30	Exophthalmos unspecified
H05.211	Displacement (lateral) of globe right eye	376.36	Lateral displacement of globe
H05.212	Displacement (lateral) of globe left eye	376.36	Lateral displacement of globe
H05.213	Displacement (lateral) of globe bilateral	376.36	Lateral displacement of globe

H05.219	Displacement (lateral) of globe unspecified eye	376.36	Lateral displacement of globe
H05.221	Edema of right orbit	376.33	Orbital edema or congestion
H05.222	Edema of left orbit	376.33	Orbital edema or congestion
H05.223	Edema of bilateral orbit	376.33	Orbital edema or congestion
H05.229	Edema of unspecified orbit	376.33	Orbital edema or congestion
H05.231	Hemorrhage of right orbit	376.32	Orbital hemorrhage
H05.232	Hemorrhage of left orbit	376.32	Orbital hemorrhage
H05.233	Hemorrhage of bilateral orbit	376.32	Orbital hemorrhage
H05.239	Hemorrhage of unspecified orbit	376.32	Orbital hemorrhage
H05.241	Constant exophthalmos right eye	376.31	Constant exophthalmos

CHAPTER 8: DISEASES OF EAR AND MASTOID PROCESS (H60-H95)

GENERAL GUIDELINES

There are no published guidelines for this chapter.

SAMPLE ICD-10-CM CODES FROM THIS CHAPTER

Note: Use an external cause code following the code for the ear condition, if applicable, to identify the cause of the ear condition

Excludes 2: certain conditions originating in the perinatal period (P04-P96)

certain infectious and parasitic diseases (A00-B99)

complications of pregnancy, childbirth and the puerperium (O00-O99)

congenital malformations, deformations and chromosomal abnormalities (Q00-Q99)

endocrine, nutritional and metabolic diseases (E00-E88)

injury, poisoning and certain other consequences of external causes (S00-T88)

neoplasms (C00-D49)

symptoms, signs and abnormal clinical and laboratory findings, not elsewhere classified (R00-R94)

This chapter contains the following blocks:	
H60-H62	Diseases of external ear
H65-H75	Diseases of middle ear and mastoid
H80-H83	Diseases of inner ear
H90-H94	Other disorders of ear
H95	Intraoperative and postprocedural complications and disorders of ear and mastoid process, not elsewhere classified

DISEASES OF EXTERNAL EAR (H60-H62)

H60   Otitis externa

H60.0 Abscess of external ear
Boil of external ear
Carbuncle of auricle or external auditory canal
Furuncle of external ear

  H60.00   Abscess of external ear, unspecified ear

  H60.01   Abscess of right external ear

  H60.02   Abscess of left external ear

  H60.03   Abscess of external ear, bilateral

H60.1 Cellulitis of external ear
Cellulitis of auricle
Cellulitis of external auditory canal

  H60.10   Cellulitis of external ear, unspecified ear

  H60.11   Cellulitis of right external ear

  H60.12   Cellulitis of left external ear

  H60.13   Cellulitis of external ear, bilateral

H60.2 Malignant otitis externa

  H60.20   Malignant otitis externa, unspecified ear

  H60.21   Malignant otitis externa, right ear

  H60.22   Malignant otitis externa, left ear

  H60.23   Malignant otitis externa, bilateral

H60.3 Other infective otitis externa

  H60.31   Diffuse otitis externa

      H60.311   Diffuse otitis externa, right ear

      H60.312   Diffuse otitis externa, left ear

      H60.313   Diffuse otitis externa, bilateral

      H60.319   Diffuse otitis externa, unspecified ear

  H60.32   Hemorrhagic otitis externa

      H60.321   Hemorrhagic otitis externa, right ear

H60.322   Hemorrhagic otitis externa, left ear

H60.323   Hemorrhagic otitis externa, bilateral

H60.329   Hemorrhagic otitis externa, unspecified ear

H60.33   Swimmer's ear

H60.331   Swimmer's ear, right ear

H60.332   Swimmer's ear, left ear

H60.333   Swimmer's ear, bilateral

H60.339   Swimmer's ear, unspecified ear

H60.39   Other infective otitis externa

H60.391   Other infective otitis externa, right ear

H60.392   Other infective otitis externa, left ear

H60.393   Other infective otitis externa, bilateral

H60.399   Other infective otitis externa, unspecified ear

H60.4   Cholesteatoma of external ear
Keratosis obturans of external ear (canal)

Excludes 2: cholesteatoma of middle ear (H71.-)
            recurrent cholesteatoma of postmastoidectomy cavity (H95.0-)

H60.40   Cholesteatoma of external ear, unspecified ear

H60.41   Cholesteatoma of right external ear

H60.42   Cholesteatoma of left external ear

H60.43   Cholesteatoma of external ear, bilateral

H60.5   Acute noninfective otitis externa

H60.50   Unspecified acute noninfective otitis externa
Acute otitis externa NOS

H60.501   Unspecified acute noninfective otitis externa, right ear

H60.502   Unspecified acute noninfective otitis externa, left ear

H60.503   Unspecified acute noninfective otitis externa, bilateral

H60.509 Unspecified acute noninfective otitis externa, unspecified ear

H60.51 **Acute actinic otitis externa**

H60.511 Acute actinic otitis externa, right ear

H60.512 Acute actinic otitis externa, left ear

H60.513 Acute actinic otitis externa, bilateral

H60.519 Acute actinic otitis externa, unspecified ear

FORWARD MAPPING SAMPLE (ICD-9-CM ➡ ICD-10-CM)			
ICD-9-CM CODE & DESCRIPTION		**ICD-10-CM CODE & DESCRIPTION**	
384.00	Acute myringitis unspecified	**H73.009**	Acute myringitis unspecified ear
384.01	Bullous myringitis	**H73.019**	Bullous myringitis unspecified ear
384.09	Other acute myringitis without otitis media	**H73.099**	Other acute myringitis unspecified ear
384.1	Chronic myringitis without otitis media	**H73.10**	Chronic myringitis unspecified ear
384.20	Perforation of tympanic membrane unspecified	**H72.90**	Unspecified perforation of tympanic membrane unspecified ear
384.21	Central perforation of tympanic membrane	**H72.00**	Central perforation of tympanic membrane unspecified ear
384.22	Attic perforation of tympanic membrane	**H72.10**	Attic perforation of tympanic membrane unspecified ear
384.23	Other marginal perforation of tympanic membrane	**H72.2x9**	Other marginal perforations of tympanic membrane unspecified ear
384.24	Multiple perforations of tympanic membrane	**H72.819**	Multiple perforations of tympanic membrane unspecified ear
384.25	Total perforation of tympanic membrane	**H72.829**	Total perforations of tympanic membrane unspecified ear
384.81	Atrophic flaccid tympanic membrane	**H73.819**	Atrophic flaccid tympanic membrane unspecified ear
384.82	Atrophic nonflaccid tympanic membrane	**H73.829**	Atrophic nonflaccid tympanic membrane unspecified ear
384.9	Unspecified disorder of tympanic membrane	**H73.93**	Unspecified disorder of tympanic membrane bilateral
385.00	Tympanosclerosis unspecified as to involvement	**H74.09**	Tympanosclerosis unspecified ear
385.01	Tympanosclerosis involving tympanic membrane only	**H74.09**	Tympanosclerosis unspecified ear
385.02	Tympanosclerosis involving tympanic membrane and ear ossicles	**H74.09**	Tympanosclerosis unspecified ear

385.03	Tympanosclerosis involving tympanic membrane ear ossicles and middle ear	H74.09	Tympanosclerosis unspecified ear
385.09	Tympanosclerosis involving other combination of structures	H74.09	Tympanosclerosis unspecified ear
385.10	Adhesive middle ear disease unspecified as to involvement	H74.19	Adhesive middle ear disease unspecified ear
385.11	Adhesions of drum head to incus	H74.19	Adhesive middle ear disease unspecified ear
385.12	Adhesions of drum head to stapes	H74.19	Adhesive middle ear disease unspecified ear
385.13	Adhesions of drum head to promontorium	H74.19	Adhesive middle ear disease unspecified ear
385.19	Other middle ear adhesions and combinations	H74.19	Adhesive middle ear disease unspecified ear
385.21	Impaired mobility of malleus	H74.319	Ankylosis of ear ossicles unspecified ear
385.22	Impaired mobility of other ear ossicles	H74.319	Ankylosis of ear ossicles unspecified ear
385.23	Discontinuity or dislocation of ear ossicles	H74.20	Discontinuity and dislocation of ear ossicles unspecified ear
385.23	Discontinuity or dislocation of ear ossicles	H74.399	Other acquired abnormalities of ear ossicles unspecified ear
385.24	Partial loss or necrosis of ear ossicles	H74.329	Partial loss of ear ossicles unspecified ear
385.30	Cholesteatoma unspecified	H71.93	Unspecified cholesteatoma bilateral
385.31	Cholesteatoma of attic	H71.03	Cholesteatoma of attic bilateral
385.32	Cholesteatoma of middle ear	H74.40	Polyp of middle ear unspecified ear
385.32	Cholesteatoma of middle ear	H71.13	Cholesteatoma of tympanum bilateral
385.33	Cholesteatoma of middle ear and mastoid	H71.23	Cholesteatoma of mastoid bilateral
385.35	Diffuse cholesteatosis of middle ear and mastoid	H71.33	Diffuse cholesteatosis bilateral
385.82	Cholesterin granuloma of middle ear	H74.8x9	Other specified disorders of middle ear and mastoid unspecified ear
385.83	Retained foreign body of middle ear	H74.8x9	Other specified disorders of middle ear and mastoid unspecified ear
385.89	Other disorders of middle ear and mastoid	H74.8x9	Other specified disorders of middle ear and mastoid unspecified ear
385.9	Unspecified disorder of middle ear and mastoid	H74.90	Unspecified disorder of middle ear and mastoid unspecified ear
386.00	Ménière's disease unspecified	H81.09	Ménière's disease unspecified ear

386.01	Active Ménière's disease cochleovestibular	H81.09	Ménière's disease unspecified ear

BACKWARD MAPPING SAMPLE (ICD-10-CM ➡ ICD-9-CM)

ICD-10-CM CODE & DESCRIPTION		ICD-9-CM CODE & DESCRIPTION	
H70.001	Acute mastoiditis without complications right ear	383.00	Acute mastoiditis without complications
H70.002	Acute mastoiditis without complications left ear	383.00	Acute mastoiditis without complications
H70.003	Acute mastoiditis without complications bilateral	383.00	Acute mastoiditis without complications
H70.009	Acute mastoiditis without complications unspecified ear	383.00	Acute mastoiditis without complications
H70.011	Subperiosteal abscess of mastoid right ear	383.01	Subperiosteal abscess of mastoid
H70.012	Subperiosteal abscess of mastoid left ear	383.01	Subperiosteal abscess of mastoid
H70.013	Subperiosteal abscess of mastoid bilateral	383.01	Subperiosteal abscess of mastoid
H70.019	Subperiosteal abscess of mastoid unspecified ear	383.01	Subperiosteal abscess of mastoid
H70.091	Acute mastoiditis with other complications right ear	383.02	Acute mastoiditis with other complications
H70.092	Acute mastoiditis with other complications left ear	383.02	Acute mastoiditis with other complications
H70.093	Acute mastoiditis with other complications bilateral	383.02	Acute mastoiditis with other complications
H70.099	Acute mastoiditis with other complications unspecified ear	383.02	Acute mastoiditis with other complications
H70.10	Chronic mastoiditis unspecified ear	383.1	Chronic mastoiditis
H70.11	Chronic mastoiditis right ear	383.1	Chronic mastoiditis
H70.12	Chronic mastoiditis left ear	383.1	Chronic mastoiditis
H70.13	Chronic mastoiditis bilateral	383.1	Chronic mastoiditis
H70.201	Unspecified petrositis right ear	383.20	Petrositis unspecified
H70.202	Unspecified petrositis left ear	383.20	Petrositis unspecified
H70.203	Unspecified petrositis bilateral	383.20	Petrositis unspecified
H70.209	Unspecified petrositis unspecified ear	383.20	Petrositis unspecified
H70.211	Acute petrositis right ear	383.21	Acute petrositis
H70.212	Acute petrositis left ear	383.21	Acute petrositis
H70.213	Acute petrositis bilateral	383.21	Acute petrositis
H70.219	Acute petrositis unspecified ear	383.21	Acute petrositis
H70.221	Chronic petrositis right ear	383.22	Chronic petrositis
H70.222	Chronic petrositis left ear	383.22	Chronic petrositis

H70.223	Chronic petrositis bilateral	383.22	Chronic petrositis
H70.229	Chronic petrositis unspecified ear	383.22	Chronic petrositis
H70.811	Postauricular fistula right ear	383.81	Postauricular fistula
H70.812	Postauricular fistula left ear	383.81	Postauricular fistula
H70.813	Postauricular fistula bilateral	383.81	Postauricular fistula
H70.819	Postauricular fistula unspecified ear	383.81	Postauricular fistula
H70.891	Other mastoiditis and related conditions right ear	383.89	Other disorders of mastoid
H70.892	Other mastoiditis and related conditions left ear	383.89	Other disorders of mastoid
H70.893	Other mastoiditis and related conditions bilateral	383.89	Other disorders of mastoid
H70.899	Other mastoiditis and related conditions unspecified ear	383.89	Other disorders of mastoid
H70.90	Unspecified mastoiditis unspecified ear	383.9	Unspecified mastoiditis
H70.91	Unspecified mastoiditis right ear	383.9	Unspecified mastoiditis
H70.92	Unspecified mastoiditis left ear	383.9	Unspecified mastoiditis
H70.93	Unspecified mastoiditis bilateral	383.9	Unspecified mastoiditis

CHAPTER 9: DISEASES OF CIRCULATORY SYSTEM (I00-I99)

GENERAL GUIDELINES

HYPERTENSION

1) **Hypertension with Heart Disease**

Heart conditions classified to I50.- or I51.4-I51.9, are assigned to, a code from category I11, Hypertensive heart disease, when a causal relationship is stated (due to hypertension) or implied (hypertensive). Use an additional code from category I50, Heart failure, to identify the type of heart failure in those patients with heart failure.

The same heart conditions (I50.-, I51.4-I51.9) with hypertension, but without a stated causal relationship, are coded separately. These codes are sequenced according to the circumstances of the admission/ encounter.

2) **Hypertensive Chronic Kidney Disease**

Assign codes from category I12, Hypertensive chronic kidney disease, when both hypertension and a condition classifiable to category N18, Chronic kidney disease (CKD), are present. Unlike hypertension with heart disease, ICD-10-CM presumes a cause-and-effect relationship and classifies chronic kidney disease with hypertension as hypertensive chronic kidney disease.

The appropriate code from category N18 should be used as a secondary code with a code from category I12 to identify the stage of chronic kidney disease.

If a patient has hypertensive chronic kidney disease and acute renal failure, an additional code for the acute renal failure is required.

3) Hypertensive Heart and Chronic Kidney Disease

Assign codes from combination category I13, Hypertensive heart and chronic kidney disease, when both hypertensive kidney disease and hypertensive heart disease are stated in the diagnosis. Assume a relationship between the hypertension and the chronic kidney disease, whether or not the condition is so designated. If heart failure is present, assign an additional code from category I50 to identify the type of heart failure.

The appropriate code from category N18, Chronic kidney disease, should be used as a secondary code with a code from category I13 to identify the stage of chronic kidney disease.

The codes in category I13, Hypertensive heart and chronic kidney disease, are combination codes that include hypertension, heart disease and chronic kidney disease. The Includes note at I13 specifies that the conditions included at I11 and I12 are included together in I13. If a patient has hypertension, heart disease and chronic kidney disease then a code from I13 should be used, not individual codes for hypertension, heart disease and chronic kidney disease, or codes from I11 or I12.

For patients with both acute renal failure and chronic kidney disease an additional code for acute renal failure is required.

4) Hypertensive Cerebrovascular Disease

For hypertensive cerebrovascular disease, first assign the appropriate code from categories I60-I69, followed by the appropriate hypertension code.

5) Hypertensive Retinopathy

Subcategory H35.0, Background retinopathy and retinal vascular changes, should be used with code I10, Essential (primary) hypertension, to include the systemic hypertension. The sequencing is based on the reason for the encounter.

6) Hypertension, Secondary

Secondary hypertension is due to an underlying condition. Two codes are required: one to identify the underlying etiology and one from category I15 to identify the hypertension. Sequencing of codes is determined by the reason for admission/encounter.

7) Hypertension, Transient

Assign code R03.0, Elevated blood pressure reading without diagnosis of hypertension, unless patient has an established diagnosis of hypertension. Assign code O13.-, Gestational [pregnancy-induced] hypertension without significant proteinuria, or O14.-, Pre-eclampsia, for transient hypertension of pregnancy.

8) Hypertension, Controlled

This diagnostic statement usually refers to an existing state of hypertension under control by therapy. Assign the appropriate code from categories I10-I15, Hypertensive diseases.

9) Hypertension, Uncontrolled

Uncontrolled hypertension may refer to untreated hypertension or hypertension not responding to current therapeutic regimen. In either case, assign the appropriate code from categories I10-I15, Hypertensive diseases.

ATHEROSCLEROTIC CORONARY ARTERY DISEASE AND ANGINA

ICD-10-CM has combination codes for atherosclerotic heart disease with angina pectoris. The subcategories for these codes are I25.11, Atherosclerotic heart disease of native coronary artery with angina pectoris and I25.7, Atherosclerosis of coronary artery bypass graft(s) and coronary artery of transplanted heart with angina pectoris.

When using one of these combination codes it is not necessary to use an additional code for angina pectoris. A causal relationship can be assumed in a patient with both atherosclerosis and angina pectoris, unless the documentation indicates the angina is due to something other than the atherosclerosis.

If a patient with coronary artery disease is admitted due to an acute myocardial infarction (AMI), the AMI should be sequenced before the coronary artery disease.

INTRAOPERATIVE AND POSTPROCEDURAL CEREBROVASCULAR ACCIDENT

Medical record documentation should clearly specify the cause- and- effect relationship between the medical intervention and the cerebrovascular accident in order to assign a code for intraoperative or postprocedural cerebrovascular accident.

Proper code assignment depends on whether it was an infarction or hemorrhage and whether it occurred intraoperatively or postoperatively. If it was a cerebral hemorrhage, code assignment depends on the type of procedure performed.

SEQUELAE OF CEREBROVASCULAR DISEASE

1) Category I69, Sequelae of Cerebrovascular disease

Category I69 is used to indicate conditions classifiable to categories I60-I67 as the causes of late effects (neurologic deficits), themselves classified elsewhere. These "late effects" include neurologic deficits that persist after initial onset of conditions classifiable to categories I60-I67. The neurologic deficits caused by cerebrovascular disease may be present from the onset or may arise at any time after the onset of the condition classifiable to categories I60-I67.

2) Codes from category I69 with codes from I60-I67

Codes from category I69 may be assigned on a health care record with codes from I60-I67, if the patient has a current cerebrovascular disease and deficits from an old cerebrovascular disease.

3) **Code Z86.73**

Assign code Z86.73, Personal history of transient ischemic attack (TIA), and cerebral infarction without residual deficits (and not a code from category I69) as an additional code for history of cerebrovascular disease when no neurologic deficits are present.

ACUTE MYOCARDIAL INFARCTION (AMI)

1) **ST elevation myocardial infarction (STEMI) and non ST elevation myocardial infarction (NSTEMI)**

The ICD-10-CM codes for acute myocardial infarction (AMI) identify the site, such as anterolateral wall or true posterior wall. Subcategories I21.0-I21.2 and code I21.4 are used for ST elevation myocardial infarction (STEMI). Code I21.4, Non-ST elevation (NSTEMI) myocardial infarction, is used for non ST elevation myocardial infarction (NSTEMI) and nontransmural MIs.

If NSTEMI evolves to STEMI, assign the STEMI code. If STEMI converts to NSTEMI due to thrombolytic therapy, it is still coded as STEMI.

When the patient requires continued care for the myocardial infarction, codes from category I21 may continue to be reported for the duration of 4 weeks (28 days) or less from onset, regardless of the healthcare setting, including when a patient is transferred from the acute care setting to the post-acute care setting if the patient is still within the four weeks time frame. For encounters after the 4 weeks time frame and the patient requires continued care related to the myocardial infarction, the appropriate aftercare code should be assigned, rather than a code from category I21. Otherwise, code I25.2, Old myocardial infarction, may be assigned for old or healed myocardial infarction not requiring further care.

2) **Acute myocardial infarction, unspecified**

Code I21.3, ST elevation (STEMI) myocardial infarction of unspecified site, is the default for the unspecified term acute myocardial infarction. If only STEMI or transmural MI without the site is documented, query the provider as to the site, or assign code I21.3.

3) **AMI documented as nontransmural or subendocardial but site provided**

If an AMI is documented as nontransmural or subendocardial, but the site is provided, it is still coded as a subendocardial AMI.

See Section I.C.21.3 for information on coding status post administration of tPA in a different facility within the last 24 hours.

4) **Subsequent acute myocardial infarction**

A code from category I22, Subsequent ST elevation (STEMI) and non ST elevation (NSTEMI) myocardial infarction, is to be used when a patient who has suffered an AMI has a new AMI within the 4 week time frame of the initial AMI. A code from category I22 must be used in conjunction with a code from category I21.

The sequencing of the I22 and I21 codes depends on the circumstances of the encounter. Should a patient who is in the hospital due to an AMI have a subsequent AMI while still in the hospital code I21 would be sequenced first as the reason for admission, with code I22 sequenced as a secondary code. Should a patient have a subsequent AMI after discharge for care of an initial AMI, and the reason for admission is the subsequent AMI, the I22 code should be sequenced first followed by the I21. An I21 code must accompany an I22 code to identify the site of the initial AMI, and to indicate that the patient is still within the 4 week time frame of healing from the initial AMI.

The guidelines for assigning the correct I22 code are the same as for the initial AMI.

SAMPLE ICD-10-CM CODES FROM THIS CHAPTER

Excludes 2: certain conditions originating in the perinatal period (P04-P96)
certain infectious and parasitic diseases (A00-B99)
complications of pregnancy, childbirth and the puerperium (O00-O99)
congenital malformations, deformations, and chromosomal abnormalities (Q00-Q99)
endocrine, nutritional and metabolic diseases (E00-E88)
injury, poisoning and certain other consequences of external causes (S00-T88)
neoplasms (C00-D49)
symptoms, signs and abnormal clinical and laboratory findings, not elsewhere classified (R00-R94)
systemic connective tissue disorders (M30-M36)
transient cerebral ischemic attacks and related syndromes (G45.-)

This chapter contains the following blocks:	
I00-I02	Acute rheumatic fever
I05-I09	Chronic rheumatic heart diseases
I10-I15	Hypertensive diseases
I20-I25	Ischemic heart diseases
I26-I28	Pulmonary heart disease and diseases of pulmonary circulation
I30-I52	Other forms of heart disease
I60-I69	Cerebrovascular diseases
I70-I79	Diseases of arteries, arterioles and capillaries
I80-I89	Diseases of veins, lymphatic vessels and lymph nodes, not elsewhere classified.
I95-I99	Other and unspecified disorders of the circulatory system

ACUTE RHEUMATIC FEVER (I00-I02)

I00   Rheumatic fever without heart involvement

Includes: arthritis, rheumatic, acute or subacute

Excludes 1: rheumatic fever with heart involvement (I01.0- I01.9)

I01   Rheumatic fever with heart involvement

Excludes 1: chronic diseases of rheumatic origin (I05-I09) unless rheumatic fever is also present or there is evidence of reactivation or activity of the rheumatic process.

I01.0   Acute rheumatic pericarditis
Any condition in I00 with pericarditis
Rheumatic pericarditis (acute)
Excludes 1: acute pericarditis not specified as rheumatic (I30.-)

I01.1   Acute rheumatic endocarditis
Any condition in I00 with endocarditis or valvulitis
Acute rheumatic valvulitis

I01.2   Acute rheumatic myocarditis
Any condition in I00 with myocarditis

I01.8   Other acute rheumatic heart disease
Any condition in I00with other or multiple types of heart involvement
Acute rheumatic pancarditis

I01.9   Acute rheumatic heart disease, unspecified
Any condition in I00 with unspecified type of heart involvement
Rheumatic carditis, acute
Rheumatic heart disease, active or acute

I02   Rheumatic chorea

Includes: Sydenham's chorea

Excludes 1: chorea NOS (G25.5)
                Huntington's chorea (G10)

I02.0   Rheumatic chorea with heart involvement
Chorea NOS with heart involvement
Rheumatic chorea with heart involvement of any type classifiable under I01.-

I02.9   Rheumatic chorea without heart involvement
Rheumatic chorea NOS

CHRONIC RHEUMATIC HEART DISEASES (I05-I09)

I05   Rheumatic mitral valve diseases

Includes: conditions classifiable to both I05.0 and I05.2-I05.9, whether specified as rheumatic or not

Excludes 1: mitral valve disease specified as nonrheumatic (I34.-)
                mitral valve disease with aortic and/or tricuspid valve involvement (I08.-)

I05.0   Rheumatic mitral stenosis
Mitral (valve) obstruction (rheumatic)

I05.1 **Rheumatic mitral insufficiency**
Rheumatic mitral incompetence
Rheumatic mitral regurgitation

Excludes 1: mitral insufficiency not specified as rheumatic (I34.0)

I05.2 **Rheumatic mitral stenosis with insufficiency**
Rheumatic mitral stenosis with incompetence or regurgitation

I05.8 **Other rheumatic mitral valve diseases**
Rheumatic mitral (valve) failure

I05.9 **Rheumatic mitral valve disease, unspecified**
Rheumatic mitral (valve) disorder (chronic) NOS

I06 **Rheumatic aortic valve diseases**

Excludes 1: aortic valve disease not specified as rheumatic (I35.-)
aortic valve disease with mitral and/or tricuspid valve involvement (I08.-)

I06.0 **Rheumatic aortic stenosis**
Rheumatic aortic (valve) obstruction

I06.1 **Rheumatic aortic insufficiency**
Rheumatic aortic incompetence
Rheumatic aortic regurgitation

I06.2 **Rheumatic aortic stenosis with insufficiency**
Rheumatic aortic stenosis with incompetence or regurgitation

I06.8 **Other rheumatic aortic valve diseases**

I06.9 **Rheumatic aortic valve disease, unspecified**
Rheumatic aortic (valve) disease NOS

I07 **Rheumatic tricuspid valve diseases**

Includes: rheumatic tricuspid valve diseases specified as rheumatic or unspecified

Excludes 1: tricuspid valve disease specified as nonrheumatic (I36.-)
tricuspid valve disease with aortic and/or mitral valve involvement (I08.-)

I07.0 **Rheumatic tricuspid stenosis**
Tricuspid (valve) stenosis (rheumatic)

I07.1 **Rheumatic tricuspid insufficiency**
Tricuspid (valve) insufficiency (rheumatic)

I07.2 **Rheumatic tricuspid stenosis and insufficiency**

I07.8 **Other rheumatic tricuspid valve diseases**

I07.9   Rheumatic tricuspid valve disease, unspecified
Rheumatic tricuspid valve disorder NOS

I08   Multiple valve diseases

Includes: multiple valve diseases specified as rheumatic or unspecified

Excludes 1: endocarditis, valve unspecified (I38)
multiple valve disease specified a nonrheumatic (I34.-, I35.-, I36.-, I37.-, I38.-, Q22.-, Q23.-, Q24.8-)
rheumatic valve disease NOS (I09.1)

I08.0   Rheumatic disorders of both mitral and aortic valves
Involvement of both mitral and aortic valves specified as rheumatic or unspecified

I08.1   Rheumatic disorders of both mitral and tricuspid valves

I08.2   Rheumatic disorders of both aortic and tricuspid valves

I08.3   Combined rheumatic disorders of mitral, aortic and tricuspid valves

I08.8   Other rheumatic multiple valve diseases

I08.9   Rheumatic multiple valve disease, unspecified

I09   Other rheumatic heart diseases

I09.0   Rheumatic myocarditis

FORWARD MAPPING SAMPLE (ICD-9-CM ➡ ICD-10-CM)

ICD-9-CM CODE & DESCRIPTION		ICD-10-CM CODE & DESCRIPTION	
415.0	Acute cor pulmonale	I26.09	Other pulmonary embolism with acute cor pulmonale
415.11	Iatrogenic pulmonary embolism and infarction	I26.99	Other pulmonary embolism without acute cor pulmonale
415.12	Septic pulmonary embolism	I26.90	Septic pulmonary embolism without acute cor pulmonale
415.19	Other pulmonary embolism and infarction	I26.99	Other pulmonary embolism without acute cor pulmonale
416.0	Primary pulmonary hypertension	I27.0	Primary pulmonary hypertension
416.1	Kyphoscoliotic heart disease	I27.1	Kyphoscoliotic heart disease
416.2	Chronic pulmonary embolism	I27.82	Chronic pulmonary embolism
416.8	Other chronic pulmonary heart diseases	I27.89	Other specified pulmonary heart diseases
416.8	Other chronic pulmonary heart diseases	I27.2	Other secondary pulmonary hypertension
416.9	Chronic pulmonary heart disease unspecified	I27.9	Pulmonary heart disease unspecified

416.9	Chronic pulmonary heart disease unspecified	I27.81	Cor pulmonale (chronic)
417.0	Arteriovenous fistula of pulmonary vessels	I28.0	Arteriovenous fistula of pulmonary vessels
417.1	Aneurysm of pulmonary artery	I28.1	Aneurysm of pulmonary artery
417.8	Other specified diseases of pulmonary circulation	I28.8	Other diseases of pulmonary vessels
417.9	Unspecified disease of pulmonary circulation	I28.9	Disease of pulmonary vessels unspecified
420.0	Acute pericarditis in diseases classified elsewhere	I32	Pericarditis in diseases classified elsewhere
420.90	Acute pericarditis unspecified	I30.9	Acute pericarditis unspecified
420.91	Acute idiopathic pericarditis	I30.0	Acute nonspecific idiopathic pericarditis
420.99	Other acute pericarditis	I30.8	Other forms of acute pericarditis
421.0	Acute and subacute bacterial endocarditis	I33.0	Acute and subacute infective endocarditis
421.1	Acute and subacute infective endocarditis in diseases classified elsewhere	I39	Endocarditis and heart valve disorders in diseases classified elsewhere
421.9	Acute endocarditis unspecified	I33.9	Acute and subacute endocarditis unspecified
422.0	Acute myocarditis in diseases classified elsewhere	I41	Myocarditis in diseases classified elsewhere
422.90	Acute myocarditis unspecified	I40.9	Acute myocarditis unspecified
422.91	Idiopathic myocarditis	I40.1	Isolated myocarditis
422.92	Septic myocarditis	I40.0	Infective myocarditis
422.93	Toxic myocarditis	I40.8	Other acute myocarditis
422.99	Other acute myocarditis	I40.8	Other acute myocarditis
423.0	Hemopericardium	I31.2	Hemopericardium not elsewhere classified
423.1	Adhesive pericarditis	I31.0	Chronic adhesive pericarditis
423.2	Constrictive pericarditis	I31.1	Chronic constrictive pericarditis
423.3	Cardiac tamponade	I31.4	Cardiac tamponade
423.8	Other specified diseases of pericardium	I31.8	Other specified diseases of pericardium
423.9	Unspecified disease of pericardium	I31.9	Disease of pericardium unspecified
424.0	Mitral valve disorders	I34.0	Nonrheumatic mitral (valve) insufficiency
424.0	Mitral valve disorders	I34.8	Other nonrheumatic mitral valve disorders
424.1	Aortic valve disorders	I35.0	Nonrheumatic aortic (valve) stenosis

424.1	Aortic valve disorders	I35.8	Other nonrheumatic aortic valve disorders
424.2	Tricuspid valve disorders specified as nonrheumatic	I36.0	Nonrheumatic tricuspid (valve) stenosis
424.2	Tricuspid valve disorders specified as nonrheumatic	I36.8	Other nonrheumatic tricuspid valve disorders

BACKWARD MAPPING SAMPLE (ICD-10-CM ➡ ICD-9-CM)

ICD-10-CM CODE & DESCRIPTION		ICD-9-CM CODE & DESCRIPTION	
I00	Rheumatic fever without heart involvement	390	Rheumatic fever without heart involvement
I01.0	Acute rheumatic pericarditis	391.0	Acute rheumatic pericarditis
I01.1	Acute rheumatic endocarditis	391.1	Acute rheumatic endocarditis
I01.2	Acute rheumatic myocarditis	391.2	Acute rheumatic myocarditis
I01.8	Other acute rheumatic heart disease	391.8	Other acute rheumatic heart disease
I01.9	Acute rheumatic heart disease unspecified	391.9	Acute rheumatic heart disease unspecified
I02.0	Rheumatic chorea with heart involvement	392.0	Rheumatic chorea with heart involvement
I02.9	Rheumatic chorea without heart involvement	392.9	Rheumatic chorea without heart involvement
I05.0	Rheumatic mitral stenosis	394.0	Mitral stenosis
I05.1	Rheumatic mitral insufficiency	394.1	Rheumatic mitral insufficiency
I05.2	Rheumatic mitral stenosis with insufficiency	394.2	Mitral stenosis with insufficiency
I05.8	Other rheumatic mitral valve diseases	394.9	Other and unspecified mitral valve diseases
I05.9	Rheumatic mitral valve disease unspecified	394.9	Other and unspecified mitral valve diseases
I06.0	Rheumatic aortic stenosis	395.0	Rheumatic aortic stenosis
I06.1	Rheumatic aortic insufficiency	395.1	Rheumatic aortic insufficiency
I06.2	Rheumatic aortic stenosis with insufficiency	395.2	Rheumatic aortic stenosis with insufficiency
I06.8	Other rheumatic aortic valve diseases	395.9	Other and unspecified rheumatic aortic diseases
I06.9	Rheumatic aortic valve disease unspecified	395.9	Other and unspecified rheumatic aortic diseases
I07.0	Rheumatic tricuspid stenosis	397.0	Diseases of tricuspid valve
I07.1	Rheumatic tricuspid insufficiency	397.0	Diseases of tricuspid valve
I07.2	Rheumatic tricuspid stenosis and insufficiency	397.0	Diseases of tricuspid valve
I07.8	Other rheumatic tricuspid valve diseases	397.0	Diseases of tricuspid valve

I07.9	Rheumatic tricuspid valve disease unspecified	397.0	Diseases of tricuspid valve
I08.0	Rheumatic disorders of both mitral and aortic valves	396.0	Mitral valve stenosis and aortic valve stenosis
I08.0	Rheumatic disorders of both mitral and aortic valves	396.1	Mitral valve stenosis and aortic valve insufficiency
I08.0	Rheumatic disorders of both mitral and aortic valves	396.2	Mitral valve insufficiency and aortic valve stenosis
I08.0	Rheumatic disorders of both mitral and aortic valves	396.3	Mitral valve insufficiency and aortic valve insufficiency
I08.1	Rheumatic disorders of both mitral and tricuspid valves	397.9	Rheumatic diseases of endocardium valve unspecified
I08.2	Rheumatic disorders of both aortic and tricuspid valves	397.9	Rheumatic diseases of endocardium valve unspecified
I08.3	Combined rheumatic disorders of mitral aortic and tricuspid valves	397.9	Rheumatic diseases of endocardium valve unspecified
I08.8	Other rheumatic multiple valve diseases	396.8	Multiple involvement of mitral and aortic valves
I08.8	Other rheumatic multiple valve diseases	397.9	Rheumatic diseases of endocardium valve unspecified
I08.9	Rheumatic multiple valve disease unspecified	396.9	Mitral and aortic valve diseases unspecified
I08.9	Rheumatic multiple valve disease unspecified	397.9	Rheumatic diseases of endocardium valve unspecified
I09.0	Rheumatic myocarditis	398.0	Rheumatic myocarditis
I09.1	Rheumatic diseases of endocardium valve unspecified	397.9	Rheumatic diseases of endocardium valve unspecified
I09.2	Chronic rheumatic pericarditis	393	Chronic rheumatic pericarditis
I09.81	Rheumatic heart failure	398.91	Rheumatic heart failure (congestive)
I09.89	Other specified rheumatic heart diseases	397.1	Rheumatic diseases of pulmonary valve
I09.89	Other specified rheumatic heart diseases	398.99	Other rheumatic heart diseases

CHAPTER 10: DISEASES OF RESPIRATORY SYSTEM (J00-J99)

GENERAL GUIDELINES

CHRONIC OBSTRUCTIVE PULMONARY DISEASE [COPD] AND ASTHMA

1) **Acute exacerbation of chronic obstructive bronchitis and asthma**

The codes in categories J44 and J45 distinguish between uncomplicated cases and those in acute exacerbation. An acute exacerbation is a worsening or a decompensation of a chronic condition. An acute exacerbation is not equivalent to an infection superimposed on a chronic condition, though an exacerbation may be triggered by an infection.

ACUTE RESPIRATORY FAILURE

1) Acute respiratory failure as principal diagnosis

A code from subcategory J96.0, Acute respiratory failure, or subcategory J96.2, Acute and chronic respiratory failure, may be assigned as a principal diagnosis when it is the condition established after study to be chiefly responsible for occasioning the admission to the hospital, and the selection is supported by the Alphabetic Index and Tabular List. However, chapter-specific coding guidelines (such as obstetrics, poisoning, HIV, newborn) that provide sequencing direction take precedence.

2) Acute respiratory failure as secondary diagnosis

Respiratory failure may be listed as a secondary diagnosis if it occurs after admission, or if it is present on admission, but does not meet the definition of principal diagnosis.

3) Sequencing of acute respiratory failure and another acute condition

When a patient is admitted with respiratory failure and another acute condition, (e.g., myocardial infarction, cerebrovascular accident, aspiration pneumonia), the principal diagnosis will not be the same in every situation. This applies whether the other acute condition is a respiratory or nonrespiratory condition. Selection of the principal diagnosis will be dependent on the circumstances of admission. If both the respiratory failure and the other acute condition are equally responsible for occasioning the admission to the hospital, and there are no chapter-specific sequencing rules, the guideline regarding two or more diagnoses that equally meet the definition for principal diagnosis may be applied in these situations.

If the documentation is not clear as to whether acute respiratory failure and another condition are equally responsible for occasioning the admission, query the provider for clarification.

INFLUENZA DUE TO CERTAIN IDENTIFIED INFLUENZA VIRUSES

Code only confirmed cases of avian influenza (code J09.0-, Influenza due to identified avian influenza virus) or novel H1N1 or swine flu, code J09.1-. This is an exception to the hospital inpatient guideline Section II, H. (Uncertain Diagnosis).

In this context, "confirmation" does not require documentation of positive laboratory testing specific for avian or novel H1N1 (H1N1 or swine flu) influenza. However, coding should be based on the provider's diagnostic statement that the patient has
avian influenza.

If the provider records "suspected or possible or probable avian influenza," the appropriate influenza code from category J11, Influenza due to unspecified influenza virus, should be assigned. A code from category J09, Influenza due to certain identified influenza viruses, should not be assigned.

VENTILATOR ASSOCIATED PNEUMONIA

1) Documentation of Ventilator associated Pneumonia

As with all procedural or postprocedural complications, code assignment is based on the provider's documentation of the relationship between the condition and the procedure.

Code J95.851, Ventilator associated pneumonia, should be assigned only when the provider has documented ventilator associated pneumonia (VAP). An additional code to identify the organism (e.g., Pseudomonas aeruginosa, code B96.5) should also be assigned. Do not assign an additional code from categories J12-J18 to identify the type of pneumonia.

Code J95.851 should not be assigned for cases where the patient has pneumonia and is on a mechanical ventilator but the provider has not specifically stated that the pneumonia is ventilator-associated pneumonia. If the documentation is unclear as to whether the patient has a pneumonia that is a complication attributable to the mechanical ventilator, query the provider.

2) Ventilator associated Pneumonia Develops after Admission

A patient may be admitted with one type of pneumonia (e.g., code J13, Pneumonia due to Streptococcus pneumonia) and subsequently develop VAP. In this instance, the principal diagnosis would be the appropriate code from categories J12-J18 for the pneumonia diagnosed at the time of admission. Code J95.851, Ventilator associated pneumonia, would be assigned as an additional diagnosis when the provider has also documented the presence of ventilator associated pneumonia.

SAMPLE ICD-10-CM CODES FROM THIS CHAPTER

Note: When a respiratory condition is described as occurring in more than one site and is not specifically indexed, it should be classified to the lower anatomic site (e.g. tracheobronchitis to bronchitis in J40).

Use additional code, where applicable, to identify:
exposure to environmental tobacco smoke (Z77.22)
exposure to tobacco smoke in the perinatal period (P96.81)
history of tobacco use (Z87.891)
occupational exposure to environmental tobacco smoke (Z57.31)
tobacco dependence (F17.-)
tobacco use (Z72.0)

Excludes 2: certain conditions originating in the perinatal period (P04-P96)
certain infectious and parasitic diseases (A00-B99)
complications of pregnancy, childbirth and the puerperium (O00-O99)
congenital malformations, deformations and chromosomal abnormalities (Q00-Q99)
endocrine, nutritional and metabolic diseases (E00-E88)
injury, poisoning and certain other consequences of external causes (S00-T88)
neoplasms (C00-D49)
smoke inhalation (T59.81-)
symptoms, signs and abnormal clinical and laboratory findings, not elsewhere classified (R00-R94)

This chapter contains the following blocks:	
J00-J06	Acute upper respiratory infections
J09-J18	Influenza and pneumonia
J20-J22	Other acute lower respiratory infections
J30-J39	Other diseases of upper respiratory tract
J40-J47	Chronic lower respiratory diseases
J60-J70	Lung diseases due to external agents
J80-J84	Other respiratory diseases principally affecting the interstitium
J85-J86	Suppurative and necrotic conditions of the lower respiratory tract
J90-J94	Other diseases of the pleura

ACUTE UPPER RESPIRATORY INFECTIONS (J00-J06)

Excludes 1: chronic obstructive pulmonary disease with acute lower respiratory infection (J44.0)
   influenza (J09-J11)

J00   Acute nasopharyngitis [common cold]
   Acute rhinitis
   Coryza (acute)
   Infective nasopharyngitis NOS
   Infective rhinitis
   Nasal catarrh, acute
   Nasopharyngitis NOS

   Excludes 1: acute pharyngitis (J02.-)
         acute sore throat NOS (J02.9)
         pharyngitis NOS (J02.9)
         rhinitis NOS (J31.0)
         sore throat NOS (J02.9)

   Excludes 2: allergic rhinitis (J30.1-J30.9)
         chronic pharyngitis (J31.2)
         chronic rhinitis (J31.0)
         chronic sore throat (J31.2)
         nasopharyngitis, chronic (J31.1)
         vasomotor rhinitis (J30.0)

J01   Acute sinusitis

   Includes: acute abscess of sinus
         acute empyema of sinus
         acute infection of sinus
         acute inflammation of sinus
         acute suppuration of sinus

   Use additional code (B95-B97) to identify infectious agent.

   Excludes 1: sinusitis NOS (J32.9)

Excludes 2: chronic sinusitis (J32.0-J32.8)

J01.0 **Acute maxillary sinusitis**
Acute antritis

    J01.00 **Acute maxillary sinusitis, unspecified**

    J01.01 **Acute recurrent maxillary sinusitis**

J01.1 **Acute frontal sinusitis**

    J01.10 **Acute frontal sinusitis, unspecified**

    J01.11 **Acute recurrent frontal sinusitis**

J01.2 **Acute ethmoidal sinusitis**

    J01.20 **Acute ethmoidal sinusitis, unspecified**

    J01.21 **Acute recurrent ethmoidal sinusitis**

J01.3 **Acute sphenoidal sinusitis**

    J01.30 **Acute sphenoidal sinusitis, unspecified**

    J01.31 **Acute recurrent sphenoidal sinusitis**

J01.4 **Acute pansinusitis**

    J01.40 **Acute pansinusitis, unspecified**

    J01.41 **Acute recurrent pansinusitis**

J01.8 **Other acute sinusitis**

    J01.80 **Other acute sinusitis**
    Acute sinusitis involving more than one sinus but not pansinusitis

    J01.81 **Other acute recurrent sinusitis**
    Acute recurrent sinusitis involving more than one sinus but not pansinusitis

J01.9 **Acute sinusitis, unspecified**

    J01.90 **Acute sinusitis, unspecified**

    J01.91 **Acute recurrent sinusitis, unspecified**

J02 **Acute pharyngitis**

Includes: acute sore throat

Excludes 1: acute laryngopharyngitis (J06.0)
          peritonsillar abscess (J36)
          pharyngeal abscess (J39.1)
          retropharyngeal abscess (J39.0)

Excludes 2: chronic pharyngitis (J31.2)

J02.0   Streptococcal pharyngitis
Septic pharyngitis
Streptococcal sore throat

     Excludes 1: scarlet fever (A38.-)

J02.8   Acute pharyngitis due to other specified organisms
Use additional code (B95-B97) to identify infectious agent

     Excludes 1: acute pharyngitis due to coxsackie virus (B08.5)
              acute pharyngitis due to gonococcus (A54.5)
              acute pharyngitis due to herpes [simplex] virus (B00.2)
              acute pharyngitis due to infectious mononucleosis (B27.-)
              acute pharyngitis due to influenza virus (J09.02, J09.12, J10.1, J11.1)
              enteroviral vesicular pharyngitis (B08.5)

J02.9   Acute pharyngitis, unspecified
Gangrenous pharyngitis (acute)
Infective pharyngitis (acute) NOS
Pharyngitis (acute) NOS
Sore throat (acute) NOS
Suppurative pharyngitis (acute)
Ulcerative pharyngitis (acute)

J03   Acute tonsillitis

Excludes 1: acute sore throat (J02.-)
          hypertrophy of tonsils (J35.1)
          peritonsillar abscess (J36)
          sore throat NOS (J02.9)
          streptococcal sore throat (J02.0)

Excludes 2: chronic tonsillitis (J35.0)

J03.0   Streptococcal tonsillitis

     J03.00   Acute streptococcal tonsillitis, unspecified

     J03.01   Acute recurrent streptococcal tonsillitis

J03.8   Acute tonsillitis due to other specified organisms
Use additional code (B95-B97) to identify infectious agent.

     Excludes 1: diphtheritic tonsillitis (A36.0)

> herpesviral pharyngotonsillitis (B00.2)
> streptococcal tonsillitis (J03.0)
> tuberculous tonsillitis (A15.8)
> Vincent's tonsillitis (A69.1)

J03.80   **Acute tonsillitis due to other specified organisms**

J03.81   **Acute recurrent tonsillitis due to other specified organisms**

J03.9   **Acute tonsillitis, unspecified**
Follicular tonsillitis (acute)
Gangrenous tonsillitis (acute)
Infective tonsillitis (acute)
Tonsillitis (acute) NOS
Ulcerative tonsillitis (acute)

J03.90   **Acute tonsillitis, unspecified**

J03.91   **Acute recurrent tonsillitis, unspecified**

FORWARD MAPPING SAMPLE (ICD-9-CM ➡ ICD-10-CM)

ICD-9-CM CODE & DESCRIPTION		ICD-10-CM CODE & DESCRIPTION	
475	Peritonsillar abscess	J36	Peritonsillar abscess
476.0	Chronic laryngitis	J37.0	Chronic laryngitis
476.1	Chronic laryngotracheitis	J37.1	Chronic laryngotracheitis
477.0	Allergic rhinitis due to pollen	J30.1	Allergic rhinitis due to pollen
477.1	Allergic rhinitis due to food	J30.5	Allergic rhinitis due to food
477.2	Allergic rhinitis due to animal (cat)(dog) hair and dander	J30.81	Allergic rhinitis due to animal (cat) (dog) hair and dander
477.8	Allergic rhinitis due to other allergen	J30.2	Other seasonal allergic rhinitis
477.8	Allergic rhinitis due to other allergen	J30.89	Other allergic rhinitis
477.9	Allergic rhinitis cause unspecified	J30.9	Allergic rhinitis unspecified
477.9	Allergic rhinitis cause unspecified	J30.0	Vasomotor rhinitis
478.0	Hypertrophy of nasal turbinates	J34.3	Hypertrophy of nasal turbinates
478.11	Nasal mucositis (ulcerative)	J34.81	Nasal mucositis (ulcerative)
478.19	Other disease of nasal cavity and sinuses	J34.0	Abscess furuncle and carbuncle of nose
478.19	Other disease of nasal cavity and sinuses	J34.1	Cyst and mucocele of nose and nasal sinus
478.19	Other disease of nasal cavity and sinuses	J34.89	Other specified disorders of nose and nasal sinuses
478.20	Unspecified disease of pharynx	J39.2	Other diseases of pharynx
478.21	Cellulitis of pharynx or nasopharynx	J39.1	Other abscess of pharynx

478.22	Parapharyngeal abscess	J39.0	Retropharyngeal and parapharyngeal abscess
478.24	Retropharyngeal abscess	J39.0	Retropharyngeal and parapharyngeal abscess
478.25	Edema of pharynx or nasopharynx	J39.2	Other diseases of pharynx
478.26	Cyst of pharynx or nasopharynx	J39.2	Other diseases of pharynx
478.29	Other diseases of pharynx or nasopharynx	J39.2	Other diseases of pharynx
478.30	Unspecified paralysis of vocal cords	J38.00	Paralysis of vocal cords and larynx unspecified
478.31	Partial unilateral paralysis of vocal cords	J38.01	Paralysis of vocal cords and larynx unilateral
478.32	Complete unilateral paralysis of vocal cords	J38.01	Paralysis of vocal cords and larynx unilateral
478.33	Partial bilateral paralysis of vocal cords	J38.02	Paralysis of vocal cords and larynx bilateral
478.34	Complete bilateral paralysis of vocal cords	J38.02	Paralysis of vocal cords and larynx bilateral
478.4	Polyp of vocal cord or larynx	J38.1	Polyp of vocal cord and larynx
478.5	Other diseases of vocal cords	J38.3	Other diseases of vocal cords
478.6	Edema of larynx	J38.4	Edema of larynx
478.70	Unspecified disease of larynx	J38.7	Other diseases of larynx
478.71	Cellulitis and perichondritis of larynx	J38.7	Other diseases of larynx
478.74	Stenosis of larynx	J38.6	Stenosis of larynx
478.75	Laryngeal spasm	J38.5	Laryngeal spasm
478.79	Other diseases of larynx	J38.7	Other diseases of larynx
478.8	Upper respiratory tract hypersensitivity reaction site unspecified	J39.3	Upper respiratory tract hypersensitivity reaction site unspecified
478.9	Other and unspecified diseases of upper respiratory tract	J39.9	Disease of upper respiratory tract unspecified
478.9	Other and unspecified diseases of upper respiratory tract	J39.8	Other specified diseases of upper respiratory tract
480.0	Pneumonia due to adenovirus	J12.0	Adenoviral pneumonia
480.1	Pneumonia due to respiratory syncytial virus	J12.1	Respiratory syncytial virus pneumonia

BACKWARD MAPPING SAMPLE (ICD-10-CM ➡ ICD-9-CM)			
ICD-10-CM CODE & DESCRIPTION		**ICD-10-CM CODE & DESCRIPTION**	
J00	Acute nasopharyngitis [common cold]	460	Acute nasopharyngitis (common cold)
J01.00	Acute maxillary sinusitis unspecified	461.0	Acute maxillary sinusitis

J01.01	Acute recurrent maxillary sinusitis	**461.0**	Acute maxillary sinusitis
J01.10	Acute frontal sinusitis unspecified	**461.1**	Acute frontal sinusitis
J01.11	Acute recurrent frontal sinusitis	**461.1**	Acute frontal sinusitis
J01.20	Acute ethmoidal sinusitis unspecified	**461.2**	Acute ethmoidal sinusitis
J01.21	Acute recurrent ethmoidal sinusitis	**461.2**	Acute ethmoidal sinusitis
J01.30	Acute sphenoidal sinusitis unspecified	**461.3**	Acute sphenoidal sinusitis
J01.31	Acute recurrent sphenoidal sinusitis	**461.3**	Acute sphenoidal sinusitis
J01.40	Acute pansinusitis unspecified	**461.8**	Other acute sinusitis
J01.41	Acute recurrent pansinusitis	**461.8**	Other acute sinusitis
J01.80	Other acute sinusitis	**461.9**	Acute sinusitis unspecified
J01.81	Other acute recurrent sinusitis	**461.9**	Acute sinusitis unspecified
J01.90	Acute sinusitis unspecified	**461.9**	Acute sinusitis unspecified
J01.91	Acute recurrent sinusitis unspecified	**461.9**	Acute sinusitis unspecified
J02.0	Streptococcal pharyngitis	**034.0**	Streptococcal sore throat
J02.8	Acute pharyngitis due to other specified organisms	**462**	Acute pharyngitis
J02.9	Acute pharyngitis unspecified	**462**	Acute pharyngitis
J03.00	Acute streptococcal tonsillitis unspecified	**034.0**	Streptococcal sore throat
J03.01	Acute recurrent streptococcal tonsillitis	**034.0**	Streptococcal sore throat
J03.80	Acute tonsillitis due to other specified organisms	**463**	Acute tonsillitis
J03.81	Acute recurrent tonsillitis due to other specified organisms	**463**	Acute tonsillitis
J03.90	Acute tonsillitis unspecified	**463**	Acute tonsillitis
J03.91	Acute recurrent tonsillitis unspecified	**463**	Acute tonsillitis
J04.0	Acute laryngitis	**464.00**	Acute laryngitis without obstruction
J04.10	Acute tracheitis without obstruction	**464.10**	Acute tracheitis without obstruction
J04.11	Acute tracheitis with obstruction	**464.11**	Acute tracheitis with obstruction
J04.2	Acute laryngotracheitis	**464.20**	Acute laryngotracheitis without obstruction
J04.30	Supraglottitis unspecified without obstruction	**464.50**	Supraglottitis, unspecified, without mention of obstruction
J04.31	Supraglottitis unspecified with obstruction	**464.51**	Supraglottitis, unspecified, with obstruction
J05.0	Acute obstructive laryngitis [croup]	**464.01**	Acute laryngitis with obstruction
J05.0	Acute obstructive laryngitis [croup]	**464.21**	Acute laryngotracheitis with obstruction

J05.0	Acute obstructive laryngitis [croup]	464.4	Croup
J05.10	Acute epiglottitis without obstruction	464.30	Acute epiglottitis without obstruction
J05.11	Acute epiglottitis with obstruction	464.31	Acute epiglottitis with obstruction
J06.0	Acute laryngopharyngitis	465.0	Acute laryngopharyngitis
J06.9	Acute upper respiratory infection unspecified	465.8	Acute upper respiratory infections of other multiple sites
J06.9	Acute upper respiratory infection unspecified	465.9	Acute upper respiratory infections of unspecified site
J09.01	Influenza due to identified avian influenza virus with pneumonia	488.0	Influenza due to identified avian influenza virus
J09.090	Influenza due to identified avian influenza virus with encephalopathy	488.0	Influenza due to identified avian influenza virus

CHAPTER 11: DISEASES OF DIGESTIVE SYSTEM (K00-K94)

GENERAL GUIDELINES

There are no published guidelines for this chapter.

SAMPLE ICD-10-CM CODES FROM THIS CHAPTER

Excludes 2: certain conditions originating in the perinatal period (P04-P96)
certain infectious and parasitic diseases (A00-B99)
complications of pregnancy, childbirth and the puerperium (O00-O99)
congenital malformations, deformations and chromosomal abnormalities (Q00-Q99)
endocrine, nutritional and metabolic diseases (E00-E88)
injury, poisoning and certain other consequences of external causes (S00-T88)
neoplasms (C00-D49)
symptoms, signs and abnormal clinical and laboratory findings, not elsewhere classified (R00-R94)

This chapter contains the following blocks:	
K00-K14	Diseases of oral cavity and salivary glands
K20-K31	Diseases of esophagus, stomach and duodenum
K35-K38	Diseases of appendix
K40-K46	Hernia
K50-K52	Noninfective enteritis and colitis
K55-K63	Other diseases of intestines
K65-K68	Diseases of peritoneum and retroperitoneum
K70-K77	Diseases of liver
K80-K87	Disorders of gallbladder, biliary tract and pancreas
K90-K94	Other diseases of the digestive system

DISEASES OF ORAL CAVITY AND SALIVARY GLANDS (K00-K14)

K00 Disorders of tooth development and eruption

Excludes 2: embedded and impacted teeth (K01.-)

K00.0 Anodontia
Hypodontia
Oligodontia

Excludes 1: acquired absence of teeth (K08.1-)

K00.1 Supernumerary teeth
Distomolar
Fourth molar
Mesiodens
Paramolar
Supplementary teeth

Excludes 2: supernumerary roots (K00.2)

K00.2 Abnormalities of size and form of teeth
Concrescence of teeth
Fusion of teeth
Gemination of teeth
Dens evaginatus
Dens in dente
Dens invaginatus
Enamel pearls
Macrodontia
Microdontia
Peg-shaped [conical] teeth
Supernumerary roots
Taurodontism
Tuberculum paramolar

Excludes 1: abnormalities of teeth due to congenital syphilis (A50.5)
tuberculum Carabelli, which is regarded as a normal variation and
should not be coded

K00.3 Mottled teeth
Dental fluorosis
Mottling of enamel
Non-fluoride enamel opacities

Excludes 2: deposits [accretions] on teeth (K03.6)

K00.4 Disturbances in tooth formation
Aplasia and hypoplasia of cementum
Dilaceration of tooth
Enamel hypoplasia (neonatal) (postnatal) (prenatal)

Regional odontodysplasia
Turner's tooth

Excludes 1: Hutchinson's teeth and mulberry molars in congenital syphilis (A50.5)

Excludes 2: mottled teeth (K00.3)

K00.5 Hereditary disturbances in tooth structure, not elsewhere classified
Amelogenesis imperfecta
Dentinogenesis imperfecta
Odontogenesis imperfecta
Dentinal dysplasia
Shell teeth

K00.6 Disturbances in tooth eruption
Dentia praecox
Natal tooth
Neonatal tooth
Premature eruption of tooth
Premature shedding of primary [deciduous] tooth
Prenatal teeth
Retained [persistent] primary tooth

Excludes 2: embedded and impacted teeth (K01.-)

K00.7 Teething syndrome

K00.8 Other disorders of tooth development
Color changes during tooth formation
Intrinsic staining of teeth NOS

Excludes 2: posteruptive color changes (K03.7)

K00.9 Disorder of tooth development, unspecified
Disorder of odontogenesis NOS

K01 Embedded and impacted teeth

Excludes 1: abnormal position of fully erupted teeth (M26.3-)

K01.0 Embedded teeth

K01.1 Impacted teeth

K02 Dental caries

Includes: dental cavities
tooth decay

K02.3 Arrested dental caries
Arrested coronal and root caries

K02.5 Dental caries on pit and fissure surface
Dental caries on chewing surface of tooth

K02.51 Dental caries on pit and fissure surface limited to enamel
White spot lesions [initial caries] on pit and fissure surface of tooth
K02.52 Dental caries on pit and fissure surface penetrating into dentin

K02.53 Dental caries on pit and fissure surface penetrating into pulp

K02.6 Dental caries on smooth surface

K02.61 Dental caries on smooth surface limited to enamel
White spot lesions [initial caries] on smooth surface of tooth
K02.62 Dental caries on smooth surface penetrating into dentin

K02.63 Dental caries on smooth surface penetrating into pulp

K02.7 Dental root caries

K02.9 Dental caries, unspecified

K03 Other diseases of hard tissues of teeth

Excludes 2: bruxism (F45.8)
            dental caries (K02.-)
            teeth-grinding NOS (F45.8)

K03.0 Excessive attrition of teeth
Approximal wear of teeth
Occlusal wear of teeth

K03.1 Abrasion of teeth
Dentifrice abrasion of teeth
Habitual abrasion of teeth
Occupational abrasion of teeth
Ritual abrasion of teeth
Traditional abrasion of teeth
Wedge defect NOS

FORWARD MAPPING SAMPLE (ICD-9-CM ➡ ICD-10-CM)			
ICD-10-CM CODE & DESCRIPTION		**ICD-10-CM CODE & DESCRIPTION**	
577.0	Acute pancreatitis	**K85.9**	Acute pancreatitis unspecified
577.1	Chronic pancreatitis	**K86.1**	Other chronic pancreatitis
577.2	Cyst and pseudocyst of pancreas	**K86.2**	Cyst of pancreas
577.2	Cyst and pseudocyst of pancreas	**K86.3**	Pseudocyst of pancreas
577.8	Other specified diseases of pancreas	**K86.8**	Other specified diseases of pancreas
577.9	Unspecified disease of pancreas	**K86.9**	Disease of pancreas unspecified
578.0	Hematemesis	**K92.0**	Hematemesis

578.1	Blood in stool	**K92.1**	Melena
578.9	Hemorrhage of gastrointestinal tract unspecified	**K92.2**	Gastrointestinal hemorrhage unspecified
579.0	Celiac disease	**K90.0**	Celiac disease
579.1	Tropical sprue	**K90.1**	Tropical sprue
579.2	Blind loop syndrome	**K90.2**	Blind loop syndrome not elsewhere classified
579.3	Other and unspecified postsurgical nonabsorption	**K91.2**	Postsurgical malabsorption not elsewhere classified
579.4	Pancreatic steatorrhea	**K90.3**	Pancreatic steatorrhea
579.8	Other specified intestinal malabsorption	**K90.89**	Other intestinal malabsorption
579.9	Unspecified intestinal malabsorption	**K90.9**	Intestinal malabsorption unspecified
580.0	Acute glomerulonephritis with lesion of proliferative glomerulonephritis	**N00.3**	Acute nephritic syndrome with diffuse mesangial proliferative glomerulonephritis
580.4	Acute glomerulonephritis with lesion of rapidly progressive glomerulonephritis	**N01.3**	Rapidly progressive nephritic syndrome with diffuse mesangial proliferative glomerulonephritis
580.81	Acute glomerulonephritis in diseases classified elsewhere	**N08**	Glomerular disorders in diseases classified elsewhere
580.89	Acute glomerulonephritis with other specified pathological lesion in kidney	**N00.8**	Acute nephritic syndrome with other morphologic changes
580.9	Acute glomerulonephritis with unspecified pathological lesion in kidney	**N00.9**	Acute nephritic syndrome with unspecified morphologic changes
581.0	Nephrotic syndrome with lesion of proliferative glomerulonephritis	**N04.4**	Nephrotic syndrome with diffuse endocapillary proliferative glomerulonephritis
581.1	Nephrotic syndrome with lesion of membranous glomerulonephritis	**N02.2**	Recurrent and persistent hematuria with diffuse membranous glomerulonephritis
581.2	Nephrotic syndrome with lesion of membranoproliferative glomerulonephritis	**N04.3**	Nephrotic syndrome with diffuse mesangial proliferative glomerulonephritis
581.3	Nephrotic syndrome with lesion of minimal change glomerulonephritis	**N04.0**	Nephrotic syndrome with minor glomerular abnormality
581.81	Nephrotic syndrome in diseases classified elsewhere	**N08**	Glomerular disorders in diseases classified elsewhere
581.89	Other nephrotic syndrome with specified pathological lesion in kidney	**N04.8**	Nephrotic syndrome with other morphologic changes

581.9	Nephrotic syndrome with unspecified pathological lesion in kidney	N04.9	Nephrotic syndrome with unspecified morphologic changes
582.0	Chronic glomerulonephritis with lesion of proliferative glomerulonephritis	N03.2	Chronic nephritic syndrome with diffuse membranous glomerulonephritis
582.1	Chronic glomerulonephritis with lesion of membranous glomerulonephritis	N03.3	Chronic nephritic syndrome with diffuse mesangial proliferative glomerulonephritis
582.2	Chronic glomerulonephritis with lesion of membranoproliferative glomerulonephritis	N03.5	Chronic nephritic syndrome with diffuse mesangiocapillary glomerulonephritis
582.4	Chronic glomerulonephritis with lesion of rapidly progressive glomerulonephritis	N03.8	Chronic nephritic syndrome with other morphologic changes
582.81	Chronic glomerulonephritis in diseases classified elsewhere	N08	Glomerular disorders in diseases classified elsewhere
582.89	Other chronic glomerulonephritis with specified pathological lesion in kidney	N03.8	Chronic nephritic syndrome with other morphologic changes
582.9	Chronic glomerulonephritis with unspecified pathological lesion in kidney	N03.9	Chronic nephritic syndrome with unspecified morphologic changes
583.0	Nephritis and nephropathy not specified as acute or chronic with lesion of proliferative glomerulonephritis	N05.9	Unspecified nephritic syndrome with unspecified morphologic changes
583.1	Nephritis and nephropathy not specified as acute or chronic with lesion of membranous glomerulonephritis	N05.2	Unspecified nephritic syndrome with diffuse membranous glomerulonephritis
583.2	Nephritis and nephropathy not specified as acute or chronic with lesion of membranoproliferative glomerulonephritis	N05.5	Unspecified nephritic syndrome with diffuse mesangiocapillary glomerulonephritis
583.4	Nephritis and nephropathy not specified as acute or chronic with lesion of rapidly progressive glomerulonephritis	N05.9	Unspecified nephritic syndrome with unspecified morphologic changes
583.6	Nephritis and nephropathy not specified as acute or chronic with lesion of renal cortical necrosis	N17.1	Acute kidney failure with acute cortical necrosis

BACKWARD MAPPING SAMPLE (ICD-10-CM ➡ ICD-9-CM)

ICD-10-CM CODE & DESCRIPTION		ICD-10-CM CODE & DESCRIPTION	
K87	Disorders of gallbladder biliary tract and pancreas in diseases classified elsewhere	577.8	Other specified diseases of pancreas
K90.0	Celiac disease	579.0	Celiac disease
K90.1	Tropical sprue	579.1	Tropical sprue
K90.2	Blind loop syndrome not elsewhere classified	579.2	Blind loop syndrome
K90.3	Pancreatic steatorrhea	579.4	Pancreatic steatorrhea
K90.4	Malabsorption due to intolerance not elsewhere classified	579.8	Other specified intestinal malabsorption
K90.81	Whipple's disease	040.2	Whipple's disease
K90.89	Other intestinal malabsorption	579.8	Other specified intestinal malabsorption
K90.9	Intestinal malabsorption unspecified	579.9	Unspecified intestinal malabsorption
K91.0	Vomiting following gastrointestinal surgery	564.3	Vomiting following gastrointestinal surgery
K91.1	Postgastric surgery syndromes	564.2	Postgastric surgery syndromes
K91.2	Postsurgical malabsorption not elsewhere classified	579.3	Other and unspecified postsurgical nonabsorption
K91.3	Postprocedural intestinal obstruction	997.4	Digestive system complications, not elsewhere classified
K91.5	Postcholecystectomy syndrome	576.0	Postcholecystectomy syndrome
K91.61	Intraoperative hemorrhage and hematoma of a digestive system organ or structure complicating a digestive system procedure	998.11	Hemorrhage complicating a procedure
K91.61	Intraoperative hemorrhage and hematoma of a digestive system organ or structure complicating a digestive system procedure	998.12	Hematoma complicating a procedure
K91.62	Intraoperative hemorrhage and hematoma of a digestive system organ or structure complicating other procedure	998.11	Hemorrhage complicating a procedure
K91.62	Intraoperative hemorrhage and hematoma of a digestive system organ or structure complicating other procedure	998.12	Hematoma complicating a procedure
K91.71	Accidental puncture and laceration of a digestive system organ or structure during a digestive system procedure	998.2	Accidental puncture or laceration during a procedure not elsewhere classified

K91.72	Accidental puncture and laceration of a digestive system organ or structure during other procedure	998.2	Accidental puncture or laceration during a procedure not elsewhere classified
K91.81	Other intraoperative complications of digestive system	997.4	Digestive system complications, not elsewhere classified
K91.82	Postprocedural hepatic failure	997.4	Digestive system complications, not elsewhere classified
K91.83	Postprocedural hepatorenal syndrome	997.4	Digestive system complications, not elsewhere classified
K91.840	Postprocedural hemorrhage and hematoma of a digestive system organ or structure following a digestive system procedure	998.11	Hemorrhage complicating a procedure
K91.840	Postprocedural hemorrhage and hematoma of a digestive system organ or structure following a digestive system procedure	998.12	Hematoma complicating a procedure
K91.841	Postprocedural hemorrhage and hematoma of a digestive system organ or structure following other procedure	998.11	Hemorrhage complicating a procedure
K91.841	Postprocedural hemorrhage and hematoma of a digestive system organ or structure following other procedure	998.12	Hematoma complicating a procedure
K91.850	Pouchitis	569.71	Pouchitis
K91.858	Other complications of intestinal pouch	569.79	Other complications of intestinal pouch
K91.89	Other postprocedural complications and disorders of digestive system	564.4	Other postoperative functional disorders
K91.89	Other postprocedural complications and disorders of digestive system	997.4	Digestive system complications, not elsewhere classified
K92.0	Hematemesis	578.0	Hematemesis
K92.1	Melena	578.1	Blood in stool
K92.2	Gastrointestinal hemorrhage unspecified	578.9	Hemorrhage of gastrointestinal tract unspecified
K92.81	Gastrointestinal mucositis (ulcerative)	569.89	Other specified disorders of intestines
K92.89	Other specified diseases of the digestive system	569.89	Other specified disorders of intestines
K92.9	Disease of digestive system unspecified	569.9	Unspecified disorder of intestine

| K94.00 | Colostomy complication unspecified | 569.60 | Colostomy and enterostomy complication unspecified |
| K94.01 | Colostomy hemorrhage | 569.69 | Other colostomy and enterostomy complication |

CHAPTER 12: DISEASES OF SKIN AND SUBCUTANEOUS TISSUE (L00-L99)

GENERAL GUIDELINES

PRESSURE ULCER STAGE CODES

1) **Pressure ulcer stages**

   Codes from category L89, Pressure ulcer, are combination codes that identify the site of the pressure ulcer as well as the stage of the ulcer.

   The ICD-10-CM classifies pressure ulcer stages based on severity, which is designated by stages 1-4, unspecified stage and unstageable.

   Assign as many codes from category L89 as needed to identify all the pressure ulcers the patient has, if applicable.

2) **Unstageable pressure ulcers**

   Assignment of the code for unstageable pressure ulcer (L89.-- 0) should be based on the clinical documentation. These codes are used for pressure ulcers whose stage cannot be clinically determined (e.g., the ulcer is covered by eschar or has been treated with a skin or muscle graft) and pressure ulcers that are documented as deep tissue injury but not documented as due to trauma. This code should not be confused with the codes for unspecified stage (L89.--9). When there is no documentation regarding the stage of the pressure ulcer, assign the appropriate code for unspecified stage (L89.--9).

3) **Documented pressure ulcer stage**

   Assignment of the pressure ulcer stage code should be guided by clinical documentation of the stage or documentation of the terms found in the Alphabetic Index. For clinical terms describing the stage that are not found in the Alphabetic Index, and there is no documentation of the stage, the provider should be queried.

4) **Patients admitted with pressure ulcers documented as healed**

   No code is assigned if the documentation states that the pressure ulcer is completely healed.

5) **Patients admitted with pressure ulcers documented as healing**

   Pressure ulcers described as healing should be assigned the appropriate pressure ulcer stage code based on the documentation in the medical record. If the documentation does not provide information about the stage of the healing pressure ulcer, assign the appropriate code for unspecified stage.

If the documentation is unclear as to whether the patient has a current (new) pressure ulcer or if the patient is being treated for a healing pressure ulcer, query the provider.

6) **Patient admitted with pressure ulcer evolving into another stage during the admission**

If a patient is admitted with a pressure ulcer at one stage and it progresses to a higher stage, assign the code for the highest stage reported for that site.

SAMPLE ICD-10-CM CODES FROM THIS CHAPTER

Excludes 2: certain conditions originating in the perinatal period (P04-P96)
certain infectious and parasitic diseases (A00-B99)
complications of pregnancy, childbirth and the puerperium (O00-O99)
congenital malformations, deformations, and chromosomal abnormalities (Q00-Q99)
endocrine, nutritional and metabolic diseases (E00-E88)
lipomelanotic reticulosis (I89.8)
neoplasms (C00-D49)
symptoms, signs and abnormal clinical and laboratory findings, not elsewhere classified (R00-R94)
systemic connective tissue disorders (M30-M36)
viral warts (B07.-)

This chapter contains the following blocks:	
L00-L08	Infections of the skin and subcutaneous tissue
L10-L14	Bullous disorders
L20-L30	Dermatitis and eczema
L40-L45	Papulosquamous disorders
L49-L54	Urticaria and erythema
L55-L59	Radiation-related disorders of the skin and subcutaneous tissue
L60-L75	Disorders of skin appendages
L76	Intraoperative and postprocedural complications of skin and subcutaneous tissue
L80-L99	Other disorders of the skin and subcutaneous tissue

INFECTIONS OF THE SKIN AND SUBCUTANEOUS TISSUE (L00-L08)

Use additional code (B95-B97) to identify infectious agent.

Excludes 2: hordeolum (H00.0)
infective dermatitis (L30.3)
local infections of skin classified in Chapter 1
lupus panniculitis (L93.2)
panniculitis NOS (M79.3)
panniculitis of neck and back (M54.0-)
Perlèche NOS (K13.0)
Perlèche due to candidiasis (B37.0)
Perlèche due to riboflavin deficiency (E53.0)

pyogenic granuloma (L98.0)
relapsing panniculitis [Weber-Christian] (M35.6)
viral warts (B07.-)
zoster (B02.-)

L00 Staphylococcal scalded skin syndrome
Ritter's disease
Use additional code to identify percentage of skin exfoliation (L49-)

Excludes 1: bullous impetigo (L01.03)
pemphigus neonatorum (L01.03)
toxic epidermal necrolysis [Lyell] (L51.2)

L01 Impetigo

Excludes 1: impetigo herpetiformis (L40.1)

L01.0 Impetigo
Impetigo contagiosa
Impetigo vulgaris

L01.00 Impetigo, unspecified
Impetigo NOS

L01.01 Non-bullous impetigo

L01.02 Bockhart's impetigo
Impetigo follicularis
Perifolliculitis NOS
Superficial pustular perifolliculitis

L01.03 Bullous impetigo
Impetigo neonatorum
Pemphigus neonatorum

L01.09 Other impetigo
Ulcerative impetigo

L01.1 Impetiginization of other dermatoses

L02 Cutaneous abscess, furuncle and carbuncle
Use additional code to identify organism (B95-B96)

Excludes 2: abscess of anus and rectal regions (K61.-)
abscess of female genital organs (external) (N76.4)
abscess of male genital organs (external) (N48.2, N49.-)

L02.0 Cutaneous abscess, furuncle and carbuncle of face

Excludes 1: abscess of ear, external (H60.0)
abscess of eyelid (H00.0)

abscess of head [any part, except face] (L02.8)
abscess of lacrimal gland (H04.0)
abscess of lacrimal passages (H04.3)
abscess of mouth (K12.2)
abscess of nose (J34.0)
abscess of orbit (H05.0)
submandibular abscess (K12.2)

L02.01   Cutaneous abscess of face

L02.02   Furuncle of face
Boil of face
Folliculitis of face

L02.03   Carbuncle of face

L02.1   Cutaneous abscess, furuncle and carbuncle of neck

L02.11   Cutaneous abscess of neck

L02.12   Furuncle of neck
Boil of neck
Folliculitis of neck

L02.13   Carbuncle of neck

L02.2   Cutaneous abscess, furuncle and carbuncle of trunk

Excludes 1: non-newborn omphalitis (L08.82)
omphalitis of newborn (P38.-)

Excludes 2: abscess of breast (N61)
abscess of buttocks (L02.3)
abscess of female external genital organs (N76.4)
abscess of male external genital organs (N48.2, N49.-)
abscess of hip (L02.4)

L02.21   Cutaneous abscess of trunk

L02.211   Cutaneous abscess of abdominal wall

L02.212   Cutaneous abscess of back [any part, except buttock]

L02.213   Cutaneous abscess of chest wall

L02.214   Cutaneous abscess of groin

L02.215   Cutaneous abscess of perineum

L02.216   Cutaneous abscess of umbilicus

          L02.219   **Cutaneous abscess of trunk, unspecified**

    L02.22   **Furuncle of trunk**
              Boil of trunk
              Folliculitis of trunk

          L02.221   **Furuncle of abdominal wall**

          L02.222   **Furuncle of back [any part, except buttock]**

          L02.223   **Furuncle of chest wall**

          L02.224   **Furuncle of groin**

          L02.225   **Furuncle of perineum**

          L02.226   **Furuncle of umbilicus**

          L02.229   **Furuncle of trunk, unspecified**

    L02.23   **Carbuncle of trunk**

          L02.231   **Carbuncle of abdominal wall**

          L02.232   **Carbuncle of back [any part, except buttock]**

          L02.233   **Carbuncle of chest wall**

          L02.234   **Carbuncle of groin**

          L02.235   **Carbuncle of perineum**

          L02.236   **Carbuncle of umbilicus**

          L02.239   **Carbuncle of trunk, unspecified**

  L02.3 **Cutaneous abscess, furuncle and carbuncle of buttock**

      Excludes 1: pilonidal cyst with abscess (L05.01)

    L02.31   **Cutaneous abscess of buttock**
              Cutaneous abscess of gluteal region

FORWARD MAPPING SAMPLE (ICD-9-CM ➡ ICD-10-CM)

ICD-9-CM CODE & DESCRIPTION		ICD-10-CM CODE & DESCRIPTION	
691.0	Diaper or napkin rash	L22	Diaper dermatitis
691.8	Other atopic dermatitis and related conditions	L20.89	Other atopic dermatitis
692.0	Contact dermatitis and other eczema due to detergents	L24.0	Irritant contact dermatitis due to detergents

692.1	Contact dermatitis and other eczema due to oils and greases	L24.1	Irritant contact dermatitis due to oils and greases
692.2	Contact dermatitis and other eczema due to solvents	L24.2	Irritant contact dermatitis due to solvents
692.3	Contact dermatitis and other eczema due to drugs and medicines in contact with skin	L25.1	Unspecified contact dermatitis due to drugs in contact with skin
692.4	Contact dermatitis and other eczema due to other chemical products	L25.3	Unspecified contact dermatitis due to other chemical products
692.5	Contact dermatitis and other eczema due to food in contact with skin	L25.4	Unspecified contact dermatitis due to food in contact with skin
692.6	Contact dermatitis and other eczema due to plants (except food)	L25.5	Unspecified contact dermatitis due to plants except food
692.70	Unspecified dermatitis due to sun	L57.8	Other skin changes due to chronic exposure to nonionizing radiation
692.71	Sunburn	L55.0	Sunburn of first degree
692.71	Sunburn	L55.9	Sunburn unspecified
692.72	Acute dermatitis due to solar radiation	L56.2	Photocontact dermatitis [berloque dermatitis]
692.72	Acute dermatitis due to solar radiation	L56.0	Drug phototoxic response
692.72	Acute dermatitis due to solar radiation	L56.1	Drug photoallergic response
692.73	Actinic reticuloid and actinic granuloma	L57.5	Actinic granuloma
692.73	Actinic reticuloid and actinic granuloma	L57.1	Actinic reticuloid
692.74	Other chronic dermatitis due to solar radiation	L57.9	Skin changes due to chronic exposure to nonionizing radiation unspecified
692.75	Disseminated superficial actinic porokeratosis (dsap)	L56.5	Disseminated superficial actinic porokeratosis (DSAP)
692.76	Sunburn of second degree	L55.1	Sunburn of second degree
692.77	Sunburn of third degree	L55.2	Sunburn of third degree
692.79	Other dermatitis due to solar radiation	L56.8	Other specified acute skin changes due to ultraviolet radiation
692.81	Dermatitis due to cosmetics	L25.0	Unspecified contact dermatitis due to cosmetics
692.82	Dermatitis due to other radiation	L58.9	Radiodermatitis unspecified
692.83	Dermatitis due to metals	L23.0	Allergic contact dermatitis due to metals
692.83	Dermatitis due to metals	L24.81	Irritant contact dermatitis due to metals

692.84	Contact dermatitis due to animal (cat) (dog) dander	L23.81	Allergic contact dermatitis due to animal (cat) (dog) dander
692.89	Contact dermatitis and other eczema due to other specified agents	L25.2	Unspecified contact dermatitis due to dyes
692.89	Contact dermatitis and other eczema due to other specified agents	L25.8	Unspecified contact dermatitis due to other agents
692.9	Contact dermatitis and other eczema unspecified cause	L25.9	Unspecified contact dermatitis unspecified cause
693.0	Dermatitis due to drugs and medicines taken internally	L27.0	Generalized skin eruption due to drugs and medicaments taken internally
693.0	Dermatitis due to drugs and medicines taken internally	L27.1	Localized skin eruption due to drugs and medicaments taken internally
693.1	Dermatitis due to food taken internally	L27.2	Dermatitis due to ingested food
693.8	Dermatitis due to other specified substances taken internally	L27.8	Dermatitis due to other substances taken internally
693.9	Dermatitis due to unspecified substance taken internally	L27.9	Dermatitis due to unspecified substance taken internally
694.0	Dermatitis herpetiformis	L13.0	Dermatitis herpetiformis
694.1	Subcorneal pustular dermatosis	L13.1	Subcorneal pustular dermatitis
694.2	Juvenile dermatitis herpetiformis	L12.2	Chronic bullous disease of childhood
694.3	Impetigo herpetiformis	L40.1	Generalized pustular psoriasis
694.4	Pemphigus	L10.0	Pemphigus vulgaris

BACKWARD MAPPING SAMPLE (ICD-10-CM ➡ ICD-9-CM)

ICD-10-CM CODE & DESCRIPTION		ICD-9-CM CODE & DESCRIPTION	
L00	Staphylococcal scalded skin syndrome	695.81	Ritter's disease
L01.00	Impetigo unspecified	684	Impetigo
L01.01	Non-bullous impetigo	684	Impetigo
L01.02	Bockhart's impetigo	684	Impetigo
L01.03	Bullous impetigo	684	Impetigo
L01.09	Other impetigo	684	Impetigo
L01.1	Impetiginization of other dermatoses	684	Impetigo
L02.01	Cutaneous abscess of face	682.0	Cellulitis and abscess of face
L02.02	Furuncle of face	680.0	Carbuncle and furuncle of face
L02.03	Carbuncle of face	680.0	Carbuncle and furuncle of face
L02.11	Cutaneous abscess of neck	682.1	Cellulitis and abscess of neck

L02.12	Furuncle of neck	680.1	Carbuncle and furuncle of neck
L02.13	Carbuncle of neck	680.1	Carbuncle and furuncle of neck
L02.211	Cutaneous abscess of abdominal wall	682.2	Cellulitis and abscess of trunk
L02.212	Cutaneous abscess of back [any part except buttock]	682.2	Cellulitis and abscess of trunk
L02.213	Cutaneous abscess of chest wall	682.2	Cellulitis and abscess of trunk
L02.214	Cutaneous abscess of groin	682.2	Cellulitis and abscess of trunk
L02.215	Cutaneous abscess of perineum	682.2	Cellulitis and abscess of trunk
L02.216	Cutaneous abscess of umbilicus	682.2	Cellulitis and abscess of trunk
L02.219	Cutaneous abscess of trunk unspecified	682.2	Cellulitis and abscess of trunk
L02.221	Furuncle of abdominal wall	680.2	Carbuncle and furuncle of trunk
L02.222	Furuncle of back [any part except buttock]	680.2	Carbuncle and furuncle of trunk
L02.223	Furuncle of chest wall	680.2	Carbuncle and furuncle of trunk
L02.224	Furuncle of groin	680.2	Carbuncle and furuncle of trunk
L02.225	Furuncle of perineum	680.2	Carbuncle and furuncle of trunk
L02.226	Furuncle of umbilicus	680.2	Carbuncle and furuncle of trunk
L02.229	Furuncle of trunk unspecified	680.2	Carbuncle and furuncle of trunk
L02.231	Carbuncle of abdominal wall	680.2	Carbuncle and furuncle of trunk
L02.232	Carbuncle of back [any part except buttock]	680.2	Carbuncle and furuncle of trunk
L02.233	Carbuncle of chest wall	680.2	Carbuncle and furuncle of trunk
L02.234	Carbuncle of groin	680.2	Carbuncle and furuncle of trunk
L02.235	Carbuncle of perineum	680.2	Carbuncle and furuncle of trunk
L02.236	Carbuncle of umbilicus	680.2	Carbuncle and furuncle of trunk
L02.239	Carbuncle of trunk unspecified	680.2	Carbuncle and furuncle of trunk
L02.31	Cutaneous abscess of buttock	682.5	Cellulitis and abscess of buttock
L02.32	Furuncle of buttock	680.5	Carbuncle and furuncle of buttock
L02.33	Carbuncle of buttock	680.5	Carbuncle and furuncle of buttock
L02.411	Cutaneous abscess of right axilla	682.3	Cellulitis and abscess of upper arm and forearm
L02.412	Cutaneous abscess of left axilla	682.3	Cellulitis and abscess of upper arm and forearm
L02.413	Cutaneous abscess of right upper limb	682.3	Cellulitis and abscess of upper arm and forearm

CHAPTER 13: DISEASES OF THE MUSCULOSKELETAL SYSTEM AND CONNECTIVE TISSUE (M00-M99)

GENERAL GUIDELINES

SITE AND LATERALITY

Most of the codes within Chapter 13 have site and laterality designations. The site represents the bone, joint or the muscle involved. For some conditions where more than one bone, joint or muscle is usually involved, such as osteoarthritis, there is a "multiple sites" code available. For categories where no multiple site code is provided and more than one bone, joint or muscle is involved, multiple codes should be used to indicate the different sites involved.

1) Bone versus joint

For certain conditions, the bone may be affected at the upper or lower end, (e.g., avascular necrosis of bone, M87, Osteoporosis, M80, M81). Though the portion of the bone affected may be at the joint, the site designation will be the bone, not the joint.

ACUTE TRAUMATIC VERSUS CHRONIC OR RECURRENT MUSCULOSKELETAL CONDITIONS

Many musculoskeletal conditions are a result of previous injury or trauma to a site, or are recurrent conditions. Bone, joint or muscle conditions that are the result of a healed injury are usually found in chapter 13. Recurrent bone, joint or muscle conditions are also usually found in chapter 13. Any current, acute injury should be coded to the appropriate injury code from chapter 19. Chronic or recurrent conditions should generally be coded with a code from chapter 13. If it is difficult to determine from the documentation in the record which code is best to describe a condition, query the provider.

CODING OF PATHOLOGIC FRACTURES

7th character A is for use as long as the patient is receiving active treatment for the fracture. Examples of active treatment are: surgical treatment, emergency department encounter, evaluation and treatment by a new physician. 7th character, D is to be used for encounters after the patient has completed active treatment. The other 7th characters, listed under each subcategory in the Tabular List, are to be used for subsequent encounters for treatment of problems associated with the healing, such as malunions, nonunions, and sequelae. Care for complications of surgical treatment for fracture repairs during the healing or recovery phase should be coded with the appropriate complication codes.

OSTEOPOROSIS

Osteoporosis is a systemic condition, meaning that all bones of the musculoskeletal system are affected. Therefore, site is not a component of the codes under category M81, Osteoporosis without current pathological fracture. The site codes under category M80, Osteoporosis with current pathological fracture, identify the site of the fracture, not the osteoporosis.

1) Osteoporosis without pathological fracture

Category M81, Osteoporosis without current pathological fracture, is for use for patients with osteoporosis who do not currently have a pathologic fracture due to the osteoporosis, even if they have had a fracture in the past. For patients with a history of osteoporosis fractures, status code Z87.310, Personal history of (healed) osteoporosis fracture, should follow the code from M81.

2) Osteoporosis with current pathological fracture

Category M80, Osteoporosis with current pathological fracture, is for patients who have a current pathologic fracture at the time of an encounter. The codes under M80 identify the site of the fracture. A code from category M80, not a traumatic fracture code, should be used for any patient with known osteoporosis who suffers a fracture, even if the patient had a minor fall or trauma, if that fall or trauma would not usually break a normal, healthy bone.

SAMPLE ICD-10-CM CODES FROM THIS CHAPTER

Note: Use an external cause code following the code for the musculoskeletal condition, if applicable, to identify the cause of the musculoskeletal condition

Excludes 2: arthropathic psoriasis (L40.5-)
certain conditions originating in the perinatal period (P04-P96)
certain infectious and parasitic diseases (A00-B99)
compartment syndrome (traumatic) (T79.A-)
complications of pregnancy, childbirth and the puerperium (O00-O99)
congenital malformations, deformations, and chromosomal abnormalities (Q00-Q99)
endocrine, nutritional and metabolic diseases (E00-E88)
injury, poisoning and certain other consequences of external causes (S00-T88)
neoplasms (C00-D49)
symptoms, signs and abnormal clinical and laboratory findings, not elsewhere classified (R00-R94)

This chapter contains the following blocks:	
M00-M02	Infectious arthropathies
M05-M14	Inflammatory polyarthropathies
M15-M19	Osteoarthritis
M20-M25	Other joint disorders
M26-M27	Dentofacial anomalies [including malocclusion] and other disorders of jaw
M30-M36	Systemic connective tissue disorders
M40-M43	Deforming dorsopathies
M45-M49	Spondylopathies
M50-M54	Other dorsopathies
M60-M63	Disorders of muscles
M65-M67	Disorders of synovium and tendon
M70-M79	Other soft tissue disorders
M80-M85	Disorders of bone density and structure

M86-M90	Other osteopathies
M91-M94	Chondropathies
M95	Other disorders of the musculoskeletal system and connective tissue
M96	Intraoperative and postprocedural complications and disorders of musculoskeletal system, not elsewhere classified
M99	Biomechanical lesions, not elsewhere classified

ARTHROPATHIES (M00-M25)

Note: Disorders affecting predominantly peripheral (limb) joints

Infectious arthropathies (M00-M02)

Note: This block comprises arthropathies due to microbiological agents. Distinction is made between the following types of etiological relationship:

a)   direct infection of joint, where organisms invade synovial tissue and microbial antigen is present in the joint;

b)   indirect infection, which may be of two types: a reactive arthropathy, where microbial infection of the body is established but neither organisms nor antigens can be identified in the joint, and a postinfective arthropathy, where microbial antigen is present but recovery of an organism is inconstant and evidence of local multiplication is lacking.

M00   Pyogenic arthritis

   M00.0   Staphylococcal arthritis and polyarthritis
   Use additional code (B95.6-B95.7) to identify bacterial agent

      M00.00   Staphylococcal arthritis, unspecified joint

      M00.01   Staphylococcal arthritis, shoulder

            M00.011   Staphylococcal arthritis, right shoulder

            M00.012   Staphylococcal arthritis, left shoulder

            M00.019   Staphylococcal arthritis, unspecified shoulder

      M00.02   Staphylococcal arthritis, elbow

            M00.021   Staphylococcal arthritis, right elbow

            M00.022   Staphylococcal arthritis, left elbow

            M00.029   Staphylococcal arthritis, unspecified elbow

      M00.03   Staphylococcal arthritis, wrist
      Staphylococcal arthritis of carpal bones

M00.031   **Staphylococcal arthritis, right wrist**

M00.032   **Staphylococcal arthritis, left wrist**

M00.039   **Staphylococcal arthritis, unspecified wrist**

M00.04 **Staphylococcal arthritis, hand**
Staphylococcal arthritis of metacarpus and phalanges

M00.041   **Staphylococcal arthritis, right hand**

M00.042   **Staphylococcal arthritis, left hand**

M00.049   **Staphylococcal arthritis, unspecified hand**

M00.05 **Staphylococcal arthritis, hip**

M00.051   **Staphylococcal arthritis, right hip**

M00.052   **Staphylococcal arthritis, left hip**

M00.059   **Staphylococcal arthritis, unspecified hip**

M00.06 **Staphylococcal arthritis, knee**

M00.061   **Staphylococcal arthritis, right knee**

M00.062   **Staphylococcal arthritis, left knee**

M00.069   **Staphylococcal arthritis, unspecified knee**

M00.07 **Staphylococcal arthritis, ankle and foot**
Staphylococcal arthritis, tarsus, metatarsus and phalanges

M00.071   **Staphylococcal arthritis, right ankle and foot**

M00.072   **Staphylococcal arthritis, left ankle and foot**

M00.079   **Staphylococcal arthritis, unspecified ankle and foot**

M00.08 **Staphylococcal arthritis, vertebrae**

M00.09 **Staphylococcal polyarthritis**

M00.1 **Pneumococcal arthritis and polyarthritis**

M00.10 **Pneumococcal arthritis, unspecified joint**

M00.11 **Pneumococcal arthritis, shoulder**

M00.111 **Pneumococcal arthritis, right shoulder**

          M00.112   **Pneumococcal arthritis, left shoulder**

          M00.119   **Pneumococcal arthritis, unspecified shoulder**

   M00.12   **Pneumococcal arthritis, elbow**

          M00.121   **Pneumococcal arthritis, right elbow**

          M00.122   **Pneumococcal arthritis, left elbow**

          M00.129   **Pneumococcal arthritis, unspecified elbow**

   M00.13   **Pneumococcal arthritis, wrist**
       Pneumococcal arthritis of carpal bones

          M00.131   **Pneumococcal arthritis, right wrist**

          M00.132   **Pneumococcal arthritis, left wrist**

          M00.139   **Pneumococcal arthritis, unspecified wrist**

   M00.14   **Pneumococcal arthritis, hand**
       Pneumococcal arthritis of metacarpus and phalanges

          M00.141   **Pneumococcal arthritis, right hand**

          M00.142   **Pneumococcal arthritis, left hand**

          M00.149   **Pneumococcal arthritis, unspecified hand**

   M00.15   **Pneumococcal arthritis, hip**

          M00.151   **Pneumococcal arthritis, right hip**

          M00.152   **Pneumococcal arthritis, left hip**

          M00.159   **Pneumococcal arthritis, unspecified hip**

   M00.16   **Pneumococcal arthritis, knee**

          M00.161   **Pneumococcal arthritis, right knee**

          M00.162   **Pneumococcal arthritis, left knee**

FORWARD MAPPING SAMPLE (ICD-9-CM ➡ ICD-10-CM)

ICD-10-CM CODE & DESCRIPTION		ICD-10-CM CODE & DESCRIPTION	
729.0	Rheumatism unspecified and fibrositis	M79.0	Rheumatism unspecified
729.1	Myalgia and myositis unspecified	M60.9	Myositis unspecified
729.1	Myalgia and myositis unspecified	M79.1	Myalgia

729.1	Myalgia and myositis unspecified	M79.7	Fibromyalgia
729.2	Neuralgia neuritis and radiculitis unspecified	M54.10	Radiculopathy site unspecified
729.2	Neuralgia neuritis and radiculitis unspecified	M79.2	Neuralgia and neuritis unspecified
729.30	Panniculitis unspecified site	M79.3	Panniculitis unspecified
729.31	Hypertrophy of fat pad knee	M79.4	Hypertrophy of (infrapatellar) fat pad
729.39	Panniculitis affecting other sites	M79.3	Panniculitis unspecified
729.4	Fasciitis unspecified	M79.3	Panniculitis unspecified
729.5	Pain in limb	M79.609	Pain in unspecified limb
729.6	Residual foreign body in soft tissue	M79.5	Residual foreign body in soft tissue
729.71	Nontraumatic compartment syndrome of upper extremity	M79.A19	Nontraumatic compartment syndrome of unspecified upper extremity
729.72	Nontraumatic compartment syndrome of lower extremity	M79.A29	Nontraumatic compartment syndrome of unspecified lower extremity
729.73	Nontraumatic compartment syndrome of abdomen	M79.A3	Nontraumatic compartment syndrome of abdomen
729.79	Nontraumatic compartment syndrome of other sites	M79.A9	Nontraumatic compartment syndrome of other sites
729.81	Swelling of limb	M79.89	Other specified soft tissue disorders
729.82	Cramp of limb	R25.2	Cramp and spasm
729.89	Other musculoskeletal symptoms referable to limbs	R29.898	Other symptoms and signs involving the musculoskeletal system
729.90	Disorders of soft tissue, unspecified	M79.9	Soft tissue disorder unspecified
729.91	Post-traumatic seroma	M70.98	Unspecified soft tissue disorder related to use overuse and pressure other
729.92	Nontraumatic hematoma of soft tissue	M79.81	Nontraumatic hematoma of soft tissue
729.99	Other disorders of soft tissue	M79.89	Other specified soft tissue disorders
730.00	Acute osteomyelitis site unspecified	M86.10	Other acute osteomyelitis unspecified site
730.00	Acute osteomyelitis site unspecified	M86.20	Subacute osteomyelitis unspecified site
730.01	Acute osteomyelitis involving shoulder region	M86.119	Other acute osteomyelitis unspecified shoulder

730.01	Acute osteomyelitis involving shoulder region	M86.219	Subacute osteomyelitis unspecified shoulder
730.02	Acute osteomyelitis involving upper arm	M86.129	Other acute osteomyelitis unspecified humerus
730.02	Acute osteomyelitis involving upper arm	M86.229	Subacute osteomyelitis unspecified humerus
730.03	Acute osteomyelitis involving forearm	M86.139	Other acute osteomyelitis unspecified radius and ulna
730.03	Acute osteomyelitis involving forearm	M86.239	Subacute osteomyelitis unspecified radius and ulna
730.04	Acute osteomyelitis involving hand	M86.249	Subacute osteomyelitis unspecified hand
730.04	Acute osteomyelitis involving hand	M86.149	Other acute osteomyelitis unspecified hand
730.05	Acute osteomyelitis involving pelvic region and thigh	M86.159	Other acute osteomyelitis unspecified femur
730.05	Acute osteomyelitis involving pelvic region and thigh	M86.259	Subacute osteomyelitis unspecified femur
730.06	Acute osteomyelitis involving lower leg	M86.169	Other acute osteomyelitis unspecified tibia and fibula
730.06	Acute osteomyelitis involving lower leg	M86.269	Subacute osteomyelitis unspecified tibia and fibula
730.07	Acute osteomyelitis involving ankle and foot	M86.179	Other acute osteomyelitis unspecified ankle and foot
730.07	Acute osteomyelitis involving ankle and foot	M86.279	Subacute osteomyelitis unspecified ankle and foot
730.08	Acute osteomyelitis involving other specified sites	M86.28	Subacute osteomyelitis other site

BACKWARD MAPPING SAMPLE (ICD-10-CM ➡ ICD-9-CM)

ICD-10-CM CODE & DESCRIPTION		ICD-10-CM CODE & DESCRIPTION	
M20.10	Hallux valgus (acquired) unspecified foot	727.1	Bunion
M20.10	Hallux valgus (acquired) unspecified foot	735.0	Hallux valgus (acquired)
M20.11	Hallux valgus (acquired) right foot	735.0	Hallux valgus (acquired)
M20.12	Hallux valgus (acquired) left foot	735.0	Hallux valgus (acquired)
M20.20	Hallux rigidus unspecified foot	735.2	Hallux rigidus
M20.21	Hallux rigidus right foot	735.2	Hallux rigidus
M20.22	Hallux rigidus left foot	735.2	Hallux rigidus
M20.30	Hallux varus (acquired) unspecified foot	735.1	Hallux varus (acquired)

M20.31	Hallux varus (acquired) right foot	735.1	Hallux varus (acquired)
M20.32	Hallux varus (acquired) left foot	735.1	Hallux varus (acquired)
M20.40	Other hammer toe(s) (acquired) unspecified foot	735.4	Other hammer toe (acquired)
M20.41	Other hammer toe(s) (acquired) right foot	735.4	Other hammer toe (acquired)
M20.42	Other hammer toe(s) (acquired) left foot	735.4	Other hammer toe (acquired)
M20.5x1	Other deformities of toe(s) (acquired) right foot	735.8	Other acquired deformities of toe
M20.5x2	Other deformities of toe(s) (acquired) left foot	735.8	Other acquired deformities of toe
M20.5x9	Other deformities of toe(s) (acquired) unspecified foot	735.8	Other acquired deformities of toe
M20.60	Acquired deformities of toe(s) unspecified, unspecified foot	735.9	Unspecified acquired deformity of toe
M20.61	Acquired deformities of toe(s) unspecified right foot	735.9	Unspecified acquired deformity of toe
M20.62	Acquired deformities of toe(s) unspecified left foot	735.9	Unspecified acquired deformity of toe
M21.00	Valgus deformity not elsewhere classified unspecified site	736.9	Acquired deformity of limb site unspecified
M21.021	Valgus deformity not elsewhere classified right elbow	736.01	Cubitus valgus (acquired)
M21.022	Valgus deformity not elsewhere classified left elbow	736.01	Cubitus valgus (acquired)
M21.029	Valgus deformity not elsewhere classified unspecified elbow	736.01	Cubitus valgus (acquired)
M21.061	Valgus deformity not elsewhere classified right knee	736.41	Genu valgum (acquired)
M21.062	Valgus deformity not elsewhere classified left knee	736.41	Genu valgum (acquired)
M21.069	Valgus deformity not elsewhere classified unspecified knee	736.41	Genu valgum (acquired)
M21.071	Valgus deformity not elsewhere classified right ankle	736.79	Other acquired deformities of ankle and foot
M21.072	Valgus deformity not elsewhere classified left ankle	736.79	Other acquired deformities of ankle and foot
M21.079	Valgus deformity not elsewhere classified unspecified ankle	736.79	Other acquired deformities of ankle and foot
M21.10	Varus deformity not elsewhere classified unspecified site	738.9	Acquired musculoskeletal deformity of unspecified site
M21.121	Varus deformity not elsewhere classified right elbow	736.02	Cubitus varus (acquired)

M21.122	Varus deformity not elsewhere classified left elbow	736.02	Cubitus varus (acquired)
M21.129	Varus deformity not elsewhere classified unspecified elbow	736.02	Cubitus varus (acquired)
M21.161	Varus deformity not elsewhere classified right knee	736.42	Genu varum (acquired)
M21.162	Varus deformity not elsewhere classified left knee	736.42	Genu varum (acquired)
M21.169	Varus deformity not elsewhere classified unspecified knee	736.42	Genu varum (acquired)
M21.171	Varus deformity not elsewhere classified right ankle	736.71	Acquired equinovarus deformity
M21.172	Varus deformity not elsewhere classified left ankle	736.71	Acquired equinovarus deformity
M21.179	Varus deformity not elsewhere classified unspecified ankle	738.9	Acquired musculoskeletal deformity of unspecified site
M21.20	Flexion deformity unspecified site	736.89	Other acquired deformity of other parts of limb

CHAPTER 14: DISEASES OF GENITOURINARY SYSTEM (N00-N99)

GENERAL GUIDELINES

CHRONIC KIDNEY DISEASE

1) **Stages of chronic kidney disease (CKD)**

The ICD-10-CM classifies CKD based on severity. The severity of CKD is designated by stages 1-5. Stage 2, code N18.2, equates to mild CKD; stage 3, code N18.3, equates to moderate CKD; and stage 4, code N18.4, equates to severe CKD. Code N18.6, End stage renal disease (ESRD), is assigned when the provider has documented end-stage-renal disease (ESRD).

If both a stage of CKD and ESRD are documented, assign code N18.6 only.

2) **Chronic kidney disease and kidney transplant status**

Patients who have undergone kidney transplant may still have some form of chronic kidney disease (CKD) because the kidney transplant may not fully restore kidney function. Therefore, the presence of CKD alone does not constitute a transplant complication. Assign the appropriate N18 code for the patient's stage of CKD and code Z94.0, Kidney transplant status. If a transplant complication such as failure or rejection or other transplant complication is documented, see section I.C.19.g for information on coding complications of a kidney transplant. If the documentation is unclear as to whether the patient has a complication of the transplant, query the provider.

3) **Chronic kidney disease with other conditions**

Patients with CKD may also suffer from other serious conditions, most commonly diabetes mellitus and hypertension. The sequencing of the CKD code in relationship to codes for other contributing conditions is based on the conventions in the Tabular List.

SAMPLE ICD-10-CM CODES FROM THIS CHAPTER

Excludes 2: certain conditions originating in the perinatal period (P04-P96)
certain infectious and parasitic diseases (A00-B99)
complications of pregnancy, childbirth and the puerperium (O00-O99)
congenital malformations, deformations and chromosomal abnormalities (Q00-Q99)
endocrine, nutritional and metabolic diseases (E00-E88)
injury, poisoning and certain other consequences of external causes (S00-T88)
neoplasms (C00-D49)
symptoms, signs and abnormal clinical and laboratory findings, not elsewhere classified (R00-R94)

This chapter contains the following blocks:	
N00-N08	Glomerular diseases
N10-N16	Renal tubulo-interstitial diseases
N17-N19	Acute kidney failure and chronic kidney disease
N20-N23	Urolithiasis
N25-N29	Other disorders of kidney and ureter
N30-N39	Other diseases of the urinary system
N40-N53	Diseases of male genital organs
N60-N65	Disorders of breast
N70-N77	Inflammatory diseases of female pelvic organs
N80-N98	Noninflammatory disorders of female genital tract
N99	Intraoperative and postprocedural complications and disorders of genitourinary system, not elsewhere classified

GLOMERULAR DISEASES (N00-N08)

Excludes 1: hypertensive chronic kidney disease (I12.-)

Code also any associated kidney failure (N17-N19).

N00 Acute nephritic syndrome

> *Includes:* acute glomerular disease
> acute glomerulonephritis
> acute nephritis

> *Excludes 1*: acute tubulo-interstitial nephritis (N10)
> nephritic syndrome NOS (N05.-)

N00.0 Acute nephritic syndrome with minor glomerular abnormality
Acute nephritic syndrome with minimal change lesion

N00.1 Acute nephritic syndrome with focal and segmental glomerular lesions
Acute nephritic syndrome with focal and segmental hyalinosis
Acute nephritic syndrome with focal and segmental sclerosis
Acute nephritic syndrome with focal glomerulonephritis

N00.2 Acute nephritic syndrome with diffuse membranous glomerulonephritis

N00.3 Acute nephritic syndrome with diffuse mesangial proliferative glomerulonephritis

N00.4 Acute nephritic syndrome with diffuse endocapillary proliferative glomerulonephritis

N00.5 Acute nephritic syndrome with diffuse mesangiocapillary glomerulonephritis
Acute nephritic syndrome with membranoproliferative glomerulonephritis, types 1 and 3, or NOS

N00.6 Acute nephritic syndrome with dense deposit disease
Acute nephritic syndrome with membranoproliferative glomerulonephritis, type 2

N00.7 Acute nephritic syndrome with diffuse crescentic glomerulonephritis
Acute nephritic syndrome with extracapillary glomerulonephritis

N00.8 Acute nephritic syndrome with other morphologic changes
Acute nephritic syndrome with proliferative glomerulonephritis NOS

N00.9 Acute nephritic syndrome with unspecified morphologic changes

N01 Rapidly progressive nephritic syndrome

Includes: rapidly progressive glomerular disease
rapidly progressive glomerulonephritis
rapidly progressive nephritis

Excludes 1: nephritic syndrome NOS (N05.-)

N01.0 Rapidly progressive nephritic syndrome with minor glomerular abnormality
Rapidly progressive nephritic syndrome with minimal change lesion

N01.1 Rapidly progressive nephritic syndrome with focal and segmental glomerular lesions
Rapidly progressive nephritic syndrome with focal and segmental hyalinosis
Rapidly progressive nephritic syndrome with focal and segmental sclerosis
Rapidly progressive nephritic syndrome with focal glomerulonephritis

N01.2 Rapidly progressive nephritic syndrome with diffuse membranous glomerulonephritis

N01.3 Rapidly progressive nephritic syndrome with diffuse mesangial proliferative glomerulonephritis

N01.4 Rapidly progressive nephritic syndrome with diffuse endocapillary proliferative glomerulonephritis

N01.5 Rapidly progressive nephritic syndrome with diffuse mesangiocapillary glomerulonephritis
Rapidly progressive nephritic syndrome with membranoproliferative glomerulonephritis, types 1and 3, or NOS

N01.6 Rapidly progressive nephritic syndrome with dense deposit disease
Rapidly progressive nephritic syndrome with membranoproliferative glomerulonephritis, type 2

N01.7 Rapidly progressive nephritic syndrome with diffuse crescentic glomerulonephritis
Rapidly progressive nephritic syndrome with extracapillary glomerulonephritis

N01.8 Rapidly progressive nephritic syndrome with other morphologic changes
Rapidly progressive nephritic syndrome with proliferative glomerulonephritis NOS

N01.9 Rapidly progressive nephritic syndrome with unspecified morphologic changes

N02 Recurrent and persistent hematuria

Excludes 1: acute cystitis with hematuria (N30.01)
acute prostatitis with hematuria (N41.01)
chronic prostatitis with hematuria (N41.11)
hematuria NOS (R31.9)
hematuria not associated with specified morphologic lesions (R31.-)

N02.0 Recurrent and persistent hematuria with minor glomerular abnormality
Recurrent and persistent hematuria with minimal change lesion

N02.1 Recurrent and persistent hematuria with focal and segmental glomerular lesions
Recurrent and persistent hematuria with focal and segmental hyalinosis
Recurrent and persistent hematuria with focal and segmental sclerosis
Recurrent and persistent hematuria with focal glomerulonephritis

N02.2 Recurrent and persistent hematuria with diffuse membranous glomerulonephritis

N02.3 Recurrent and persistent hematuria with diffuse mesangial proliferative glomerulonephritis

N02.4 Recurrent and persistent hematuria with diffuse endocapillary proliferative glomerulonephritis

N02.5 Recurrent and persistent hematuria with diffuse mesangiocapillary glomerulonephritis
Recurrent and persistent hematuria with membranoproliferative glomerulonephritis, types 1and 3, or NOS

N02.6 Recurrent and persistent hematuria with dense deposit disease
Recurrent and persistent hematuria with membranoproliferative glomerulonephritis, type 2

N02.7 Recurrent and persistent hematuria with diffuse crescentic glomerulonephritis
Recurrent and persistent hematuria with extracapillary glomerulonephritis

N02.8 Recurrent and persistent hematuria with other morphologic changes
Recurrent and persistent hematuria with proliferative glomerulonephritis NOS

N02.9 Recurrent and persistent hematuria with unspecified morphologic changes

N03 Chronic nephritic syndrome

Includes: chronic glomerular disease
chronic glomerulonephritis
chronic nephritis

Excludes 1: chronic tubulo-interstitial nephritis (N11.-)
diffuse sclerosing glomerulonephritis (N05.8-)
nephritic syndrome NOS (N05.-)

N03.0 Chronic nephritic syndrome with minor glomerular abnormality
Chronic nephritic syndrome with minimal change lesion

N03.1 Chronic nephritic syndrome with focal and segmental glomerular lesions
Chronic nephritic syndrome with focal and segmental hyalinosis
Chronic nephritic syndrome with focal and segmental sclerosis
Chronic nephritic syndrome with focal glomerulonephritis

FORWARD MAPPING SAMPLE (ICD-9-CM ➡ ICD-10-CM)			
ICD-10-CM CODE & DESCRIPTION		**ICD-10-CM CODE & DESCRIPTION**	
586	Renal failure unspecified	N19	Unspecified kidney failure
587	Renal sclerosis unspecified	N26.9	Renal sclerosis unspecified
588.0	Renal osteodystrophy	N25.0	Renal osteodystrophy
588.1	Nephrogenic diabetes insipidus	N25.1	Nephrogenic diabetes insipidus
588.81	Secondary hyperparathyroidism (of renal origin)	N25.81	Secondary hyperparathyroidism of renal origin
588.89	Other specified disorders resulting from impaired renal function	N25.89	Other disorders resulting from impaired renal tubular function
588.9	Unspecified disorder resulting from impaired renal function	N25.9	Disorder resulting from impaired renal tubular function unspecified
589.0	Unilateral small kidney	N27.0	Small kidney unilateral

589.1	Bilateral small kidneys	N27.1	Small kidney bilateral
589.9	Small kidney unspecified	N27.9	Small kidney unspecified
590.00	Chronic pyelonephritis without lesion of renal medullary necrosis	N11.8	Other chronic tubulo-interstitial nephritis
590.01	Chronic pyelonephritis with lesion of renal medullary necrosis	N11.1	Chronic obstructive pyelonephritis
590.10	Acute pyelonephritis without lesion of renal medullary necrosis	N10	Acute tubulo-interstitial nephritis
590.11	Acute pyelonephritis with lesion of renal medullary necrosis	N10	Acute tubulo-interstitial nephritis
590.2	Renal and perinephric abscess	N15.1	Renal and perinephric abscess
590.3	Pyeloureteritis cystica	N28.85	Pyeloureteritis cystica
590.80	Pyelonephritis unspecified	N11.9	Chronic tubulo-interstitial nephritis unspecified
590.81	Pyelitis or pyelonephritis in diseases classified elsewhere	N16	Renal tubulo-interstitial disorders in diseases classified elsewhere
590.9	Infection of kidney unspecified	N15.9	Renal tubulo-interstitial disease unspecified
591	Hydronephrosis	N13.30	Unspecified hydronephrosis
592.0	Calculus of kidney	N20.0	Calculus of kidney
592.1	Calculus of ureter	N20.1	Calculus of ureter
592.9	Urinary calculus unspecified	N20.9	Urinary calculus unspecified
593.0	Nephroptosis	N28.83	Nephroptosis
593.1	Hypertrophy of kidney	N28.81	Hypertrophy of kidney
593.2	Cyst of kidney acquired	N28.1	Cyst of kidney acquired
593.3	Stricture or kinking of ureter	N13.5	Crossing vessel and stricture of ureter without hydronephrosis
593.4	Other ureteric obstruction	N13.8	Other obstructive and reflux uropathy
593.5	Hydroureter	N13.4	Hydroureter
593.6	Postural proteinuria	R80.2	Orthostatic proteinuria unspecified
593.70	Vesicoureteral reflux unspecified or without reflux nephropathy	N13.70	Vesicoureteral-reflux unspecified
593.70	Vesicoureteral reflux unspecified or without reflux nephropathy	N13.71	Vesicoureteral-reflux without reflux nephropathy
593.71	Vesicoureteral reflux with reflux nephropathy unilateral	N13.721	Vesicoureteral-reflux with reflux nephropathy without hydroureter unilateral
593.72	Vesicoureteral reflux with reflux nephropathy bilateral	N13.722	Vesicoureteral-reflux with reflux nephropathy without hydroureter bilateral

593.73	Other vesicoureteral reflux with reflux nephropathy nos	N13.729	Vesicoureteral-reflux with reflux nephropathy without hydroureter unspecified
593.81	Vascular disorders of kidney	N28.0	Ischemia and infarction of kidney
593.82	Ureteral fistula	N28.89	Other specified disorders of kidney and ureter
593.89	Other specified disorders of kidney and ureter	N28.89	Other specified disorders of kidney and ureter
593.9	Unspecified disorder of kidney and ureter	N28.9	Disorder of kidney and ureter unspecified
594.0	Calculus in diverticulum of bladder	N21.0	Calculus in bladder

BACKWARD MAPPING SAMPLE (ICD-10-CM ➡ ICD-9-CM)

ICD-10-CM CODE & DESCRIPTION		ICD-10-CM CODE & DESCRIPTION	
N19	Unspecified kidney failure	586	Renal failure unspecified
N20.0	Calculus of kidney	592.0	Calculus of kidney
N20.1	Calculus of ureter	592.1	Calculus of ureter
N20.2	Calculus of kidney with calculus of ureter	592.0	Calculus of kidney
N20.9	Urinary calculus unspecified	592.9	Urinary calculus unspecified
N21.0	Calculus in bladder	594.0	Calculus in diverticulum of bladder
N21.0	Calculus in bladder	594.1	Other calculus in bladder
N21.1	Calculus in urethra	594.2	Calculus in urethra
N21.8	Other lower urinary tract calculus	594.8	Other lower urinary tract calculus
N21.9	Calculus of lower urinary tract unspecified	594.9	Calculus of lower urinary tract unspecified
N22	Calculus of urinary tract in diseases classified elsewhere	592.9	Urinary calculus unspecified
N23	Unspecified renal colic	788.0	Renal colic
N25.0	Renal osteodystrophy	588.0	Renal osteodystrophy
N25.1	Nephrogenic diabetes insipidus	588.1	Nephrogenic diabetes insipidus
N25.81	Secondary hyperparathyroidism of renal origin	588.81	Secondary hyperparathyroidism (of renal origin)
N25.89	Other disorders resulting from impaired renal tubular function	588.89	Other specified disorders resulting from impaired renal function
N25.9	Disorder resulting from impaired renal tubular function unspecified	588.9	Unspecified disorder resulting from impaired renal function
N26.1	Atrophy of kidney (terminal)	587	Renal sclerosis unspecified
N26.2	Page kidney	405.91	Unspecified renovascular hypertension
N26.9	Renal sclerosis unspecified	587	Renal sclerosis unspecified
N27.0	Small kidney unilateral	589.0	Unilateral small kidney

N27.1	Small kidney bilateral	589.1	Bilateral small kidneys
N27.9	Small kidney unspecified	589.9	Small kidney unspecified
N28.0	Ischemia and infarction of kidney	593.81	Vascular disorders of kidney
N28.1	Cyst of kidney acquired	593.2	Cyst of kidney acquired
N28.81	Hypertrophy of kidney	593.1	Hypertrophy of kidney
N28.82	Megaloureter	593.89	Other specified disorders of kidney and ureter
N28.83	Nephroptosis	593.0	Nephroptosis
N28.84	Pyelitis cystica	593.89	Other specified disorders of kidney and ureter
N28.85	Pyeloureteritis cystica	590.3	Pyeloureteritis cystica
N28.86	Ureteritis cystica	593.89	Other specified disorders of kidney and ureter
N28.89	Other specified disorders of kidney and ureter	593.82	Ureteral fistula
N28.89	Other specified disorders of kidney and ureter	593.89	Other specified disorders of kidney and ureter
N28.9	Disorder of kidney and ureter unspecified	593.9	Unspecified disorder of kidney and ureter
N29	Other disorders of kidney and ureter in diseases classified elsewhere	593.9	Unspecified disorder of kidney and ureter
N30.00	Acute cystitis without hematuria	595.0	Acute cystitis
N30.01	Acute cystitis with hematuria	595.0	Acute cystitis
N30.10	Interstitial cystitis (chronic) without hematuria	595.1	Chronic interstitial cystitis
N30.11	Interstitial cystitis (chronic) with hematuria	595.1	Chronic interstitial cystitis
N30.20	Other chronic cystitis without hematuria	595.2	Other chronic cystitis

CHAPTER 15: PREGNANCY, CHILDBIRTH, AND THE PUERPERIUM (O00-O94)

GENERAL GUIDELINES FOR OBSTETRIC CASES

1) **Codes from chapter 15 and sequencing priority**

Obstetric cases require codes from chapter 15, codes in the range O00-O9A, Pregnancy, Childbirth, and the Puerperium. Chapter 15 codes have sequencing priority over codes from other chapters. Additional codes from other chapters may be used in conjunction with chapter 15 codes to further specify conditions. Should the provider document that the pregnancy is incidental to the encounter, then code Z33.1, Pregnant state, incidental, should be used in place of any chapter 15 codes. It is the provider's responsibility to state that the condition being treated is not affecting the pregnancy.

2) Chapter 15 codes used only on the maternal record

Chapter 15 codes are to be used only on the maternal record, never on the record of the newborn.

3) Final character for trimester

The majority of codes in Chapter 15 have a final character indicating the trimester of pregnancy. The timeframes for the trimesters are indicated at the beginning of the chapter. If trimester is not a component of a code it is because the condition always occurs in a specific trimester, or the concept of trimester of pregnancy is not applicable. Certain codes have characters for only certain trimesters because the condition does not occur in all trimesters, but it may occur in more than just one.

Assignment of the final character for trimester should be based on the provider's documentation of the trimester (or number of weeks) for the current admission/encounter. This applies to the assignment of trimester for pre-existing conditions as well as those that develop during or are due to the pregnancy. The provider's documentation of the number of weeks may be used to assign the appropriate code identifying the trimester.

Whenever delivery occurs during the current admission, and there is an "in childbirth" option for the obstetric complication being coded, the "in childbirth" code should be assigned.

4) Selection of trimester for inpatient admissions that encompass more than one trimesters

In instances when a patient is admitted to a hospital for complications of pregnancy during one trimester and remains in the hospital into a subsequent trimester, the trimester character for the antepartum complication code should be assigned on the basis of the trimester when the complication developed, not the trimester of the discharge. If the condition developed prior to the current admission/encounter or represents a pre-existing condition, the trimester character for the trimester at the time of the admission/encounter should be assigned.

5) Unspecified trimester

Each category that includes codes for trimester has a code for "unspecified trimester." The "unspecified trimester" code should rarely be used, such as when the documentation in the record is insufficient to determine the trimester and it is not possible to obtain clarification.

6) Fetal Extensions

Where applicable, a 7th character is to be assigned for certain categories (O31, O32, O33.3 - O33.6, O35, O36, O40, O41, O60.1, O60.2, O64, and O69) to identify the fetus for which the complication code applies.

Assign 7th character "0":

- For single gestations
- When the documentation in the record is insufficient to determine the fetus affected and it is not possible to obtain clarification.
- When it is not possible to clinically determine which fetus is affected.

SELECTION OF OB PRINCIPAL OR FIRST-LISTED DIAGNOSIS

1) Routine outpatient prenatal visits

For routine outpatient prenatal visits when no complications are present, a code from category Z34, Encounter for supervision of normal pregnancy, should be used as the first-listed diagnosis. These codes should not be used in conjunction with chapter 15 codes.

2) Prenatal outpatient visits for high-risk patients

For routine prenatal outpatient visits for patients with high-risk pregnancies, a code from category O09, Supervision of high-risk pregnancy, should be used as the first-listed diagnosis. Secondary chapter 15 codes may be used in conjunction with these codes if appropriate.

3) Episodes when no delivery occurs

In episodes when no delivery occurs, the principal diagnosis should correspond to the principal complication of the pregnancy which necessitated the encounter. Should more than one complication exist, all of which are treated or monitored, any of the complications codes may be sequenced first.

4) When a delivery occurs

When a delivery occurs, the principal diagnosis should correspond to the main circumstances or complication of the delivery. In cases of cesarean delivery, the selection of the principal diagnosis should be the condition established after study that was responsible for the patient's admission. If the patient was admitted with a condition that resulted in the performance of a cesarean procedure, that condition should be selected as the principal diagnosis. If the reason for the admission/ encounter was unrelated to the condition resulting in the cesarean delivery, the condition related to the reason for the admission/encounter should be selected as the principal diagnosis.

5) Outcome of delivery

A code from category Z37, Outcome of delivery, should be included on every maternal record when a delivery has occurred. These codes are not to be used on subsequent records or on the newborn record.

PRE-EXISTING CONDITIONS VERSUS CONDITIONS DUE TO THE PREGNANCY

Certain categories in Chapter 15 distinguish between conditions of the mother that existed prior to pregnancy (pre-existing) and those that are a direct result of pregnancy. When assigning codes from Chapter 15, it is important to assess if a condition was pre-existing prior to pregnancy or developed during or due to the pregnancy in order to assign the correct code.

Categories that do not distinguish between pre-existing and pregnancy- related conditions may be used for either. It is acceptable to use codes specifically for the puerperium with codes complicating pregnancy and childbirth if a condition arises postpartum during the delivery encounter.

PRE-EXISTING HYPERTENSION IN PREGNANCY

Category O10, Pre-existing hypertension complicating pregnancy, childbirth and the puerperium, includes codes for hypertensive heart and hypertensive chronic kidney disease. When assigning one of the O10 codes that includes hypertensive heart disease or hypertensive chronic kidney disease, it is necessary to add a secondary code from the appropriate hypertension category to specify the type of heart failure or chronic kidney disease.

FETAL CONDITIONS AFFECTING THE MANAGEMENT OF THE MOTHER

1) Codes from categories O35 and O36

Codes from categories O35, Maternal care for known or suspected fetal abnormality and damage, and O36, Maternal care for other fetal problems, are assigned only when the fetal condition is actually responsible for modifying the management of the mother, i.e., by requiring diagnostic studies, additional observation, special care, or termination of pregnancy. The fact that the fetal condition exists does not justify assigning a code from this series to the mother's record.

2) In utero surgery

In cases when surgery is performed on the fetus, a diagnosis code from category O35, Maternal care for known or suspected fetal abnormality and damage, should be assigned identifying the fetal condition. Assign the appropriate procedure code for the procedure performed.

No code from Chapter 16, the perinatal codes, should be used on the mother's record to identify fetal conditions. Surgery performed in utero on a fetus is still to be coded as an obstetric encounter.

HIV INFECTION IN PREGNANCY, CHILDBIRTH AND THE PUERPERIUM

During pregnancy, childbirth or the puerperium, a patient admitted because of an HIV-related illness should receive a principal diagnosis from subcategory O98.7-, Human immunodeficiency [HIV] disease complicating pregnancy, childbirth and the puerperium, followed by the code(s) for the HIV-related illness(es).

Patients with asymptomatic HIV infection status admitted during pregnancy, childbirth, or the puerperium should receive codes of O98.7- and Z21, Asymptomatic human immunodeficiency virus [HIV] infection status.

DIABETES MELLITUS IN PREGNANCY

Diabetes mellitus is a significant complicating factor in pregnancy. Pregnant women who are diabetic should be assigned a code from category O24, Diabetes mellitus in pregnancy, childbirth, and the puerperium, first, followed by the appropriate diabetes code(s) (E08- E13) from Chapter 4.

LONG TERM USE OF INSULIN

Code Z79.4, Long-term (current) use of insulin, should also be assigned if the diabetes mellitus is being treated with insulin.

GESTATIONAL (PREGNANCY INDUCED) DIABETES

Gestational (pregnancy induced) diabetes can occur during the second and third trimester of pregnancy in women who were not diabetic prior to pregnancy. Gestational diabetes can cause complications in the pregnancy similar to those of pre-existing diabetes mellitus. It also puts the woman at greater risk of developing diabetes after the pregnancy. Codes for gestational diabetes are in subcategory O24.4, Gestational diabetes mellitus. No other code from category O24, Diabetes mellitus in pregnancy, childbirth, and the puerperium, should be used with a code from O24.4

The codes under subcategory O24.4 include diet controlled and insulin controlled. If a patient with gestational diabetes is treated with both diet and insulin, only the code for insulin-controlled is required. Code Z79.4, Long-term (current) use of insulin, should not be assigned with codes from subcategory O24.4.

An abnormal glucose tolerance in pregnancy is assigned a code from subcategory O99.81, Abnormal glucose complicating pregnancy, childbirth, and the puerperium.

SEPSIS AND SEPTIC SHOCK COMPLICATING ABORTION, PREGNANCY, CHILDBIRTH AND THE PUERPERIUM

When assigning a chapter 15 code for sepsis complicating abortion, pregnancy, childbirth, and the puerperium, a code for the specific type of infection should be assigned as an additional diagnosis. If severe sepsis is present, a code from subcategory R65.2, Severe sepsis, and code(s) for associated organ dysfunction(s) should also be assigned as additional diagnoses.

PUERPERAL SEPSIS

Code O85, Puerperal sepsis, should be assigned with a secondary code to identify the causal organism (e.g., for a bacterial infection, assign a code from category B95-B96, Bacterial infections in conditions classified elsewhere). A code from category A40, Streptococcal sepsis, or A41, Other sepsis, should not be used for puerperal sepsis. If applicable, use additional codes to identify severe sepsis (R65.2-) and any associated acute organ dysfunction.

ALCOHOL AND TOBACCO USE DURING PREGNANCY, CHILDBIRTH AND THE PUERPERIUM

1) **Alcohol use during pregnancy, childbirth and the puerperium**

   Codes under subcategory O99.31, Alcohol use complicating pregnancy, childbirth, and the puerperium, should be assigned for any pregnancy case when a mother uses alcohol during the pregnancy or postpartum. A secondary code from category F10, Alcohol related disorders, should also be assigned to identify manifestations of the alcohol use.

2) **Tobacco use during pregnancy, childbirth and the puerperium**

   Codes under subcategory O99.33, Smoking (tobacco) complicating pregnancy, childbirth, and the puerperium, should be assigned for any pregnancy case when a mother uses any type of tobacco product during the pregnancy or postpartum. A secondary code from category F17, Nicotine dependence, or code Z72.0, Tobacco use, should also be assigned to identify the type of nicotine dependence.

POISONING, TOXIC EFFECTS, ADVERSE EFFECTS AND UNDERDOSING IN A PREGNANT PATIENT

A code from subcategory O9A.2, Injury, poisoning and certain other consequences of external causes complicating pregnancy, childbirth, and the puerperium, should be sequenced first, followed by the appropriate poisoning, toxic effect, adverse effect or underdosing code, and then the additional code(s) that specifies the condition caused by the poisoning, toxic effect, adverse effect or underdosing.

NORMAL DELIVERY, CODE O80

1) Encounter for full term uncomplicated delivery

Code O80 should be assigned when a woman is admitted for a full-term normal delivery and delivers a single, healthy infant without any complications antepartum, during the delivery, or postpartum during the delivery episode. Code O80 is always a principal diagnosis. It is not to be used if any other code from chapter 15 is needed to describe a current complication of the antenatal, delivery, or perinatal period. Additional codes from other chapters may be used with code O80 if they are not related to or are in any way complicating the pregnancy.

2) Uncomplicated delivery with resolved antepartum complication

Code O80 may be used if the patient had a complication at some point during the pregnancy, but the complication is not present at the time of the admission for delivery.

3) Outcome of delivery for O80

Z37.0, Single live birth, is the only outcome of delivery code appropriate for use with O80.

THE PERIPARTUM AND POSTPARTUM PERIODS

1) Peripartum and Postpartum periods

The postpartum period begins immediately after delivery and continues for six weeks following delivery. The peripartum period is defined as the last month of pregnancy to five months postpartum.

2) Peripartum and postpartum complication

A postpartum complication is any complication occurring within the six-week period.

3) Pregnancy-related complications after 6 week period

Chapter 15 codes may also be used to describe pregnancy-related complications after the peripartum or postpartum period if the provider documents that a condition is pregnancy related.

4) Admission for routine postpartum care following delivery outside hospital

When the mother delivers outside the hospital prior to admission and is admitted for routine postpartum care and no complications are noted, code Z39.0, Encounter for care and examination of mother immediately after delivery, should be assigned as the principal diagnosis.

5) Pregnancy associated cardiomyopathy

Pregnancy associated cardiomyopathy, code O90.3, is unique in that it may be diagnosed in the third trimester of pregnancy but may continue to progress months after delivery. For this reason, it is referred to as peripartum cardiomyopathy. Code O90.3 is only for use when the cardiomyopathy develops as a result of pregnancy in a woman who did not have pre-existing heart disease.

CODE O94, SEQUELAE OF COMPLICATION OF PREGNANCY, CHILDBIRTH, AND THE PUERPERIUM

1) Code O94

Code O94, Sequelae of complication of pregnancy, childbirth, and the puerperium, is for use in those cases when an initial complication of a pregnancy develops a sequelae requiring care or treatment at a future date.

2) After the initial postpartum period

This code may be used at any time after the initial postpartum period.

3) Sequencing of Code O94

This code, like all late effect codes, is to be sequenced following the code describing the sequelae of the complication.

ABORTIONS

1) Abortion with Liveborn Fetus

When an attempted termination of pregnancy results in a liveborn fetus, assign a code from subcategory O60.1, Preterm labor with preterm delivery, and a code from category Z37, Outcome of Delivery. The procedure code for the attempted termination of pregnancy should also be assigned.

2) Retained Products of Conception following an abortion

Subsequent encounters for retained products of conception following a spontaneous abortion or elective termination of pregnancy are assigned the appropriate code from category O03, Spontaneous abortion, or codes O07.4, Failed attempted termination of pregnancy without complication and Z33.2, Encounter for elective termination of pregnancy. This advice is appropriate even when the patient was discharged previously with a discharge diagnosis of complete abortion.

ABUSE IN A PREGNANT PATIENT

For suspected or confirmed cases of abuse of a pregnant patient, a code(s) from subcategories O9A.3, Physical abuse complicating pregnancy, childbirth, and the puerperium, O9A.4, Sexual abuse complicating pregnancy, childbirth, and the puerperium, and O9A.5, Psychological abuse complicating pregnancy, childbirth, and the puerperium, should be sequenced first, followed by the appropriate codes (if applicable) to identify any associated current injury due to physical abuse, sexual abuse, and the perpetrator of abuse.

SAMPLE ICD-10-CM CODES FROM THIS CHAPTER

NOTE: CODES FROM THIS CHAPTER ARE FOR USE ONLY ON MATERNAL RECORDS, NEVER ON NEWBORN RECORDS

Codes from this chapter are for use for conditions related to or aggravated by the pregnancy, childbirth, or by the puerperium (maternal causes or obstetric causes).

Trimesters are counted from the first day of the last menstrual period. They are defined as follows:

1st trimester- less than 14 weeks 0 days
2nd trimester- 14 weeks 0 days to less than 28 weeks 0 days
3rd trimester- 28 weeks 0 days until delivery

Excludes 1: supervision of normal pregnancy (Z34.-)

Excludes 2: mental and behavioral disorders associated with the puerperium (F53)
        obstetrical tetanus (A34)
        postpartum necrosis of pituitary gland (E23.0)
        puerperal osteomalacia (M83.0)

This chapter contains the following blocks:	
O00-O08	Pregnancy with abortive outcome
O09	Supervision of high risk pregnancy
O10-O16	Edema, proteinuria and hypertensive disorders in pregnancy, childbirth and the puerperium
O20-O29	Other maternal disorders predominantly related to pregnancy
O30-O48	Maternal care related to the fetus and amniotic cavity and possible delivery problems
O60-O77	Complications of labor and delivery
O80-O82	Encounter for delivery
O85-O92	Complications predominantly related to the puerperium
O94-O9A	Other obstetric conditions, not elsewhere classified

PREGNANCY WITH ABORTIVE OUTCOME (O00-O08)

Excludes 1: continuing pregnancy in multiple gestation after abortion of one fetus or more
        (O31.1-, O31.3-)

O00   Ectopic pregnancy

    Includes: ruptured ectopic pregnancy

Use additional code from category O08 to identify any associated complication

O00.0 Abdominal pregnancy

Excludes 1: maternal care for viable fetus in abdominal pregnancy (O36.7-)

O00.1 Tubal pregnancy
Fallopian pregnancy
Rupture of (fallopian) tube due to pregnancy
Tubal abortion

O00.2 Ovarian pregnancy

O00.8 Other ectopic pregnancy
Cervical pregnancy
Cornual pregnancy
Intraligamentous pregnancy
Mural pregnancy

O00.9 Ectopic pregnancy, unspecified

O01 Hydatidiform mole
Use additional code from category O08 to identify any associated complication.

Excludes 1: chorioadenoma (destruens) (D39.2)
malignant hydatidiform mole (D39.2)

O01.0 Classical hydatidiform mole
Complete hydatidiform mole

O01.1 Incomplete and partial hydatidiform mole

O01.9 Hydatidiform mole, unspecified
Trophoblastic disease NOS
Vesicular mole NOS

O02 Other abnormal products of conception
Use additional code from category O08 to identify any associated complication.

Excludes 1: papyraceous fetus (O31.0-)

O02.0 Blighted ovum and non-hydatidiform mole
Carneous mole
Fleshy mole
Intrauterine mole NOS
Molar pregnancy NEC
Pathological ovum

O02.1 Missed abortion
Early fetal death, before completion of 20 weeks of gestation, with retention of dead fetus

Excludes 1: failed induced abortion (O07.-)
  fetal death (intrauterine) (late) (O36.4)
  missed abortion with blighted ovum (O02.0)
  missed abortion with hydatidiform mole (O01.-)
  missed abortion with non-hydatidiform (O02.0)
  missed delivery (O36.4)
  stillbirth (P95)

O02.8 Other specified abnormal products of conception

Excludes 1: abnormal products of conception with blighted ovum (O02.0)
  abnormal products of conception with hydatidiform mole (O01.-)
  abnormal products of conception with non-hydatidiform mole (O02.0)

O02.9 Abnormal product of conception, unspecified

O03 Spontaneous abortion
Note: Incomplete abortion includes retained products of conception following spontaneous abortion

Includes: miscarriage

O03.0 Genital tract and pelvic infection following incomplete spontaneous abortion
Endometritis following incomplete spontaneous abortion
Oophoritis following incomplete spontaneous abortion
Parametritis following incomplete spontaneous abortion
Pelvic peritonitis following incomplete spontaneous abortion
Salpingitis following incomplete spontaneous abortion
Salpingo-oophoritis following incomplete spontaneous abortion

Excludes 1: sepsis following incomplete spontaneous abortion (O03.37)
  urinary tract infection following incomplete spontaneous abortion (O03.38)

O03.1 Delayed or excessive hemorrhage following incomplete spontaneous abortion
Afibrinogenemia following incomplete spontaneous abortion
Defibrination syndrome following incomplete spontaneous abortion
Hemolysis following incomplete spontaneous abortion
Intravascular coagulation following incomplete spontaneous abortion

O03.2 Embolism following incomplete spontaneous abortion
Air embolism following incomplete spontaneous abortion
Amniotic fluid embolism following incomplete spontaneous abortion
Blood-clot embolism following incomplete spontaneous abortion
Embolism NOS following incomplete spontaneous abortion
Fat embolism following incomplete spontaneous abortion
Pulmonary embolism following incomplete spontaneous abortion
Pyemic embolism following incomplete spontaneous abortion
Septic or septicopyemic embolism following incomplete spontaneous abortion
Soap embolism following incomplete spontaneous abortion

O03.3 Other and unspecified complications following incomplete spontaneous abortion

O03.30 Unspecified complication following incomplete spontaneous abortion

O03.31 Shock following incomplete spontaneous abortion
Circulatory collapse following incomplete spontaneous abortion
Shock (postprocedural) following incomplete spontaneous abortion

Excludes 1: shock due to infection following incomplete spontaneous abortion (O03.37)

O03.32 Renal failure following incomplete spontaneous abortion
Kidney failure (acute) following incomplete spontaneous abortion
Oliguria following incomplete spontaneous abortion
Renal shutdown following incomplete spontaneous abortion
Renal tubular necrosis following incomplete spontaneous abortion
Uremia following incomplete spontaneous abortion

O03.33 Metabolic disorder following incomplete spontaneous abortion

O03.34 Damage to pelvic organs following incomplete spontaneous abortion
Laceration, perforation, tear or chemical damage of bladder following incomplete spontaneous abortion
Laceration, perforation, tear or chemical damage of bowel following incomplete spontaneous abortion
Laceration, perforation, tear or chemical damage of broad ligament following incomplete spontaneous abortion
Laceration, perforation, tear or chemical damage of cervix following incomplete spontaneous abortion
Laceration, perforation, tear or chemical damage of periurethral tissue following incomplete spontaneous abortion
Laceration, perforation, tear or chemical damage of uterus following incomplete spontaneous abortion
Laceration, perforation, tear or chemical damage of vagina following incomplete spontaneous abortion

O03.35 Other venous complications following incomplete spontaneous abortion

O03.36 Cardiac arrest following incomplete spontaneous abortion

O03.37 Sepsis following incomplete spontaneous abortion
Use additional code (B95-B97), to identify infectious agent
Use additional code (R65.2-) to identify severe sepsis, if applicable

Excludes 1: septic or septicopyemic embolism following incomplete spontaneous abortion (O03.2)

O03.38 Urinary tract infection following incomplete spontaneous abortion
Cystitis following incomplete spontaneous abortion

FORWARD MAPPING SAMPLE (ICD-9-CM ➡ ICD-10-CM)

ICD-10-CM CODE & DESCRIPTION		ICD-10-CM CODE & DESCRIPTION	
640.00	Threatened abortion unspecified as to episode of care	O20.0	Threatened abortion
640.01	Threatened abortion delivered	O20.0	Threatened abortion
640.03	Threatened abortion antepartum	O20.0	Threatened abortion
640.80	Other specified hemorrhage in early pregnancy unspecified as to episode of care	O20.8	Other hemorrhage in early pregnancy
640.81	Other specified hemorrhage in early pregnancy delivered	O20.8	Other hemorrhage in early pregnancy
640.83	Other specified hemorrhage in early pregnancy antepartum	O20.8	Other hemorrhage in early pregnancy
640.90	Unspecified hemorrhage in early pregnancy unspecified as to episode of care	O20.9	Hemorrhage in early pregnancy unspecified
640.91	Unspecified hemorrhage in early pregnancy delivered	O20.9	Hemorrhage in early pregnancy unspecified
640.93	Unspecified hemorrhage in early pregnancy antepartum	O20.9	Hemorrhage in early pregnancy unspecified
641.00	Placenta previa without hemorrhage unspecified as to episode of care	O44.00	Placenta previa specified as without hemorrhage unspecified trimester
641.01	Placenta previa without hemorrhage with delivery	O44.03	Placenta previa specified as without hemorrhage third trimester
641.01	Placenta previa without hemorrhage with delivery	O44.01	Placenta previa specified as without hemorrhage first trimester
641.01	Placenta previa without hemorrhage with delivery	O44.02	Placenta previa specified as without hemorrhage second trimester
641.03	Placenta previa without hemorrhage antepartum	O44.03	Placenta previa specified as without hemorrhage third trimester
641.03	Placenta previa without hemorrhage antepartum	O44.01	Placenta previa specified as without hemorrhage first trimester
641.03	Placenta previa without hemorrhage antepartum	O44.02	Placenta previa specified as without hemorrhage second trimester
641.10	Hemorrhage from placenta previa unspecified as to episode of care	O44.10	Placenta previa with hemorrhage unspecified trimester
641.11	Hemorrhage from placenta previa with delivery	O44.11	Placenta previa with hemorrhage first trimester
641.11	Hemorrhage from placenta previa with delivery	O44.12	Placenta previa with hemorrhage second trimester

641.11	Hemorrhage from placenta previa with delivery	O44.13	Placenta previa with hemorrhage third trimester
641.13	Hemorrhage from placenta previa antepartum	O44.12	Placenta previa with hemorrhage second trimester
641.13	Hemorrhage from placenta previa antepartum	O44.13	Placenta previa with hemorrhage third trimester
641.13	Hemorrhage from placenta previa antepartum	O44.11	Placenta previa with hemorrhage first trimester
641.20	Premature separation of placenta unspecified as to episode of care	O45.8x9	Other premature separation of placenta unspecified trimester
641.21	Premature separation of placenta with delivery	O45.8x1	Other premature separation of placenta first trimester
641.21	Premature separation of placenta with delivery	O45.8x2	Other premature separation of placenta second trimester
641.21	Premature separation of placenta with delivery	O45.8x3	Other premature separation of placenta third trimester
641.21	Premature separation of placenta with delivery	O45.91	Premature separation of placenta unspecified first trimester
641.21	Premature separation of placenta with delivery	O45.92	Premature separation of placenta unspecified second trimester
641.21	Premature separation of placenta with delivery	O45.93	Premature separation of placenta unspecified third trimester
641.23	Premature separation of placenta antepartum	O45.8x3	Other premature separation of placenta third trimester
641.23	Premature separation of placenta antepartum	O45.91	Premature separation of placenta unspecified first trimester
641.23	Premature separation of placenta antepartum	O45.93	Premature separation of placenta unspecified third trimester
641.23	Premature separation of placenta antepartum	O45.92	Premature separation of placenta unspecified second trimester
641.23	Premature separation of placenta antepartum	O45.8x1	Other premature separation of placenta first trimester
641.23	Premature separation of placenta antepartum	O45.8x2	Other premature separation of placenta second trimester
641.30	Antepartum hemorrhage associated with coagulation defects unspecified as to episode of care	O46.009	Antepartum hemorrhage with coagulation defect unspecified, unspecified trimester
641.30	Antepartum hemorrhage associated with coagulation defects unspecified as to episode of care	O46.019	Antepartum hemorrhage with afibrinogenemia unspecified trimester
641.30	Antepartum hemorrhage associated with coagulation defects unspecified as to episode of care	O46.029	Antepartum hemorrhage with disseminated intravascular coagulation unspecified trimester

BACKWARD MAPPING SAMPLE (ICD-10-CM ➤ ICD-9-CM)

ICD-10-CM CODE & DESCRIPTION		ICD-10-CM CODE & DESCRIPTION	
O76	Abnormality in fetal heart rate and rhythm complicating labor and delivery	659.71	Abnormality in fetal heart rate or rhythm delivered with or without antepartum condition
O77.0	Labor and delivery complicated by meconium in amniotic fluid	656.81	Other specified fetal and placental problems affecting management of mother delivered
O77.1	Fetal stress in labor or delivery due to drug administration	656.81	Other specified fetal and placental problems affecting management of mother delivered
O77.8	Labor and delivery complicated by other evidence of fetal stress	656.81	Other specified fetal and placental problems affecting management of mother delivered
O77.9	Labor and delivery complicated by fetal stress unspecified	656.81	Other specified fetal and placental problems affecting management of mother delivered
O80	Encounter for full-term uncomplicated delivery	650	Normal delivery
O82	Encounter for cesarean delivery without indication	669.71	Cesarean delivery without indication delivered with or without antepartum condition
O85	Puerperal sepsis	670.22	Puerperal sepsis, delivered, with mention of postpartum complication
O85	Puerperal sepsis	670.24	Puerperal sepsis, postpartum condition or complication
O86.0	Infection of obstetric surgical wound	674.32	Other complications of obstetrical surgical wounds with delivery with postpartum complication
O86.0	Infection of obstetric surgical wound	674.34	Other complications of obstetrical surgical wounds postpartum condition or complication
O86.11	Cervicitis following delivery	646.64	Postpartum infections of genitourinary tract
O86.12	Endometritis following delivery	670.12	Puerperal endometritis, delivered, with mention of postpartum complication
O86.12	Endometritis following delivery	670.14	Puerperal endometritis, postpartum condition or complication
O86.13	Vaginitis following delivery	646.64	Postpartum infections of genitourinary tract
O86.19	Other infection of genital tract following delivery	646.64	Postpartum infections of genitourinary tract
O86.20	Urinary tract infection following delivery unspecified	646.64	Postpartum infections of genitourinary tract

O86.21	Infection of kidney following delivery	646.64	Postpartum infections of genitourinary tract
O86.22	Infection of bladder following delivery	646.64	Postpartum infections of genitourinary tract
O86.29	Other urinary tract infection following delivery	646.64	Postpartum infections of genitourinary tract
O86.4	Pyrexia of unknown origin following delivery	672.02	Puerperal pyrexia of unknown origin delivered with postpartum complication
O86.4	Pyrexia of unknown origin following delivery	672.04	Puerperal pyrexia of unknown origin postpartum
O86.81	Puerperal septic thrombophlebitis	670.32	Puerperal septic thrombophlebitis, delivered, with mention of postpartum complication
O86.81	Puerperal septic thrombophlebitis	670.34	Puerperal septic thrombophlebitis, postpartum condition or complication
O86.89	Other specified puerperal infections	670.82	Other major puerperal infection, delivered, with mention of postpartum complication
O86.89	Other specified puerperal infections	670.84	Other major puerperal infection, postpartum condition or complication
O87.0	Superficial thrombophlebitis in the puerperium	671.22	Superficial thrombophlebitis with delivery with postpartum complication
O87.0	Superficial thrombophlebitis in the puerperium	671.24	Postpartum superficial thrombophlebitis
O87.1	Deep phlebothrombosis in the puerperium	671.42	Deep phlebothrombosis postpartum with delivery
O87.1	Deep phlebothrombosis in the puerperium	671.44	Deep phlebothrombosis postpartum
O87.2	Hemorrhoids in the puerperium	671.82	Other venous complications with delivery with postpartum complication
O87.2	Hemorrhoids in the puerperium	671.84	Other postpartum venous complications
O87.3	Cerebral venous thrombosis in the puerperium	671.52	Other phlebitis and thrombosis with delivery with postpartum complication
O87.3	Cerebral venous thrombosis in the puerperium	671.54	Other postpartum phlebitis and thrombosis
O87.4	Varicose veins of lower extremity in the puerperium	671.02	Varicose veins of legs with delivery with postpartum complication

O87.4	Varicose veins of lower extremity in the puerperium	671.04	Postpartum varicose veins of legs
O87.8	Other venous complications in the puerperium	671.82	Other venous complications with delivery with postpartum complication
O87.8	Other venous complications in the puerperium	671.84	Other postpartum venous complications
O87.9	Venous complication in the puerperium unspecified	671.92	Unspecified venous complication with delivery with postpartum complication
O87.9	Venous complication in the puerperium unspecified	671.94	Unspecified postpartum venous complication

CHAPTER 16: NEWBORN (PERINATAL) GUIDELINES (P00-P96)

GENERAL GUIDELINES

For coding and reporting purposes the perinatal period is defined as before birth through the 28th day following birth. The following guidelines are provided for reporting purposes.

1) **Use of Chapter 16 Codes**

Codes in this chapter are <u>never</u> for use on the maternal record. Codes from Chapter 15, the obstetric chapter, are never permitted on the newborn record. Chapter 16 codes may be used throughout the life of the patient if the condition is still present.

2) **Principal Diagnosis for Birth Record**

When coding the birth episode in a newborn record, assign a code from category Z38, Liveborn infants according to place of birth and type of delivery, as the principal diagnosis. A code from category Z38 is assigned only once, to a newborn at the time of birth. If a newborn is transferred to another institution, a code from category Z38 should not be used at the receiving hospital.

A code from category Z38 is used only on the newborn record, not on the mother's record.

3) **Use of Codes from other Chapters with Codes from Chapter 16**

Codes from other chapters may be used with codes from chapter 16 if the codes from the other chapters provide more specific detail. Codes for signs and symptoms may be assigned when a definitive diagnosis has not been established. If the reason for the encounter is a perinatal condition, the code from chapter 16 should be sequenced first.

4) **Use of Chapter 16 Codes after the Perinatal Period**

Should a condition originate in the perinatal period, and continue throughout the life of the patient, the perinatal code should continue to be used regardless of the patient's age.

5) Birth process or community acquired conditions

If a newborn has a condition that may be either due to the birth process or community acquired and the documentation does not indicate which it is, the default is due to the birth process and the code from Chapter 16 should be used. If the condition is community-acquired, a code from Chapter 16 should not be assigned.

6) Code all clinically significant conditions

All clinically significant conditions noted on routine newborn examination should be coded. A condition is clinically significant if it requires:

- clinical evaluation; or
- therapeutic treatment; or
- diagnostic procedures; or
- extended length of hospital stay; or
- increased nursing care and/or monitoring; or
- has implications for future health care needs

Note: The perinatal guidelines listed above are the same as the general coding guidelines for "additional diagnoses", except for the final point regarding implications for future health care needs. Codes should be assigned for conditions that have been specified by the provider as having implications for future health care needs.

OBSERVATION AND EVALUATION OF NEWBORNS FOR SUSPECTED CONDITIONS NOT FOUND

Assign a code from categories P00-P04 to identify those instances when a healthy newborn is evaluated for a suspected condition that is determined after study not to be present. Do not use a code from categories P00-P04 when the patient has identified signs or symptoms of a suspected problem; in such cases, code the sign or symptom.

CODING ADDITIONAL PERINATAL DIAGNOSES

1) Assigning codes for conditions that require treatment

Assign codes for conditions that require treatment or further investigation, prolong the length of stay, or require resource utilization.

2) Codes for conditions specified as having implications for future health care needs

Assign codes for conditions that have been specified by the provider as having implications for future health care needs.

Note: This guideline should not be used for adult patients.

PREMATURITY AND FETAL GROWTH RETARDATION

Providers utilize different criteria in determining prematurity. A code for prematurity should not be assigned unless it is documented. Assignment of codes in categories P05, Disorders of newborn related to slow fetal growth and fetal malnutrition, and P07, Disorders of newborn related to short gestation and low birth weight, not elsewhere classified, should be based on the recorded birth weight and estimated gestational age. Codes from category P05 should not be assigned with codes from category P07.

When both birth weight and gestational age are available, two codes from category P07 should be assigned, with the code for birth weight sequenced before the code for gestational age.

LOW BIRTH WEIGHT AND IMMATURITY STATUS

Codes from category P07, Disorders of newborn related to short gestation and low birth weight, not elsewhere classified, are for use for a child or adult who was premature or had a low birth weight as a newborn and this is affecting the patient's current health status.

BACTERIAL SEPSIS OF NEWBORN

Category P36, Bacterial sepsis of newborn, includes congenital sepsis. If a perinate is documented as having sepsis without documentation of congenital or community acquired, the default is congenital and a code from category P36 should be assigned. If the P36 code includes the causal organism, an additional code from category B95, Streptococcus, Staphylococcus, and Enterococcus as the cause of diseases classified elsewhere, or B96, Other bacterial agents as the cause of diseases classified elsewhere, should not be assigned. If the P36 code does not include the causal organism, assign an additional code from category B96. If applicable, use additional codes to identify severe sepsis (R65.2-) and any associated acute organ dysfunction.

STILLBIRTH

Code P95, Stillbirth, is only for use in institutions that maintain separate records for stillbirths. No other code should be used with P95. Code P95 should not be used on the mother's record.

SAMPLE ICD-10-CM CODES FROM THIS CHAPTER

Note: Codes from this chapter are for use on newborn records only, never on maternal records

Includes: conditions that have their origin in the fetal or perinatal period (before birth through the first 28 days after birth) even if morbidity occurs later

Excludes 2: congenital malformations, deformations and chromosomal abnormalities (Q00-Q99)
endocrine, nutritional and metabolic diseases (E00-E88)
injury, poisoning and certain other consequences of external causes (S00-T88)
neoplasms (C00-D49)
tetanus neonatorum (A33)

This chapter contains the following blocks:	
P00-P04	Newborn affected by maternal factors and by complications of pregnancy, labor, and delivery
P05-P08	Disorders of newborn related to length of gestation and fetal growth
P09	Abnormal findings on neonatal screening

P10-P15	Birth trauma
P19-P29	Respiratory and cardiovascular disorders specific to the perinatal period
P35-P39	Infections specific to the perinatal period
P50-P61	Hemorrhagic and hematological disorders of newborn
P70-P74	Transitory endocrine and metabolic disorders specific to newborn
P76-P78	Digestive system disorders of newborn
P80-P83	Conditions involving the integument and temperature regulation of newborn
P84	Other problems with newborn
P90-P96	Other disorders originating in the perinatal period

NEWBORN AFFECTED BY MATERNAL FACTORS AND BY COMPLICATIONS OF PREGNANCY, LABOR, AND DELIVERY (P00-P04)

Note: These codes are for use when the listed maternal conditions are specified as the cause of confirmed morbidity or potential morbidity which have their origin in the perinatal period (before birth through the first 28 days after birth).

Codes from these categories are also for use for newborns who are suspected of having an abnormal condition resulting from exposure from the mother or the birth process, but without signs or symptoms, and, which after examination and observation, is found not to exist. These codes may be used even if treatment is begun for a suspected condition that is ruled out.

P00   **Newborn (suspected to be) affected by maternal conditions that may be unrelated to present pregnancy**
Code first any current condition in newborn

   Excludes 2: newborn (suspected to be) affected by maternal complications of pregnancy
(P01.-)
newborn affected by maternal endocrine and metabolic disorders (P70-P74)
newborn affected by noxious substances transmitted via placenta or breast milk
(P04.-)

   P00.0   **Newborn (suspected to be) affected by maternal hypertensive disorders**
Newborn (suspected to be) affected by maternal conditions classifiable to O10-O11, O13-O16

   P00.1   **Newborn (suspected to be) affected by maternal renal and urinary tract diseases**
Newborn (suspected to be) affected by maternal conditions classifiable to N00-N39

   P00.2   **Newborn (suspected to be) affected by maternal infectious and parasitic diseases**
Newborn (suspected to be) affected by maternal infectious disease classifiable to A00-B99, J09 and J10

      Excludes 1: infections specific to the perinatal period (P35-P39)
maternal genital tract or other localized infections (P00.8)

P00.3 Newborn (suspected to be) affected by other maternal circulatory and respiratory diseases
Newborn (suspected to be) affected by maternal conditions classifiable to I00-I99, J00-J99, Q20-Q34and not included in P00.0, P00.2

P00.4 Newborn (suspected to be) affected by maternal nutritional disorders
Newborn (suspected to be) affected by maternal disorders classifiable to E40-E64
Maternal malnutrition NOS

P00.5 Newborn (suspected to be) affected by maternal injury
Newborn (suspected to be) affected by maternal conditions classifiable to O97.2

P00.6 Newborn (suspected to be) affected by surgical procedure on mother
Newborn (suspected to be) affected by amniocentesis

Excludes 1: Cesarean delivery for present delivery (P03.4)
damage to placenta from amniocentesis, Cesarean delivery or surgical induction (P02.1)
previous surgery to uterus or pelvic organs (P03.89)

Excludes 2: newborn affected by complication of (fetal) intrauterine procedure (P96.5)

P00.7 Newborn (suspected to be) affected by other medical procedures on mother, not elsewhere classified
Newborn (suspected to be) affected by radiation to mother

Excludes 1: damage to placenta from amniocentesis, cesarean delivery or surgical induction (P02.1)
newborn affected by other complications of labor and delivery (P03.-)

P00.8 Newborn (suspected to be) affected by other maternal conditions

P00.81 Newborn (suspected to be) affected by periodontal disease in mother

P00.89 Newborn (suspected to be) affected by other maternal conditions
Newborn (suspected to be) affected by conditions classifiable to T80-T88
Newborn (suspected to be) affected by maternal genital tract or other localized infections
Newborn (suspected to be) affected by maternal systemic lupus erythematosus

P00.9 Newborn (suspected to be) affected by unspecified maternal condition

P01 Newborn (suspected to be) affected by maternal complications of pregnancy
Code first any current condition in newborn

P01.0 Newborn (suspected to be) affected by incompetent cervix

P01.1 Newborn (suspected to be) affected by premature rupture of membranes

P01.2 Newborn (suspected to be) affected by oligohydramnios

Excludes 1: oligohydramnios due to premature rupture of membranes (P01.1)

P01.3 Newborn (suspected to be) affected by polyhydramnios
Newborn (suspected to be) affected by hydramnios

P01.4 Newborn (suspected to be) affected by ectopic pregnancy
Newborn (suspected to be) affected by abdominal pregnancy

P01.5 Newborn (suspected to be) affected by multiple pregnancy
Newborn (suspected to be) affected by triplet (pregnancy)
Newborn (suspected to be) affected by twin (pregnancy)

P01.6 Newborn (suspected to be) affected by maternal death

P01.7 Newborn (suspected to be) affected by malpresentation before labor
Newborn (suspected to be) affected by breech presentation before labor
Newborn (suspected to be) affected by external version before labor
Newborn (suspected to be) affected by face presentation before labor
Newborn (suspected to be) affected by transverse lie before labor
Newborn (suspected to be) affected by unstable lie before labor

P01.8 Newborn (suspected to be) affected by other maternal complications of pregnancy

P01.9 Newborn (suspected to be) affected by maternal complication of pregnancy, unspecified

P02 Newborn (suspected to be) affected by complications of placenta, cord and membranes
Code first any current condition in newborn

P02.0 Newborn (suspected to be) affected by placenta previa

P02.1 Newborn (suspected to be) affected by other forms of placental separation and hemorrhage
Newborn (suspected to be) affected by abruptio placenta
Newborn (suspected to be) affected by accidental hemorrhage
Newborn (suspected to be) affected by antepartum hemorrhage
Newborn (suspected to be) affected by damage to placenta from amniocentesis, cesarean delivery or surgical induction
Newborn (suspected to be) affected by maternal blood loss
Newborn (suspected to be) affected by premature separation of placenta

P02.2 Newborn (suspected to be) affected by other and unspecified morphological and functional abnormalities of placenta

P02.20 Newborn (suspected to be) affected by unspecified morphological and functional abnormalities of placenta

FORWARD MAPPING SAMPLE (ICD-9-CM ➡ ICD-10-CM)

ICD-10-CM CODE & DESCRIPTION		ICD-10-CM CODE & DESCRIPTION	
776.0	Hemorrhagic disease of newborn	P53	Hemorrhagic disease of newborn
776.1	Transient neonatal thrombocytopenia	P61.0	Transient neonatal thrombocytopenia
776.2	Disseminated intravascular coagulation in newborn	P60	Disseminated intravascular coagulation of newborn
776.3	Other transient neonatal disorders of coagulation	P61.6	Other transient neonatal disorders of coagulation
776.4	Polycythemia neonatorum	P61.1	Polycythemia neonatorum
776.5	Congenital anemia	P61.4	Other congenital anemias not elsewhere classified
776.5	Congenital anemia	P61.3	Congenital anemia from fetal blood loss
776.6	Anemia of prematurity	P61.2	Anemia of prematurity
776.7	Transient neonatal neutropenia	P61.5	Transient neonatal neutropenia
776.8	Other specified transient hematological disorders of fetus or newborn	P61.8	Other specified perinatal hematological disorders
776.9	Unspecified hematological disorder specific to newborn	P61.9	Perinatal hematological disorder unspecified
777.1	Meconium obstruction in fetus or newborn	P76.0	Meconium plug syndrome
777.2	Intestinal obstruction in newborn due to inspissated milk	P76.2	Intestinal obstruction due to inspissated milk
777.3	Hematemesis and melena of newborn due to swallowed maternal blood	P78.2	Neonatal hematemesis and melena due to swallowed maternal blood
777.4	Transitory ileus of newborn	P76.1	Transitory ileus of newborn
777.50	Necrotizing enterocolitis in newborn, unspecified	P77.9	Necrotizing enterocolitis in newborn unspecified
777.51	Stage i necrotizing enterocolitis in newborn	P77.1	Stage 1 necrotizing enterocolitis in newborn
777.52	Stage ii necrotizing enterocolitis in newborn	P77.2	Stage 2 necrotizing enterocolitis in newborn
777.53	Stage iii necrotizing enterocolitis in newborn	P77.3	Stage 3 necrotizing enterocolitis in newborn
777.6	Perinatal intestinal perforation	P78.0	Perinatal intestinal perforation
777.8	Other specified perinatal disorders of digestive system	P78.89	Other specified perinatal digestive system disorders
777.9	Unspecified perinatal disorder of digestive system	P78.9	Perinatal digestive system disorder unspecified
778.0	Hydrops fetalis not due to isoimmunization	P83.2	Hydrops fetalis not due to hemolytic disease

778.1	Sclerema neonatorum	P83.0	Sclerema neonatorum
778.2	Cold injury syndrome of newborn	P80.0	Cold injury syndrome
778.3	Other hypothermia of newborn	P80.8	Other hypothermia of newborn
778.4	Other disturbances of temperature regulation of newborn	P81.0	Environmental hyperthermia of newborn
778.4	Other disturbances of temperature regulation of newborn	P81.8	Other specified disturbances of temperature regulation of newborn
778.5	Other and unspecified edema of newborn	P83.30	Unspecified edema specific to newborn
778.5	Other and unspecified edema of newborn	P83.39	Other edema specific to newborn
778.6	Congenital hydrocele	P83.5	Congenital hydrocele
778.7	Breast engorgement in newborn	P83.4	Breast engorgement of newborn
778.8	Other specified conditions involving the integument of fetus and newborn	P83.8	Other specified conditions of integument specific to newborn
778.9	Unspecified condition involving the integument and temperature regulation of fetus and newborn	P83.9	Condition of the integument specific to newborn unspecified
779.0	Convulsions in newborn	P90	Convulsions of newborn
779.1	Other and unspecified cerebral irritability in newborn	P91.9	Disturbance of cerebral status of newborn unspecified
779.1	Other and unspecified cerebral irritability in newborn	P91.8	Other specified disturbances of cerebral status of newborn
779.2	Cerebral depression coma and other abnormal cerebral signs in fetus or newborn	P91.4	Neonatal cerebral depression
779.2	Cerebral depression coma and other abnormal cerebral signs in fetus or newborn	P91.5	Neonatal coma
779.31	Feeding problems in newborn	P92.1	Regurgitation and rumination of newborn

BACKWARD MAPPING SAMPLE (ICD-10-CM ➡ ICD-9-CM)			
ICD-10-CM CODE & DESCRIPTION		**ICD-10-CM CODE & DESCRIPTION**	
P60	Disseminated intravascular coagulation of newborn	776.2	Disseminated intravascular coagulation in newborn
P61.0	Transient neonatal thrombocytopenia	776.1	Transient neonatal thrombocytopenia
P61.1	Polycythemia neonatorum	776.4	Polycythemia neonatorum
P61.2	Anemia of prematurity	776.6	Anemia of prematurity
P61.3	Congenital anemia from fetal blood loss	776.5	Congenital anemia
P61.4	Other congenital anemias not elsewhere classified	776.5	Congenital anemia

P61.5	Transient neonatal neutropenia	776.7	Transient neonatal neutropenia
P61.6	Other transient neonatal disorders of coagulation	776.3	Other transient neonatal disorders of coagulation
P61.8	Other specified perinatal hematological disorders	776.8	Other specified transient hematological disorders of fetus or newborn
P61.9	Perinatal hematological disorder unspecified	776.9	Unspecified hematological disorder specific to newborn
P70.0	Syndrome of infant of mother with gestational diabetes	775.0	Syndrome of 'infant of a diabetic mother'
P70.1	Syndrome of infant of a diabetic mother	775.0	Syndrome of 'infant of a diabetic mother'
P70.2	Neonatal diabetes mellitus	775.1	Neonatal diabetes mellitus
P70.3	Iatrogenic neonatal hypoglycemia	775.6	Neonatal hypoglycemia
P70.4	Other neonatal hypoglycemia	775.6	Neonatal hypoglycemia
P70.8	Other transitory disorders of carbohydrate metabolism of newborn	775.89	Other neonatal endocrine and metabolic disturbances
P70.9	Transitory disorder of carbohydrate metabolism of newborn unspecified	775.9	Unspecified endocrine and metabolic disturbances specific to the fetus and newborn
P71.0	Cow's milk hypocalcemia in newborn	775.4	Hypocalcemia and hypomagnesaemia of newborn
P71.1	Other neonatal hypocalcemia	775.4	Hypocalcemia and hypomagnesaemia of newborn
P71.2	Neonatal hypomagnesemia	775.4	Hypocalcemia and hypomagnesaemia of newborn
P71.3	Neonatal tetany without calcium or magnesium deficiency	775.4	Hypocalcemia and hypomagnesaemia of newborn
P71.4	Transitory neonatal hypoparathyroidism	775.4	Hypocalcemia and hypomagnesaemia of newborn
P71.8	Other transitory neonatal disorders of calcium and magnesium metabolism	775.4	Hypocalcemia and hypomagnesaemia of newborn
P71.9	Transitory neonatal disorder of calcium and magnesium metabolism unspecified	775.4	Hypocalcemia and hypomagnesaemia of newborn
P72.0	Neonatal goiter not elsewhere classified	775.89	Other neonatal endocrine and metabolic disturbances
P72.1	Transitory neonatal hyperthyroidism	775.3	Neonatal thyrotoxicosis
P72.2	Other transitory neonatal disorders of thyroid function not elsewhere classified	775.89	Other neonatal endocrine and metabolic disturbances
P72.8	Other specified transitory neonatal endocrine disorders	775.89	Other neonatal endocrine and metabolic disturbances

P72.9	Transitory neonatal endocrine disorder unspecified	775.9	Unspecified endocrine and metabolic disturbances specific to the fetus and newborn
P74.0	Late metabolic acidosis of newborn	775.7	Late metabolic acidosis of newborn
P74.1	Dehydration of newborn	775.5	Other transitory neonatal electrolyte disturbances
P74.2	Disturbances of sodium balance of newborn	775.5	Other transitory neonatal electrolyte disturbances
P74.3	Disturbances of potassium balance of newborn	775.5	Other transitory neonatal electrolyte disturbances
P74.4	Other transitory electrolyte disturbances of newborn	775.5	Other transitory neonatal electrolyte disturbances
P74.5	Transitory tyrosinemia of newborn	775.89	Other neonatal endocrine and metabolic disturbances
P74.6	Transitory hyperammonemia of newborn	775.89	Other neonatal endocrine and metabolic disturbances
P74.8	Other transitory metabolic disturbances of newborn	775.89	Other neonatal endocrine and metabolic disturbances
P74.9	Transitory metabolic disturbance of newborn unspecified	775.9	Unspecified endocrine and metabolic disturbances specific to the fetus and newborn
P76.0	Meconium plug syndrome	777.1	Meconium obstruction in fetus or newborn

CHAPTER 17: CONGENITAL MALFORMATIONS, DEFORMATIONS, AND CHROMOSOMAL ABNORMALITIES (Q00-Q99)

GENERAL GUIDELINES

Assign an appropriate code(s) from categories Q00-Q99, Congenital malformations, deformations, and chromosomal abnormalities when a malformation/deformation or chromosomal abnormality is documented. A malformation/ deformation/or chromosomal abnormality may be the principal/ first-listed diagnosis on a record or a secondary diagnosis.

When a malformation/deformation/or chromosomal abnormality does not have a unique code assignment, assign additional code(s) for any manifestations that may be present.

When the code assignment specifically identifies the malformation/ deformation/or chromosomal abnormality, manifestations that are an inherent component of the anomaly should not be coded separately. Additional codes should be assigned for manifestations that are not an inherent component.

Codes from Chapter 17 may be used throughout the life of the patient. If a congenital malformation or deformity has been corrected, a personal history code should be used to identify the history of the malformation or deformity. Although present at birth, malformation/

deformation/or chromosomal abnormality may not be identified until later in life. Whenever the condition is diagnosed by the physician, it is appropriate to assign a code from codes Q00-Q99.

For the birth admission, the appropriate code from category Z38, Liveborn infants, according to place of birth and type of delivery, should be sequenced as the principal diagnosis, followed by any congenital anomaly codes, Q00- Q99.

SAMPLE ICD-10-CM CODES FROM THIS CHAPTER

Note: Codes from this chapter are not for use on maternal or fetal records

Excludes 1: inborn errors of metabolism (E70-E88)

This chapter contains the following blocks:	
Q00-Q07	Congenital malformations of the nervous system
Q10-Q18	Congenital malformations of eye, ear, face and neck
Q20-Q28	Congenital malformations of the circulatory system
Q30-Q34	Congenital malformations of the respiratory system
Q35-Q37	Cleft lip and cleft palate
Q38-Q45	Other congenital malformations of the digestive system
Q50-Q56	Congenital malformations of genital organs
Q60-Q64	Congenital malformations of the urinary system
Q65-Q79	Congenital malformations and deformations of the musculoskeletal system
Q80-Q89	Other congenital malformations
Q90-Q99	Chromosomal abnormalities, not elsewhere classified

CONGENITAL MALFORMATIONS OF THE NERVOUS SYSTEM (Q00-Q07)

Q00   Anencephaly and similar malformations

Q00.0 Anencephaly
Acephaly
Acrania
Amyelencephaly
Hemianencephaly
Hemicephaly

Q00.1 Craniorachischisis

Q00.2 Iniencephaly

Q01   Encephalocele

Includes: Arnold-Chiari syndrome, type III
encephalocystocele
encephalomyelocele
hydroencephalocele
hydromeningocele, cranial

meningocele, cerebral
meningoencephalocele

Excludes 1: Meckel-Gruber syndrome (Q61.9)

Q01.0 Frontal encephalocele

Q01.1 Nasofrontal encephalocele

Q01.2 Occipital encephalocele

Q01.8 Encephalocele of other sites

Q01.9 Encephalocele, unspecified

Q02   Microcephaly

Includes: hydromicrocephaly
micrencephalon

Excludes 1: Meckel-Gruber syndrome (Q61.9)

Q03   Congenital hydrocephalus

Includes: hydrocephalus in newborn

Excludes 1: Arnold-Chiari syndrome, type II (Q07.0-)
acquired hydrocephalus (G91.-)
hydrocephalus due to congenital toxoplasmosis (P37.1)
hydrocephalus with spina bifida (Q05.0-Q05.4)

Q03.0 Malformations of aqueduct of Sylvius
Anomaly of aqueduct of Sylvius
Obstruction of aqueduct of Sylvius, congenital
Stenosis of aqueduct of Sylvius

Q03.1 Atresia of foramina of Magendie and Luschka
Dandy-Walker syndrome

Q03.8 Other congenital hydrocephalus

Q03.9 Congenital hydrocephalus, unspecified

Q04   Other congenital malformations of brain

Excludes 1: cyclopia (Q87.0)
macrocephaly (Q75.3)

Q04.0 Congenital malformations of corpus callosum
Agenesis of corpus callosum

Q04.1 Arhinencephaly

Q04.2 Holoprosencephaly

Q04.3 Other reduction deformities of brain
Absence of part of brain
Agenesis of part of brain
Agyria
Aplasia of part of brain
Hydranencephaly
Hypoplasia of part of brain
Lissencephaly
Microgyria
Pachygyria
Excludes 1: congenital malformations of corpus callosum (Q04.0)

Q04.4 Septo-optic dysplasia of brain

Q04.5 Megalencephaly

Q04.6 Congenital cerebral cysts
Porencephaly
Schizencephaly

Excludes 1: acquired porencephalic cyst (G93.0)

Q04.8 Other specified congenital malformations of brain
Arnold-Chiari syndrome, type IV
Macrogyria

Q04.9 Congenital malformation of brain, unspecified
Congenital anomaly NOS of brain
Congenital deformity NOS of brain
Congenital disease or lesion NOS of brain
Multiple anomalies NOS of brain, congenital

Q05 Spina bifida

Includes: hydromeningocele (spinal)
meningocele (spinal)
meningomyelocele
myelocele
myelomeningocele
rachischisis
spina bifida (aperta)(cystica)
syringomyelocele

Use additional code for any associated paraplegia (paraparesis) (G82.2-)

Excludes 1: Arnold-Chiari syndrome, type II (Q07.0-)
spina bifida occulta (Q76.0)

Q05.0 **Cervical spina bifida with hydrocephalus**

Q05.1 **Thoracic spina bifida with hydrocephalus**
Dorsal spina bifida with hydrocephalus
Thoracolumbar spina bifida with hydrocephalus

FORWARD MAPPING SAMPLE (ICD-9-CM ➡ ICD-10-CM)

ICD-10-CM CODE & DESCRIPTION		ICD-10-CM CODE & DESCRIPTION	
740.0	Anencephalus	Q00.0	Anencephaly
740.1	Craniorachischisis	Q00.1	Craniorachischisis
740.2	Iniencephaly	Q00.2	Iniencephaly
741.00	Spina bifida unspecified region with hydrocephalus	Q05.4	Unspecified spina bifida with hydrocephalus
741.01	Spina bifida cervical region with hydrocephalus	Q05.0	Cervical spina bifida with hydrocephalus
741.02	Spina bifida dorsal (thoracic) region with hydrocephalus	Q05.1	Thoracic spina bifida with hydrocephalus
741.03	Spina bifida lumbar region with hydrocephalus	Q05.2	Lumbar spina bifida with hydrocephalus
741.90	Spina bifida unspecified region without hydrocephalus	Q05.8	Sacral spina bifida without hydrocephalus
741.91	Spina bifida cervical region without hydrocephalus	Q05.5	Cervical spina bifida without hydrocephalus
741.92	Spina bifida dorsal (thoracic) region without hydrocephalus	Q05.6	Thoracic spina bifida without hydrocephalus
741.93	Spina bifida lumbar region without hydrocephalus	Q05.7	Lumbar spina bifida without hydrocephalus
742.0	Encephalocele	Q01.9	Encephalocele unspecified
742.1	Microcephalus	Q02	Microcephaly
742.2	Congenital reduction deformities of brain	Q04.1	Arhinencephaly
742.2	Congenital reduction deformities of brain	Q04.2	Holoprosencephaly
742.2	Congenital reduction deformities of brain	Q04.3	Other reduction deformities of brain
742.3	Congenital hydrocephalus	Q03.0	Malformations of aqueduct of Sylvius
742.3	Congenital hydrocephalus	Q03.1	Atresia of foramina of Magendie and Luschka
742.3	Congenital hydrocephalus	Q03.8	Other congenital hydrocephalus
742.4	Other specified congenital anomalies of brain	Q04.5	Megalencephaly
742.4	Other specified congenital anomalies of brain	Q04.8	Other specified congenital malformations of brain

742.4	Other specified congenital anomalies of brain	Q04.6	Congenital cerebral cysts
742.51	Diastematomyelia	Q06.2	Diastematomyelia
742.53	Hydromyelia	Q06.4	Hydromyelia
742.59	Other specified congenital anomalies of spinal cord	Q06.0	Amyelia
742.59	Other specified congenital anomalies of spinal cord	Q06.1	Hypoplasia and dysplasia of spinal cord
742.59	Other specified congenital anomalies of spinal cord	Q06.3	Other congenital cauda equina malformations
742.59	Other specified congenital anomalies of spinal cord	Q06.8	Other specified congenital malformations of spinal cord
742.8	Other specified congenital anomalies of nervous system	Q07.8	Other specified congenital malformations of nervous system
742.8	Other specified congenital anomalies of nervous system	G90.1	Familial dysautonomia [Riley-Day]
742.9	Unspecified congenital anomaly of brain spinal cord and nervous system	Q07.9	Congenital malformation of nervous system unspecified
743.00	Clinical anophthalmos unspecified	Q11.1	Other anophthalmos
743.03	Cystic eyeball congenital	Q11.0	Cystic eyeball
743.06	Cryptophthalmos	Q11.2	Microphthalmos
743.10	Microphthalmos unspecified	Q11.2	Microphthalmos
743.11	Simple microphthalmos	Q11.2	Microphthalmos
743.12	Microphthalmos associated with other anomalies of eye and adnexa	Q11.2	Microphthalmos
743.20	Buphthalmos unspecified	Q15.0	Congenital glaucoma
743.21	Simple buphthalmos	Q15.0	Congenital glaucoma
743.22	Buphthalmos associated with other ocular anomalies	Q15.0	Congenital glaucoma

BACKWARD MAPPING SAMPLE (ICD-10-CM ➡ ICD-9-CM)			
ICD-10-CM CODE & DESCRIPTION		**ICD-10-CM CODE & DESCRIPTION**	
Q00.0	Anencephaly	740.0	Anencephalus
Q00.1	Craniorachischisis	740.1	Craniorachischisis
Q00.2	Iniencephaly	740.2	Iniencephaly
Q01.0	Frontal encephalocele	742.0	Encephalocele
Q01.1	Nasofrontal encephalocele	742.0	Encephalocele
Q01.2	Occipital encephalocele	742.0	Encephalocele
Q01.8	Encephalocele of other sites	742.0	Encephalocele
Q01.9	Encephalocele unspecified	742.0	Encephalocele
Q02	Microcephaly	742.1	Microcephalus

Q03.0	Malformations of aqueduct of Sylvius	742.3	Congenital hydrocephalus
Q03.1	Atresia of foramina of Magendie and Luschka	742.3	Congenital hydrocephalus
Q03.8	Other congenital hydrocephalus	742.3	Congenital hydrocephalus
Q03.9	Congenital hydrocephalus unspecified	742.3	Congenital hydrocephalus
Q04.0	Congenital malformations of corpus callosum	742.2	Congenital reduction deformities of brain
Q04.1	Arhinencephaly	742.2	Congenital reduction deformities of brain
Q04.2	Holoprosencephaly	742.2	Congenital reduction deformities of brain
Q04.3	Other reduction deformities of brain	742.2	Congenital reduction deformities of brain
Q04.4	Septo-optic dysplasia of brain	742.4	Other specified congenital anomalies of brain
Q04.5	Megalencephaly	742.4	Other specified congenital anomalies of brain
Q04.6	Congenital cerebral cysts	742.4	Other specified congenital anomalies of brain
Q04.8	Other specified congenital malformations of brain	742.4	Other specified congenital anomalies of brain
Q04.9	Congenital malformation of brain unspecified	742.4	Other specified congenital anomalies of brain
Q05.0	Cervical spina bifida with hydrocephalus	741.01	Spina bifida cervical region with hydrocephalus
Q05.1	Thoracic spina bifida with hydrocephalus	741.02	Spina bifida dorsal (thoracic) region with hydrocephalus
Q05.2	Lumbar spina bifida with hydrocephalus	741.03	Spina bifida lumbar region with hydrocephalus
Q05.3	Sacral spina bifida with hydrocephalus	741.03	Spina bifida lumbar region with hydrocephalus
Q05.4	Unspecified spina bifida with hydrocephalus	741.00	Spina bifida unspecified region with hydrocephalus
Q05.5	Cervical spina bifida without hydrocephalus	741.91	Spina bifida cervical region without hydrocephalus
Q05.6	Thoracic spina bifida without hydrocephalus	741.92	Spina bifida dorsal (thoracic) region without hydrocephalus
Q05.7	Lumbar spina bifida without hydrocephalus	741.93	Spina bifida lumbar region without hydrocephalus
Q05.8	Sacral spina bifida without hydrocephalus	741.90	Spina bifida unspecified region without hydrocephalus

Q05.9	Spina bifida unspecified	741.90	Spina bifida unspecified region without hydrocephalus
Q06.0	Amyelia	742.59	Other specified congenital anomalies of spinal cord
Q06.1	Hypoplasia and dysplasia of spinal cord	742.59	Other specified congenital anomalies of spinal cord
Q06.2	Diastematomyelia	742.51	Diastematomyelia
Q06.3	Other congenital cauda equina malformations	742.59	Other specified congenital anomalies of spinal cord
Q06.4	Hydromyelia	742.53	Hydromyelia
Q06.8	Other specified congenital malformations of spinal cord	742.59	Other specified congenital anomalies of spinal cord
Q06.9	Congenital malformation of spinal cord unspecified	742.59	Other specified congenital anomalies of spinal cord
Q07.00	Arnold-Chiari syndrome without spina bifida or hydrocephalus	741.90	Spina bifida unspecified region without hydrocephalus

CHAPTER 18: SYMPTOMS, SIGNS, AND ABNORMAL CLINICAL AND LABORATORY FINDINGS, NOT ELSEWHERE CLASSIFIED (R00-R99)

GENERAL GUIDELINES

Chapter 18 includes symptoms, signs, abnormal results of clinical or other investigative procedures, and ill-defined conditions regarding which no diagnosis classifiable elsewhere is recorded. Signs and symptoms that point to a specific diagnosis have been assigned to a category in other chapters of the classification.

USE OF SYMPTOM CODES

Codes that describe symptoms and signs are acceptable for reporting purposes when a related definitive diagnosis has not been established (confirmed) by the provider.

USE OF A SYMPTOM CODE WITH A DEFINITIVE DIAGNOSIS CODE

Codes for signs and symptoms may be reported in addition to a related definitive diagnosis when the sign or symptom is not routinely associated with that diagnosis, such as the various signs and symptoms associated with complex syndromes. The definitive diagnosis code should be sequenced before the symptom code.

Signs or symptoms that are associated routinely with a disease process should not be assigned as additional codes, unless otherwise instructed by the classification.

COMBINATION CODES THAT INCLUDE SYMPTOMS

ICD-10-CM contains a number of combination codes that identify both the definitive diagnosis and common symptoms of that diagnosis. When using one of these combination codes, an additional code should not be assigned for the symptom.

REPEATED FALLS

Code R29.6, Repeated falls, is for use for encounters when a patient has recently fallen and the reason for the fall is being investigated.

Code Z91.81, History of falling, is for use when a patient has fallen in the past and is at risk for future falls. When appropriate, both codes R29.6 and Z91.81 may be assigned together.

COMA SCALE

The coma scale codes (R40.2-) can be used in conjunction with traumatic brain injury codes, acute cerebrovascular disease or sequelae of cerebrovascular disease codes. These codes are primarily for use by trauma registries, but they may be used in any setting where this information is collected. The coma scale codes should be sequenced after the diagnosis code(s).

These codes, one from each subcategory, are needed to complete the scale. The 7th character indicates when the scale was recorded. The 7th character should match for all three codes.

At a minimum, report the initial score documented on presentation at your facility. This may be a score from the emergency medicine technician (EMT) or in the emergency department. If desired, a facility may choose to capture multiple Glasgow coma scale scores.

FUNCTIONAL QUADRIPLEGIA

Functional quadriplegia (code R53.2) is the lack of ability to use one's limbs or to ambulate due to extreme debility. It is not associated with neurologic deficit or injury, and code R53.2 should not be used for cases of neurologic quadriplegia. It should only be assigned if functional quadriplegia is specifically documented in the medical record.

SIRS DUE TO NON-INFECTIOUS PROCESS

The systemic inflammatory response syndrome (SIRS) can develop as a result of certain non-infectious disease processes, such as trauma, malignant neoplasm, or pancreatitis. When SIRS is documented with a noninfectious condition, and no subsequent infection is documented, the code for the underlying condition, such as an injury, should be assigned, followed by code R65.10, Systemic inflammatory response syndrome (SIRS) of non-infectious origin without acute organ dysfunction, or code R65.11, Systemic inflammatory response syndrome (SIRS) of non-infectious origin with acute organ dysfunction. If an associated acute organ dysfunction is documented, the appropriate code(s) for the specific type of organ dysfunction(s) should be assigned in addition to code R65.11. If acute organ dysfunction is documented, but it cannot be determined if the acute organ dysfunction is associated with SIRS or due to another condition (e.g., directly due to the trauma), the provider should be queried.

DEATH NOS

Code R99, Ill-defined and unknown cause of mortality, is only for use in the very limited circumstance when a patient who has already died is brought into an emergency department or other healthcare facility and is pronounced dead upon arrival. It does not represent the discharge disposition of death.

SAMPLE ICD-10-CM CODES FROM THIS CHAPTER

Note: This chapter includes symptoms, signs, abnormal results of clinical or other investigative procedures, and ill-defined conditions regarding which no diagnosis classifiable elsewhere is recorded.

Signs and symptoms that point rather definitely to a given diagnosis have been assigned to a category in other chapters of the classification. In general, categories in this chapter include the less well-defined conditions and symptoms that, without the necessary study of the case to establish a final diagnosis, point perhaps equally to two or more diseases or to two or more systems of the body. Practically all categories in the chapter could be designated 'not otherwise specified', 'unknown etiology' or 'transient'. The Alphabetical Index should be consulted to determine which symptoms and signs are to be allocated here and which to other chapters. The residual subcategories, numbered .8, are generally provided for other relevant symptoms that cannot be allocated elsewhere in the classification.

The conditions and signs or symptoms included in categories R00-R94 consist of: (a) cases for which no more specific diagnosis can be made even after all the facts bearing on the case have been investigated: (b) signs or symptoms existing at the time of initial encounter that proved to be transient and whose causes could not be determined; (c) provisional diagnosis in a patient who failed to return for further investigation or care;(d) cases referred elsewhere for investigation or treatment before the diagnosis was made; (e) cases in which a more precise diagnosis was not available for any other reason; (f) certain symptoms, for which supplementary information is provided, that represent important problems in medical care in their own right.

Excludes 2: abnormal findings on antenatal screening of mother (O28.-)
certain conditions originating in the perinatal period (P04-P96)
signs and symptoms classified in the body system chapters
signs and symptoms of breast (N63, N64.5)

This chapter contains the following blocks:	
R00-R09	Symptoms and signs involving the circulatory and respiratory systems
R10-R19	Symptoms and signs involving the digestive system and abdomen
R20-R23	Symptoms and signs involving the skin and subcutaneous tissue
R25-R29	Symptoms and signs involving the nervous and musculoskeletal systems
R30-R39	Symptoms and signs involving the genitourinary system
R40-R46	Symptoms and signs involving cognition, perception, emotional state and behavior
R47-R49	Symptoms and signs involving speech and voice
R50-R69	General symptoms and signs
R70-R79	Abnormal findings on examination of blood, without diagnosis

R80-R82	Abnormal findings on examination of urine, without diagnosis
R83-R89	Abnormal findings on examination of other body fluids, substances and tissues, without diagnosis
R90-R94	Abnormal findings on diagnostic imaging and in function studies, without diagnosis
R97	Abnormal tumor markers
R99	Ill-defined and unknown cause of mortality

SYMPTOMS AND SIGNS INVOLVING THE CIRCULATORY AND RESPIRATORY SYSTEMS (R00-R09)

R00 **Abnormalities of heart beat**

Excludes 1: abnormalities originating in the perinatal period (P29.1)
specified arrhythmias (I47-I49)

R00.0 **Tachycardia, unspecified**
Rapid heart beat
Sinoauricular tachycardia NOS
Sinus [sinusal] tachycardia NOS

Excludes 1: neonatal tachycardia (P29.11)
paroxysmal tachycardia (I47.-)

R00.1 **Bradycardia, unspecified**
Sinoatrial bradycardia
Sinus bradycardia
Slow heart beat
Vagal bradycardia

Excludes 1: neonatal bradycardia (P29.12)

R00.2 **Palpitations**
Awareness of heart beat

R00.8 **Other abnormalities of heart beat**

R00.9 **Unspecified abnormalities of heart beat**

R01 **Cardiac murmurs and other cardiac sounds**

Excludes 1: cardiac murmurs and sounds originating in the perinatal period (P29.8)

R01.0 **Benign and innocent cardiac murmurs**
Functional cardiac murmur

R01.1 **Cardiac murmur, unspecified**
Cardiac bruit NOS
Heart murmur NOS

R01.2 **Other cardiac sounds**

Cardiac dullness, increased or decreased
Precordial friction

R03   Abnormal blood-pressure reading, without diagnosis

R03.0 Elevated blood-pressure reading, without diagnosis of hypertension
Note: This category is to be used to record an episode of elevated blood pressure in a patient in whom no formal diagnosis of hypertension has been made, or as an isolated incidental finding.

R03.1 Nonspecific low blood-pressure reading

Excludes 1: hypotension (I95.-)
         maternal hypotension syndrome (O26.5-)
         neurogenic orthostatic hypotension (G90.3)

R04   Hemorrhage from respiratory passages

R04.0 Epistaxis
Hemorrhage from nose
Nosebleed

R04.1 Hemorrhage from throat

Excludes 2: hemoptysis (R04.2)

R04.2 Hemoptysis
Blood-stained sputum
Cough with hemorrhage

R04.8 Hemorrhage from other sites in respiratory passages

R04.81   Acute idiopathic pulmonary hemorrhage in infants
AIPHI
Acute idiopathic hemorrhage in infants over 28 days old

Excludes 1: perinatal pulmonary hemorrhage (P26.-)
         von Willebrand's disease (D68.0)

R04.89   Hemorrhage from other sites in respiratory passages
Pulmonary hemorrhage NOS

R04.9 Hemorrhage from respiratory passages, unspecified

R05   Cough

Excludes 1: cough with hemorrhage (R04.2)
    smoker's cough (J41.0)

R06   Abnormalities of breathing

Excludes 1: acute respiratory distress syndrome (J80)
  respiratory arrest (R09.2)
  respiratory arrest of newborn (P28.81)
  respiratory distress syndrome of newborn (P22.-)
  respiratory failure (J96.-)
  respiratory failure of newborn (P28.5)

R06.0 Dyspnea

Excludes 1: tachypnea NOS (R06.82)
  transient tachypnea of newborn (P22.1)

R06.00	**Dyspnea, unspecified**
R06.01	**Orthopnea**
R06.02	**Shortness of breath**
R06.09	**Other forms of dyspnea**

R06.1 Stridor

Excludes 1: congenital laryngeal stridor (P28.89)
  laryngismus (stridulus) (J38.5)

R06.2 Wheezing

Excludes 1: Asthma (J45.-)

R06.3 Periodic breathing
Cheyne-Stokes breathing

R06.4 Hyperventilation

Excludes 1: psychogenic hyperventilation (F45.8)

R06.5 Mouth breathing

Excludes 2: dry mouth NOS (R68.2)

R06.6 Hiccough

Excludes 1: psychogenic hiccough (F45.8)

R06.7 Sneezing

R06.8 Other abnormalities of breathing

R06.81 Apnea, not elsewhere classified
Apnea NOS
Excludes 1: apnea (of) newborn (P28.4)
  sleep apnea (G47.3-)
  sleep apnea of newborn (primary) (P28.3)

R06.82 Tachypnea, not elsewhere classified
Tachypnea NOS
Excludes 1: transitory tachypnea of newborn (P22.1)

R06.83 **Snoring**

R06.89 **Other abnormalities of breathing**
Breath-holding (spells)
Sighing

R06.9 **Unspecified abnormalities of breathing**

R07 **Pain in throat and chest**

Excludes 1: epidemic myalgia (B33.0)

Excludes 2: jaw pain R68.84
pain in breast (N64.4)

R07.0 **Pain in throat**

Excludes 1: chronic sore throat (J31.2)
sore throat (acute) NOS (J02.9)

Excludes 2: dysphagia (R13.1-)

FORWARD MAPPING SAMPLE (ICD-9-CM ➡ ICD-10-CM)			
ICD-9-CM CODE & DESCRIPTION		**ICD-10-CM CODE & DESCRIPTION**	
785.0	Tachycardia unspecified	R00.0	Tachycardia unspecified
785.1	Palpitations	R00.2	Palpitations
785.2	Undiagnosed cardiac murmurs	R01.1	Cardiac murmur unspecified
785.3	Other abnormal heart sounds	R01.2	Other cardiac sounds
785.4	Gangrene	I96	Gangrene not elsewhere classified
785.50	Shock unspecified	R57.9	Shock unspecified
785.51	Cardiogenic shock	R57.0	Cardiogenic shock
785.52	Septic shock	R65.21	Severe sepsis with septic shock
785.59	Other shock without trauma	R57.1	Hypovolemic shock
785.59	Other shock without trauma	R57.8	Other shock
785.6	Enlargement of lymph nodes	R59.1	Generalized enlarged lymph nodes
785.9	Other symptoms involving cardiovascular system	R09.89	Other specified symptoms and signs involving the circulatory and respiratory systems
786.00	Respiratory abnormality unspecified	R06.9	Unspecified abnormalities of breathing
786.01	Hyperventilation	R06.4	Hyperventilation
786.02	Orthopnea	R06.01	Orthopnea
786.03	Apnea	R06.81	Apnea not elsewhere classified
786.04	Cheyne-stokes respiration	R06.3	Periodic breathing
786.05	Shortness of breath	R06.02	Shortness of breath
786.06	Tachypnea	R06.82	Tachypnea not elsewhere classified

786.07	Wheezing	R06.2	Wheezing
786.09	Respiratory abnormality other	R06.09	Other forms of dyspnea
786.09	Respiratory abnormality other	R06.89	Other abnormalities of breathing
786.09	Respiratory abnormality other	R06.00	Dyspnea unspecified
786.1	Stridor	R06.1	Stridor
786.2	Cough	R05	Cough
786.3	Hemoptysis	R04.2	Hemoptysis
786.3	Hemoptysis	R04.8	Hemorrhage from other sites in respiratory passages
786.4	Abnormal sputum	R09.3	Abnormal sputum
786.50	Unspecified chest pain	R07.9	Chest pain unspecified
786.51	Precordial pain	R07.2	Precordial pain
786.52	Painful respiration	R07.1	Chest pain on breathing
786.59	Other chest pain	R07.89	Other chest pain
786.6	Swelling mass or lump in chest	R22.2	Localized swelling mass and lump trunk
786.7	Abnormal chest sounds	R09.89	Other specified symptoms and signs involving the circulatory and respiratory systems
786.8	Hiccough	R06.6	Hiccough
786.9	Other symptoms involving respiratory system and chest	R06.89	Other abnormalities of breathing
787.01	Nausea with vomiting	R11.2	Nausea with vomiting unspecified
787.02	Nausea alone	R11.0	Nausea
787.03	Vomiting alone	R11.12	Projectile vomiting
787.03	Vomiting alone	R11.11	Vomiting without nausea

BACKWARD MAPPING SAMPLE (ICD-10-CM ➡ ICD-9-CM)			
ICD-9-CM CODE & DESCRIPTION		**ICD-10-CM CODE & DESCRIPTION**	
R00.0	Tachycardia unspecified	785.0	Tachycardia unspecified
R00.1	Bradycardia unspecified	427.89	Other specified cardiac dysrhythmias
R00.2	Palpitations	785.1	Palpitations
R00.8	Other abnormalities of heart beat	785.3	Other abnormal heart sounds
R00.9	Unspecified abnormalities of heart beat	785.3	Other abnormal heart sounds
R01.0	Benign and innocent cardiac murmurs	785.2	Undiagnosed cardiac murmurs
R01.1	Cardiac murmur unspecified	785.2	Undiagnosed cardiac murmurs
R01.2	Other cardiac sounds	785.3	Other abnormal heart sounds
R03.0	Elevated blood-pressure reading without diagnosis of hypertension	796.2	Elevated blood pressure reading without diagnosis of hypertension

R03.1	Nonspecific low blood-pressure reading	796.3	Nonspecific low blood pressure reading
R04.0	Epistaxis	784.7	Epistaxis
R04.1	Hemorrhage from throat	784.8	Hemorrhage from throat
R04.2	Hemoptysis	786.3	Hemoptysis
R04.8	Hemorrhage from other sites in respiratory passages	786.3	Hemoptysis
R04.9	Hemorrhage from respiratory passages unspecified	786.3	Hemoptysis
R05	Cough	786.2	Cough
R06.00	Dyspnea unspecified	786.09	Respiratory abnormality other
R06.01	Orthopnea	786.02	Orthopnea
R06.02	Shortness of breath	786.05	Shortness of breath
R06.09	Other forms of dyspnea	786.09	Respiratory abnormality other
R06.1	Stridor	786.1	Stridor
R06.2	Wheezing	786.07	Wheezing
R06.3	Periodic breathing	786.04	Cheyne-stokes respiration
R06.4	Hyperventilation	786.01	Hyperventilation
R06.5	Mouth breathing	784.99	Other symptoms involving head and neck
R06.6	Hiccough	786.8	Hiccough
R06.7	Sneezing	784.99	Other symptoms involving head and neck
R06.81	Apnea not elsewhere classified	786.03	Apnea
R06.82	Tachypnea not elsewhere classified	786.06	Tachypnea
R06.83	Snoring	784.99	Other symptoms involving head and neck
R06.89	Other abnormalities of breathing	784.99	Other symptoms involving head and neck
R06.89	Other abnormalities of breathing	786.09	Respiratory abnormality other
R06.89	Other abnormalities of breathing	786.9	Other symptoms involving respiratory system and chest
R06.9	Unspecified abnormalities of breathing	786.00	Respiratory abnormality unspecified
R07.0	Pain in throat	784.1	Throat pain
R07.1	Chest pain on breathing	786.52	Painful respiration
R07.2	Precordial pain	786.51	Precordial pain
R07.81	Pleurodynia	786.59	Other chest pain
R07.82	Intercostal pain	786.59	Other chest pain
R07.89	Other chest pain	786.59	Other chest pain

CHAPTER 19: INJURY, POISONING, AND CERTAIN OTHER CONSEQUENCES OF EXTERNAL CAUSES (S00-T88)

GENERAL GUIDELINES

CODE EXTENSIONS

Most categories in chapter 19 have 7th character extensions that are required for each applicable code. Most categories in this chapter have three extensions (with the exception of fractures): A, initial encounter, D, subsequent encounter and S, sequela.

Extension "A", initial encounter is used while the patient is receiving active treatment for the injury. Examples of active treatment are: surgical treatment, emergency department encounter, and evaluation and treatment by a new physician.

Extension "D" subsequent encounter is used for encounters after the patient has received active treatment of the injury and is receiving routine care for the injury during the healing or recovery phase. Examples of subsequent care are: cast change or removal, removal of external **or** internal fixation device, medication adjustment, other aftercare and follow up visits following injury treatment.

The aftercare Z codes should not be used for aftercare for injuries. For aftercare of an injury, assign the acute injury code with the 7th character "D" (subsequent encounter).

Extension "S", sequela, is for use for complications or conditions that arise as a direct result of an injury, such as scar formation after a burn. The scars are sequelae of the burn. When using extension "S", it is necessary to use both the injury code that precipitated the sequela and the code for the sequela itself. The "S" is added only to the injury code, not the sequela code. The "S" extension identifies the injury responsible for the sequela. The specific type of sequela (e.g. scar) is sequenced first, followed by the injury code.

CODING OF INJURIES

When coding injuries, assign separate codes for each injury unless a combination code is provided, in which case the combination code is assigned. Code T07, Unspecified multiple injuries should not be assigned unless information for a more specific code is not available. Traumatic injury codes (S00-T14.9) are not to be used for normal, healing surgical wounds or to identify complications of surgical wounds.

The code for the most serious injury, as determined by the provider and the focus of treatment, is sequenced first.

1) **Superficial injuries**

   Superficial injuries such as abrasions or contusions are not coded when associated with more severe injuries of the same site.

2) **Primary injury with damage to nerves/blood vessels**

   When a primary injury results in minor damage to peripheral nerves or blood vessels, the primary injury is sequenced first with additional code(s) for injuries to nerves and spinal cord (such as category S04), and/or injury to blood vessels (such as category S15). When the primary injury is to the blood vessels or nerves, that injury should be sequenced first.

CODING OF TRAUMATIC FRACTURES

The principles of multiple coding of injuries should be followed in coding fractures. Fractures of specified sites are coded individually by site in accordance with both the provisions within categories S02, S12, S22, S32, S42, S49, S52, S59, S62, S72, S79, S82, S89, S92 and the level of detail furnished by medical record content.

A fracture not indicated as open or closed should be coded to closed. A fracture not indicated whether displaced or not displaced should be coded to displaced.

More specific guidelines are as follows:

1) Initial vs. Subsequent Encounter for Fractures

Traumatic fractures are coded using the appropriate 7th character extension for initial encounter (A, B, C) while the patient is receiving active treatment for the fracture. Examples of active treatment are: surgical treatment, emergency department encounter, and evaluation and treatment by a new physician. The appropriate 7th character for initial encounter should also be assigned for a patient who delayed seeking treatment for the fracture or nonunion.

Fractures are coded using the appropriate 7th character extension for subsequent care for encounters after the patient has completed active treatment of the fracture and is receiving routine care for the fracture during the healing or recovery phase. Examples of fracture aftercare are: cast change or removal, removal of external or internal fixation device, medication adjustment, and follow-up visits following fracture treatment.

Care for complications of surgical treatment for fracture repairs during the healing or recovery phase should be coded with the appropriate complication codes.

Care of complications of fractures, such as malunion and nonunion, should be reported with the appropriate 7th character extensions for subsequent care with nonunion (K, M, N,) or subsequent care with malunion (P, Q, R).

A code from category M80, not a traumatic fracture code, should be used for any patient with known osteoporosis who suffers a fracture, even if the patient had a minor fall or trauma, if that fall or trauma would not usually break a normal, healthy bone.
The aftercare Z codes should not be used for aftercare for traumatic fractures. For aftercare of a traumatic fracture, assign the acute fracture code with the appropriate 7th character.

2) Multiple fractures sequencing

Multiple fractures are sequenced in accordance with the severity of the fracture.

CODING OF BURNS AND CORROSIONS

The ICD-10-CM makes a distinction between burns and corrosions. The burn codes are for thermal burns, except sunburns, that come from a heat source, such as a fire or hot appliance. The burn codes are also for burns resulting from electricity and radiation. Corrosions are burns due to chemicals. The guidelines are the same for burns and corrosions.

Current burns (T20-T25) are classified by depth, extent and by agent (X code). Burns are classified by depth as first degree (erythema), second degree (blistering), and third degree (full-thickness involvement). Burns of the eye and internal organs (T26-T28) are classified by site, but not by degree.

1) **Sequencing of burn and related condition codes**

Sequence first the code that reflects the highest degree of burn when more than one burn is present.

(a) When the reason for the admission or encounter is for treatment of external multiple burns, sequence first the code that reflects the burn of the highest degree.

(b) When a patient has both internal and external burns, the circumstances of admission govern the selection of the principal diagnosis or first-listed diagnosis.

(c) When a patient is admitted for burn injuries and other related conditions such as smoke inhalation and/or respiratory failure, the circumstances of admission govern the selection of the principal or first-listed diagnosis.

2) **Burns of the same local site**

Classify burns of the same local site (three-character category level, T20-T28) but of different degrees to the subcategory identifying the highest degree recorded in the diagnosis.

3) **Non-healing burns**

Non-healing burns are coded as acute burns.

Necrosis of burned skin should be coded as a non-healed burn.

4) **Infected Burn**

For any documented infected burn site, use an additional code for the infection.

5) **Assign separate codes for each burn site**

When coding burns, assign separate codes for each burn site. Category T30, Burn and corrosion, body region unspecified is extremely vague and should rarely be used.

6) **Burns and Corrosions Classified According to Extent of Body Surface Involved**

Assign codes from category T31, Burns classified according to extent of body surface involved, or T32, Corrosions classified according to extent of body surface involved, when the site of the burn is not specified or when there is a need for additional data. It is advisable to use category T31 as additional coding when needed to provide data for evaluating burn mortality, such as that needed by burn units. It is also advisable to use category T31 as an additional code for reporting purposes when there is mention of a third-degree burn involving 20 percent or more of the body surface.

Categories T31 and T32 are based on the classic "rule of nines" in estimating body surface involved: head and neck are assigned nine percent, each arm nine percent, each leg 18 percent, the anterior trunk 18 percent, posterior trunk 18 percent, and genitalia one percent. Providers may change these percentage assignments where necessary to accommodate infants and children who have proportionately larger heads than adults, and patients who have large buttocks, thighs, or abdomen that involve burns.

7) Encounters for treatment of late effects of burns

Encounters for the treatment of the late effects of burns or corrosions (i.e., scars or joint contractures) should be coded with a burn or corrosion code with the 7th character "S" for sequela.

8) Sequelae with a late effect code and current burn

When appropriate, both a code for a current burn or corrosion with 7th character extension "A" or "D" and a burn or corrosion code with extension "S" may be assigned on the same record (when both a current burn and sequelae of an old burn exist). Burns and corrosions do not heal at the same rate and a current healing wound may still exist with sequela of a healed burn or corrosion.

9) Use of an external cause code with burns and corrosions

An external cause code should be used with burns and corrosions to identify the source and intent of the burn, as well as the place where it occurred.

ADVERSE EFFECTS, POISONING, UNDERDOSING AND TOXIC EFFECTS

Codes in categories T36-T65 are combination codes that include the substances related to adverse effects, poisonings, toxic effects and underdosing, as well as the external cause. No additional external cause code is required for poisonings, toxic effects, adverse effects and underdosing codes.

A code from categories T36-T65 is sequenced first, followed by the code(s) that specify the nature of the adverse effect, poisoning, or toxic effect. Note: This sequencing instruction does not apply to underdosing codes (fifth or sixth character "6", for example T36.0x6-).

1) Do not code directly from the Table of Drugs

Do not code directly from the Table of Drugs and Chemicals. Always refer back to the Tabular List.

2) Use as many codes as necessary to describe

Use as many codes as necessary to describe completely all drugs, medicinal or biological substances.

3) If the same code would describe the causative agent

If the same code would describe the causative agent for more than one adverse reaction, poisoning, toxic effect or underdosing, assign the code only once.

4) If two or more drugs, medicinal or biological substances

If two or more drugs, medicinal or biological substances are reported, code each individually unless **a** combination code is listed in the Table of Drugs and Chemicals.

5) The occurrence of drug toxicity is classified in ICD-10- CM as follows:

(a) Adverse Effect

Assign the appropriate code for adverse effect (for example, T36.0x5-) when the drug was correctly prescribed and properly administered. Use additional code(s) for all manifestations of adverse effects. Examples of manifestations are tachycardia, delirium, gastrointestinal hemorrhaging, vomiting, hypokalemia, hepatitis, renal failure, or respiratory failure.

(b) Poisoning

When coding a poisoning or reaction to the improper use of a medication (e.g., overdose, wrong substance given or taken in error, wrong route of administration), assign the appropriate code from categories T36-T50. Poisoning codes have an associated intent: accidental, intentional self-harm, assault and undetermined. Use additional code(s) for all manifestations of poisonings.

If there is also a diagnosis of abuse or dependence on the substance, the abuse or dependence is coded as an additional code.

Examples of poisoning include:

(i) Error was made in drug prescription Errors made in drug prescription or in the administration of the drug by provider, nurse, patient, or other person.

(ii) Overdose of a drug intentionally taken

If an overdose of a drug was intentionally taken or administered and resulted in drug toxicity, it would be coded as a poisoning.

(iii) Nonprescribed drug taken with correctly prescribed and properly administered drug
If a nonprescribed drug or medicinal agent was taken in combination with a correctly prescribed and properly administered drug, any drug toxicity or other reaction resulting from the interaction of the two drugs would be classified as a poisoning.

(iv) Interaction of drug(s) and alcohol

When a reaction results from the interaction of a drug(s) and alcohol, this would be classified as poisoning.

(c) Underdosing

Underdosing refers to taking less of a medication than is prescribed by a provider or a manufacturer's instruction. For underdosing, assign the code from categories T36-T50 (fifth or sixth character "6").

Codes for underdosing should never be assigned as principal or first-listed codes. If a patient has a relapse or exacerbation of the medical condition for which the drug is prescribed because of the reduction in dose, then the medical condition itself should be coded.

Noncompliance (Z91.12-, Z91.13-) or complication of care (Y63.61, Y63.8-Y63.9) codes are to be used with an underdosing code to indicate intent, if known.

(d) Toxic Effects

When a harmful substance is ingested or comes in contact with a person, this is classified as a toxic effect. The toxic effect codes are in categories T51-T65.

Toxic effect codes have an associated intent: accidental, intentional self-harm, assault and undetermined.

ADULT AND CHILD ABUSE, NEGLECT AND OTHER MALTREATMENT

Sequence first the appropriate code from categories T74.- (Adult and child abuse, neglect and other maltreatment, confirmed) or T76 - (Adult and child abuse, neglect and other maltreatment, suspected) for abuse, neglect and other maltreatment, followed by any accompanying mental health or injury code(s).

If the documentation in the medical record states abuse or neglect it is coded as confirmed (T74.-). It is coded as suspected if it is documented as suspected (T76.-).

For cases of confirmed abuse or neglect an external cause code from the assault section (X92-Y08) should be added to identify the cause of any physical injuries. A perpetrator code (Y07) should be added when the perpetrator of the abuse is known. For suspected cases of abuse or neglect, do not report external cause or perpetrator code.

If a suspected case of abuse, neglect or mistreatment is ruled out during an encounter code Z04.71, Suspected adult physical and sexual abuse, ruled out, or code Z04.72, Suspected child physical and sexual abuse, ruled out, should be used, not a code from T76.

COMPLICATIONS OF CARE

1) **Complications of care**

(a) Documentation of complications of care

As with all procedural or postprocedural complications, code assignment is based on the provider's documentation of the relationship between the condition and the procedure.

2) Pain due to medical devices

Pain associated with devices, implants or grafts left in a surgical site (for example painful hip prosthesis) is assigned to the appropriate code(s) found in Chapter 19, Injury, poisoning, and certain other consequences of external causes. Specific codes for pain due to medical devices are found in the T code section of the ICD-10-CM. Use additional code(s) from category G89 to identify acute or chronic pain due to presence of the device, implant or graft (G89.18 or G89.28).

3) Transplant complications

(a) Transplant complications other than kidney
Codes under category T86, Complications of transplanted organs and tissues, are for use for both complications and rejection of transplanted organs. A transplant complication code is only assigned if the complication affects the function of the transplanted organ. Two codes are required to fully describe a transplant complication: the appropriate code from category T86 and a secondary code that identifies the complication.

Pre-existing conditions or conditions that develop after the transplant are not coded as complications unless they affect the function of the transplanted organs.

See I.C.21.c.3 for transplant organ removal status See I.C.2.r for malignant neoplasm associated with transplanted organ.

(b) Chronic kidney disease and kidney transplant complications

Patients who have undergone kidney transplant may still have some form of chronic kidney disease (CKD) because the kidney transplant may not fully restore kidney function. Code T86.1- should be assigned for documented complications of a kidney transplant, such as transplant failure or rejection or other transplant complication. Code T86.1- should not be assigned for post kidney transplant patients who have chronic kidney (CKD) unless a transplant complication such as transplant failure or rejection is documented. If the documentation is unclear as to whether the patient has a complication of the transplant, query the provider.

For patients with CKD following a kidney transplant, but who do not have a complication such as failure or rejection, *see section I.C.14. Chronic kidney disease and kidney transplant status.*

4) Complication codes that include the external cause

As with certain other T codes, some of the complications of care codes have the external cause included in the code. The code includes the nature of the complication as well as the type of procedure that caused the complication. No external cause code indicating the type of procedure is necessary for these codes.

5) Complications of care codes within the body system chapters

Intraoperative and postprocedural complication codes are found within the body system chapters with codes specific to the organs and structures of that body system. These codes should be sequenced first, followed by a code(s) for the specific complication, if applicable.

SAMPLES ICD-10-CM CODES FROM THIS CHAPTER

Use additional code to identify any retained foreign body, if applicable (Z18.-)

Excludes 1: birth trauma (P10-P15)
          obstetric trauma (O70-O71)

This chapter contains the following blocks:	
S00-S09	Injuries to the head
S10-S19	Injuries to the neck
S20-S29	Injuries to the thorax
S30-S39	Injuries to the abdomen, lower back, lumbar spine, pelvis and external genitals
S40-S49	Injuries to the shoulder and upper arm
S50-S59	Injuries to the elbow and forearm
S60-S69	Injuries to the wrist, hand and fingers
S70-S79	Injuries to the hip and thigh
S80-S89	Injuries to the knee and lower leg
S90-S99	Injuries to the ankle and foot
T07	Injuries involving multiple body regions
T14	Injury of unspecified body region
T15-T19	Effects of foreign body entering through natural orifice
T20-T25	Burns and corrosions of external body surface, specified by site
T26-T28	Burns and corrosions confined to eye and internal organs
T30-T32	Burns and corrosions of multiple and unspecified body regions
T33-T34	Frostbite
T36-T50	Poisoning by, adverse effects of and underdosing of drugs, medicaments and biological substances
T51-T65	Toxic effects of substances chiefly nonmedicinal as to source
T66-T78	Other and unspecified effects of external causes
T79	Certain early complications of trauma
T80-T88	Complications of surgical and medical care, not elsewhere classified

Note: Use secondary code(s) from Chapter 20, External causes of morbidity, to indicate cause of injury. Codes within the T section that include the external cause do not require an additional external cause code. The chapter uses the S-section for coding different types of injuries related to single body regions and the T-section to cover injuries to unspecified body regions as well as poisoning and certain other consequences of external causes.

INJURIES TO THE HEAD (S00-S09)

Includes: injuries of ear
               injuries of eye
               injuries of face [any part]

injuries of gum
injuries of jaw
injuries of oral cavity
injuries of palate
injuries of periocular area
injuries of scalp
injuries of temporomandibular joint area
injuries of tongue
injuries of tooth

Excludes 2: burns and corrosions (T20-T32)
effects of foreign body in ear (T16)
effects of foreign body in larynx (T17.3)
effects of foreign body in mouth NOS (T18.0)
effects of foreign body in nose (T17.0-T17.1)
effects of foreign body in pharynx (T17.2)
effects of foreign body on external eye (T15.-)
frostbite (T33-T34)
insect bite or sting, venomous (T63.4)
Code also for any associated infection

S00 Superficial injury of head

Excludes 1: diffuse cerebral contusion (S06.2-)
focal cerebral contusion (S06.3-)
injury of eye and orbit (S05.-)
open wound of head (S01.-)

The appropriate 7th character is to be added to each code from category S00

A - initial encounter
D - subsequent encounter
S - sequela

S00.0 Superficial injury of scalp

S00.00 Unspecified superficial injury of scalp

S00.01 Abrasion of scalp

S00.02 Blister (nonthermal) of scalp

S00.03 Contusion of scalp
Bruise of scalp
Hematoma of scalp

S00.04 External constriction of part of scalp

S00.05 Superficial foreign body of scalp
Splinter in the scalp

S00.06   **Insect bite (nonvenomous) of scalp**

S00.07   **Other superficial bite of scalp**
Excludes 1: open bite of scalp (S01.05)

S00.1   **Contusion of eyelid and periocular area**
Black eye

Excludes 2: contusion of eyeball and orbital tissues (S05.1)

S00.10   **Contusion of unspecified eyelid and periocular area**

S00.11   **Contusion of right eyelid and periocular area**

S00.12   **Contusion of left eyelid and periocular area**

S00.2   **Other and unspecified superficial injuries of eyelid and periocular area**

Excludes 2: superficial injury of conjunctiva and cornea (S05.0-)

S00.20   **Unspecified superficial injury of eyelid and periocular area**
     S00.201   **Unspecified superficial injury of right eyelid and periocular area**

     S00.202   **Unspecified superficial injury of left eyelid and periocular area**

     S00.209   **Unspecified superficial injury of unspecified eyelid and periocular area**

S00.21   **Abrasion of eyelid and periocular area**

     S00.211   **Abrasion of right eyelid and periocular area**

     S00.212   **Abrasion of left eyelid and periocular area**

     S00.219   **Abrasion of unspecified eyelid and periocular area**

S00.22   **Blister (nonthermal) of eyelid and periocular area**

     S00.221   **Blister (nonthermal) of right eyelid and periocular area**

     S00.222   **Blister (nonthermal) of left eyelid and periocular area**

     S00.229   **Blister (nonthermal) of unspecified eyelid and periocular area**

S00.24   **External constriction of eyelid and periocular area**

     S00.241   **External constriction of right eyelid and periocular area**

> **S00.242**   **External constriction of left eyelid and periocular area**
>
> **S00.249**   **External constriction of unspecified eyelid and periocular area**

S00.25   **Superficial foreign body of eyelid and periocular area**
Splinter of eyelid and periocular area

Excludes 2: retained foreign body in eyelid (H02.81-)

> **S00.251**   **Superficial foreign body of right eyelid and periocular area**
>
> **S00.252**   **Superficial foreign body of left eyelid and periocular area**
>
> **S00.259**   **Superficial foreign body of unspecified eyelid and periocular area**

S00.26   **Insect bite (nonvenomous) of eyelid and periocular area**

> **S00.261**   **Insect bite (nonvenomous) of right eyelid and periocular area**

FORWARD MAPPING SAMPLE (ICD-9-CM ➡ ICD-10-CM)			
ICD-9-CM CODE & DESCRIPTION		**ICD-10-CM CODE & DESCRIPTION**	
805.00	Closed fracture of cervical vertebra unspecified level	S12.9xxA	Fracture of neck unspecified initial encounter
805.01	Closed fracture of first cervical vertebra	S12.000A	Unspecified displaced fracture of first cervical vertebra initial encounter for closed fracture
805.01	Closed fracture of first cervical vertebra	S12.001A	Unspecified nondisplaced fracture of first cervical vertebra initial encounter for closed fracture
805.02	Closed fracture of second cervical vertebra	S12.101A	Unspecified nondisplaced fracture of second cervical vertebra initial encounter for closed fracture
805.02	Closed fracture of second cervical vertebra	S12.100A	Unspecified displaced fracture of second cervical vertebra initial encounter for closed fracture
805.03	Closed fracture of third cervical vertebra	S12.201A	Unspecified nondisplaced fracture of third cervical vertebra initial encounter for closed fracture
805.03	Closed fracture of third cervical vertebra	S12.200A	Unspecified displaced fracture of third cervical vertebra initial encounter for closed fracture

805.04	Closed fracture of fourth cervical vertebra	S12.300A	Unspecified displaced fracture of fourth cervical vertebra initial encounter for closed fracture
805.04	Closed fracture of fourth cervical vertebra	S12.301A	Unspecified nondisplaced fracture of fourth cervical vertebra initial encounter for closed fracture
805.05	Closed fracture of fifth cervical vertebra	S12.400A	Unspecified displaced fracture of fifth cervical vertebra initial encounter for closed fracture
805.05	Closed fracture of fifth cervical vertebra	S12.401A	Unspecified nondisplaced fracture of fifth cervical vertebra initial encounter for closed fracture
805.06	Closed fracture of sixth cervical vertebra	S12.501A	Unspecified nondisplaced fracture of sixth cervical vertebra initial encounter for closed fracture
805.06	Closed fracture of sixth cervical vertebra	S12.500A	Unspecified displaced fracture of sixth cervical vertebra initial encounter for closed fracture
805.07	Closed fracture of seventh cervical vertebra	S12.600A	Unspecified displaced fracture of seventh cervical vertebra initial encounter for closed fracture
805.07	Closed fracture of seventh cervical vertebra	S12.601A	Unspecified nondisplaced fracture of seventh cervical vertebra initial encounter for closed fracture
805.08	Closed fracture of multiple cervical vertebrae	S12.9xxA	Fracture of neck unspecified initial encounter
805.10	Open fracture of cervical vertebra unspecified level	S12.9xxA	Fracture of neck unspecified initial encounter
805.11	Open fracture of first cervical vertebra	S12.000B	Unspecified displaced fracture of first cervical vertebra initial encounter for open fracture
805.11	Open fracture of first cervical vertebra	S12.001B	Unspecified nondisplaced fracture of first cervical vertebra initial encounter for open fracture
805.12	Open fracture of second cervical vertebra	S12.100B	Unspecified displaced fracture of second cervical vertebra initial encounter for open fracture
805.12	Open fracture of second cervical vertebra	S12.101B	Unspecified nondisplaced fracture of second cervical vertebra initial encounter for open fracture

805.13	Open fracture of third cervical vertebra	S12.200B	Unspecified displaced fracture of third cervical vertebra initial encounter for open fracture
805.13	Open fracture of third cervical vertebra	S12.201B	Unspecified nondisplaced fracture of third cervical vertebra initial encounter for open fracture
805.14	Open fracture of fourth cervical vertebra	S12.300B	Unspecified displaced fracture of fourth cervical vertebra initial encounter for open fracture
805.14	Open fracture of fourth cervical vertebra	S12.301B	Unspecified nondisplaced fracture of fourth cervical vertebra initial encounter for open fracture
805.15	Open fracture of fifth cervical vertebra	S12.400B	Unspecified displaced fracture of fifth cervical vertebra initial encounter for open fracture
805.15	Open fracture of fifth cervical vertebra	S12.401B	Unspecified nondisplaced fracture of fifth cervical vertebra initial encounter for open fracture
805.16	Open fracture of sixth cervical vertebra	S12.500B	Unspecified displaced fracture of sixth cervical vertebra initial encounter for open fracture
805.16	Open fracture of sixth cervical vertebra	S12.501B	Unspecified nondisplaced fracture of sixth cervical vertebra initial encounter for open fracture
805.17	Open fracture of seventh cervical vertebra	S12.600B	Unspecified displaced fracture of seventh cervical vertebra initial encounter for open fracture
805.17	Open fracture of seventh cervical vertebra	S12.601B	Unspecified nondisplaced fracture of seventh cervical vertebra initial encounter for open fracture
805.18	Open fracture of multiple cervical vertebrae	S12.9xxA	Fracture of neck unspecified initial encounter
805.2	Closed fracture of dorsal (thoracic) vertebra without spinal cord injury	S22.009A	Unspecified fracture of unspecified thoracic vertebra initial encounter for closed fracture
805.3	Open fracture of dorsal (thoracic) vertebra without spinal cord injury	S22.009B	Unspecified fracture of unspecified thoracic vertebra initial encounter for open fracture
805.4	Closed fracture of lumbar vertebra without spinal cord injury	S32.009A	Unspecified fracture of unspecified lumbar vertebra initial encounter for closed fracture

805.5	Open fracture of lumbar vertebra without spinal cord injury	S32.009B	Unspecified fracture of unspecified lumbar vertebra initial encounter for open fracture
805.6	Closed fracture of sacrum and coccyx without spinal cord injury	S32.10xA	Unspecified fracture of sacrum initial encounter for closed fracture
805.6	Closed fracture of sacrum and coccyx without spinal cord injury	S32.2xxA	Fracture of coccyx initial encounter for closed fracture
805.7	Open fracture of sacrum and coccyx without spinal cord injury	S32.10xB	Unspecified fracture of sacrum initial encounter for open fracture
805.7	Open fracture of sacrum and coccyx without spinal cord injury	S32.2xxB	Fracture of coccyx initial encounter for open fracture

BACKWARD MAPPING SAMPLE (ICD-10-CM ➡ ICD-9-CM)

ICD-9-CM CODE & DESCRIPTION		ICD-10-CM CODE & DESCRIPTION	
S22.000A	Wedge compression fracture of unspecified thoracic vertebra initial encounter for closed fracture	805.2	Closed fracture of dorsal (thoracic) vertebra without spinal cord injury
S22.000B	Wedge compression fracture of unspecified thoracic vertebra initial encounter for open fracture	805.3	Open fracture of dorsal (thoracic) vertebra without spinal cord injury
S22.000D	Wedge compression fracture of unspecified thoracic vertebra subsequent encounter for fracture with routine healing	V54.17	Aftercare for healing traumatic fracture of vertebrae
S22.000G	Wedge compression fracture of unspecified thoracic vertebra subsequent encounter for fracture with delayed healing	V54.17	Aftercare for healing traumatic fracture of vertebrae
S22.000K	Wedge compression fracture of unspecified thoracic vertebra subsequent encounter for fracture with nonunion	733.82	Nonunion of fracture
S22.000S	Wedge compression fracture of unspecified thoracic vertebra sequela	905.1	Late effect of fracture of spine and trunk without spinal cord lesion
S22.001A	Stable burst fracture of unspecified thoracic vertebra initial encounter for closed fracture	805.2	Closed fracture of dorsal (thoracic) vertebra without spinal cord injury
S22.001B	Stable burst fracture of unspecified thoracic vertebra initial encounter for open fracture	805.3	Open fracture of dorsal (thoracic) vertebra without spinal cord injury

S22.001D	Stable burst fracture of unspecified thoracic vertebra subsequent encounter for fracture with routine healing	V54.17	Aftercare for healing traumatic fracture of vertebrae
S22.001G	Stable burst fracture of unspecified thoracic vertebra subsequent encounter for fracture with delayed healing	V54.17	Aftercare for healing traumatic fracture of vertebrae
S22.001K	Stable burst fracture of unspecified thoracic vertebra subsequent encounter for fracture with nonunion	733.82	Nonunion of fracture
S22.001S	Stable burst fracture of unspecified thoracic vertebra sequela	905.1	Late effect of fracture of spine and trunk without spinal cord lesion
S22.002A	Unstable burst fracture of unspecified thoracic vertebra initial encounter for closed fracture	805.2	Closed fracture of dorsal (thoracic) vertebra without spinal cord injury
S22.002B	Unstable burst fracture of unspecified thoracic vertebra initial encounter for open fracture	805.3	Open fracture of dorsal (thoracic) vertebra without spinal cord injury
S22.002D	Unstable burst fracture of unspecified thoracic vertebra subsequent encounter for fracture with routine healing	V54.17	Aftercare for healing traumatic fracture of vertebrae
S22.002G	Unstable burst fracture of unspecified thoracic vertebra subsequent encounter for fracture with delayed healing	V54.17	Aftercare for healing traumatic fracture of vertebrae
S22.002K	Unstable burst fracture of unspecified thoracic vertebra subsequent encounter for fracture with nonunion	733.82	Nonunion of fracture
S22.002S	Unstable burst fracture of unspecified thoracic vertebra sequela	905.1	Late effect of fracture of spine and trunk without spinal cord lesion
S22.008A	Other fracture of unspecified thoracic vertebra initial encounter for closed fracture	805.2	Closed fracture of dorsal (thoracic) vertebra without spinal cord injury
S22.008B	Other fracture of unspecified thoracic vertebra initial encounter for open fracture	805.3	Open fracture of dorsal (thoracic) vertebra without spinal cord injury
T07	Unspecified multiple injuries	959.8	Other and unspecified injury to other specified sites including multiple

T14.8	Other injury of unspecified body region	959.9	Other and unspecified injury to unspecified site
T14.90	Injury unspecified	959.9	Other and unspecified injury to unspecified site
T14.91	Suicide attempt	959.9	Other and unspecified injury to unspecified site
T14.91	Suicide attempt	E95.89	Suicide and self-inflicted injury by unspecified means
T15.00xA	Foreign body in cornea unspecified eye initial encounter	930.0	Corneal foreign body
T15.00xA	Foreign body in cornea unspecified eye initial encounter	E91.4	Foreign body accidentally entering eye and adnexa
T15.00xD	Foreign body in cornea unspecified eye subsequent encounter	V58.89	Other specified aftercare
T15.00xS	Foreign body in cornea unspecified eye sequela	908.5	Late effect of foreign body in orifice
T15.01xA	Foreign body in cornea right eye initial encounter	930.0	Corneal foreign body
T15.01xA	Foreign body in cornea right eye initial encounter	E91.4	Foreign body accidentally entering eye and adnexa
T15.01xD	Foreign body in cornea right eye subsequent encounter	V58.89	Other specified aftercare
T15.01xS	Foreign body in cornea right eye sequela	908.5	Late effect of foreign body in orifice
T15.02xA	Foreign body in cornea left eye initial encounter	930.0	Corneal foreign body
T15.02xA	Foreign body in cornea left eye initial encounter	E91.4	Foreign body accidentally entering eye and adnexa
T15.02xD	Foreign body in cornea left eye subsequent encounter	V58.89	Other specified aftercare
T15.02xS	Foreign body in cornea left eye sequela	908.5	Late effect of foreign body in orifice
T15.10xA	Foreign body in conjunctival sac unspecified eye initial encounter	930.1	Foreign body in conjunctival sac
T15.10xA	Foreign body in conjunctival sac unspecified eye initial encounter	E91.4	Foreign body accidentally entering eye and adnexa
T15.10xD	Foreign body in conjunctival sac unspecified eye subsequent encounter	V58.89	Other specified aftercare

CHAPTER 20: EXTERNAL CAUSES OF MORBIDITY (V01-Y99)

GENERAL GUIDELINES

Introduction: These guidelines are provided for the reporting of external causes of morbidity codes in order that there will be standardization in the process. These codes are secondary codes for use in any health care setting.

External cause codes are intended to provide data for injury research and evaluation of injury prevention strategies. These codes capture how the injury or health condition happened (cause), the intent (unintentional or accidental; or intentional, such as suicide or assault), the place where the event occurred the activity of the patient at the time of the event, and the person's status (e.g., civilian, military).

1) **Used with any code in the range of A00.0-T88.9, Z00-Z99**

   An external cause code may be used with any code in the range of A00.0-T88.9, Z00-Z99, classification that is a health condition due to an external cause. Though they are most applicable to injuries, they are also valid for use with such things as infections or diseases due to an external source, and other health conditions, such as a heart attack that occurs during strenuous physical activity.

2) **External cause code used for length of treatment**

   Assign the external cause code, with the appropriate 7th character (initial encounter, subsequent encounter or sequela) for each encounter for which the injury or condition is being treated.

3) **Use the full range of external cause codes**

   Use the full range of external cause codes to completely describe the cause, the intent, the place of occurrence, and if applicable, the activity of the patient at the time of the event, and the patient's status, for all injuries, and other health conditions due to an external cause.

4) **Assign as many external cause codes as necessary**

   Assign as many external cause codes as necessary to fully explain each cause. If only one external code can be recorded, assign the code most related to the principal diagnosis.

5) **The selection of the appropriate external cause code**

   The selection of the appropriate external cause code is guided by the Alphabetic Index of External Causes and by Inclusion and Exclusion notes in the Tabular List.

6) **External cause code can never be a principal diagnosis**

   An external cause code can never be a principal (first-listed) diagnosis.

7) Combination external cause codes

Certain of the external cause codes are combination codes that identify sequential events that result in an injury, such as a fall which results in striking against an object. The injury may be due to either event or both. The combination external cause code used should correspond to the sequence of events regardless of which caused the most serious injury.

8) No external cause code needed in certain circumstances

No external cause code from Chapter 20 is needed if the external cause and intent are included in a code from another chapter (e.g. T36.0x1- Poisoning by penicillins, accidental (unintentional)).

PLACE OF OCCURRENCE GUIDELINE

Codes from category Y92, Place of occurrence of the external cause, are secondary codes for use after other external cause codes to identify the location of the patient at the time of injury or other condition.

A place of occurrence code is used only once, at the initial encounter for treatment. No 7th characters are used for Y92. Only one code from Y92 should be recorded on a medical record. A place of occurrence code should be used in conjunction with an activity code, Y93.

Do not use place of occurrence code Y92.9 if the place is not stated or is not applicable.

ACTIVITY CODE

Assign a code from category Y93, Activity code, to describe the activity of the patient at the time the injury or other health condition occurred.

An activity code is used only once, at the initial encounter for treatment. Only one code from Y93 should be recorded on a medical record. An activity code should be used in conjunction with a place of occurrence code, Y92.

The activity codes are not applicable to poisonings, adverse effects, misadventures or late effects.

Do not assign Y93.9, Unspecified activity, if the activity is not stated.

A code from category Y93 is appropriate for use with external cause and intent codes if identifying the activity provides additional information about the event.

PLACE OF OCCURRENCE, ACTIVITY, AND STATUS CODES USED WITH OTHER EXTERNAL CAUSE CODE

When applicable, place of occurrence, activity, and external cause status codes are sequenced after the main external cause code(s). Regardless of the number of external cause codes assigned, there should be only one place of occurrence code, one activity code, and one external cause status code assigned to an encounter.

IF THE REPORTING FORMAT LIMITS THE NUMBER OF EXTERNAL CAUSE CODES

If the reporting format limits the number of external cause codes that can be used in reporting clinical data, report the code for the cause/intent most related to the principal diagnosis. If the format permits capture of additional external cause codes, the cause/intent, including medical misadventures, of the additional events should be reported rather than the codes for place, activity, or external status.

MULTIPLE EXTERNAL CAUSE CODING GUIDELINES

More than one external cause code is required to fully describe the external cause of an illness or injury. The assignment of external cause codes should be sequenced in the following priority:

- If two or more events cause separate injuries, an external cause code should be assigned for each cause. The first-listed external cause code will be selected in the following order:

- External codes for child and adult abuse take priority over all other external cause codes.

- External cause codes for terrorism events take priority over all other external cause codes except child and adult abuse.

- External cause codes for cataclysmic events take priority over all other external cause codes except child and adult abuse and terrorism.

- External cause codes for transport accidents take priority over all other external cause codes except cataclysmic events, child and adult abuse and terrorism.

- Activity and external cause status codes are assigned following all causal (intent) external cause codes.

- The first-listed external cause code should correspond to the cause of the most serious diagnosis due to an assault, accident, or self-harm, following the order of hierarchy listed above.

CHILD AND ADULT ABUSE GUIDELINE

Adult and child abuse, neglect and maltreatment are classified as assault. Any of the assault codes may be used to indicate the external cause of any injury resulting from the confirmed abuse.

For confirmed cases of abuse, neglect and maltreatment, when the perpetrator is known, a code from Y07, Perpetrator of maltreatment and neglect, should accompany any other assault codes.

UNKNOWN OR UNDETERMINED INTENT GUIDELINE

If the intent (accident, self-harm, assault) of the cause of an injury or other condition is unknown or unspecified, code the intent as accidental intent. All transport accident categories assume accidental intent.

1) **Use of undetermined intent**

External cause codes for events of undetermined intent are only for use if the documentation in the record specifies that the intent cannot be determined.

LATE EFFECTS OF EXTERNAL CAUSE GUIDELINES

1) Late effect external cause codes

Late effects are reported using the external cause code with the 7th character extension "S" for sequela. These codes should be used with any report of a late effect or sequela resulting from a previous injury.

2) Late effect external cause code with a related current injury

A late effect external cause code should never be used with a related current nature of injury code.

3) Use of late effect external cause codes for subsequent visits

Use a late effect external cause code for subsequent visits when a late effect of the initial injury is being treated. Do not use a late effect external cause code for subsequent visits for follow- up care (e.g., to assess healing, to receive rehabilitative therapy) of the injury when no late effect of the injury has been documented.

TERRORISM GUIDELINES

1) Cause of injury identified by the Federal Government (FBI) as terrorism

When the cause of an injury is identified by the Federal Government (FBI) as terrorism, the first-listed external cause code should be a code from category Y38, Terrorism. The definition of terrorism employed by the FBI is found at the inclusion note at the beginning of category Y38. Use additional code for place of occurrence (Y92.-). More than one Y38 code may be assigned if the injury is the result of more than one mechanism of terrorism.

2) Cause of an injury is suspected to be the result of terrorism

When the cause of an injury is suspected to be the result of terrorism a code from category Y38 should not be assigned. Suspected cases should be classified as assault.

3) Code Y38.9, Terrorism, secondary effects

Assign code Y38.9, Terrorism, secondary effects, for conditions occurring subsequent to the terrorist event. This code should not be assigned for conditions that are due to the initial terrorist act.

It is acceptable to assign code Y38.9 with another code from Y38 if there is an injury due to the initial terrorist event and an injury that is a subsequent result of the terrorist event.

EXTERNAL CAUSE STATUS

A code from category Y99, External cause status, should be assigned whenever any other external cause code is assigned for an encounter, including an Activity code, except for the events noted below. Assign a code from category Y99, External cause status, to indicate the work status of the person at the time the event occurred. The status code indicates whether the event occurred during military activity, whether a non-military person was at work, whether an individual including a student or volunteer was involved in a non-work activity at the time of the causal event.

A code from Y99, External cause status, should be assigned, when applicable, with other external cause codes, such as transport accidents and falls. The external cause status codes are not applicable to poisonings, adverse effects, misadventures or late effects. Do not assign a code from category Y99 if no other external cause codes (cause, activity) are applicable for the encounter.

An external cause status code is used only once, at the initial encounter for treatment. Only one code from Y99 should be recorded on a medical record.

Do not assign code Y99.9, Unspecified external cause status, if the status is not stated.

SAMPLE ICD-10-CM CODES FROM THIS CHAPTER

Note: This chapter permits the classification of environmental events and circumstances as the cause of injury, and other adverse effects. Where a code from this section is applicable, it is intended that it shall be used secondary to a code from another chapter of the Classification indicating the nature of the condition. Most often, the condition will be classifiable to Chapter 19, Injury, poisoning and certain other consequences of external causes (S00-T88). Other conditions that may be stated to be due to external causes are classified in Chapters I to XVIII. For these conditions, codes from Chapter 20 should be used to provide additional information as to the cause of the condition.

This chapter contains the following blocks:	
V00-V09	Pedestrian injured in transport accident
V10-V19	Pedal cycle rider injured in transport accident
V20-V29	Motorcycle rider injured in transport accident
V30-V39	Occupant of three-wheeled motor vehicle injured in transport accident
V40-V49	Car occupant injured in transport accident
V50-V59	Occupant of pick-up truck or van injured in transport accident
V60-V69	Occupant of heavy transport vehicle injured in transport accident
V70-V79	Bus occupant injured in transport accident
V80-V89	Other land transport accidents
V90-V94	Water transport accidents
V95-V97	Air and space transport accidents
V98-V99	Other and unspecified transport accidents
W00-W19	Slipping, tripping, stumbling and falls
W20-W49	Exposure to inanimate mechanical forces
W50-W64	Exposure to animate mechanical forces
W65-W74	Accidental non-transport drowning and submersion
W85-W99	Exposure to electric current, radiation and extreme ambient air temperature and pressure

X00-X08	Exposure to smoke, fire and flames
X10-X19	Contact with heat and hot substances
X30-X39	Exposure to forces of nature
X52-X58	Accidental exposure to other specified factors
X71-X83	Intentional self-harm
X92-Y09	Assault
Y21-Y33	Event of undetermined intent
Y35-Y38	Legal intervention, operations of war, military operations, and terrorism
Y62-Y69	Misadventures to patients during surgical and medical care
Y70-Y82	Medical devices associated with adverse incidents in diagnostic and therapeutic use
Y83-Y84	Surgical and other medical procedures as the cause of abnormal reaction of the patient, or of later complication, without mention of misadventure at the time of the procedure
Y90-Y99	Supplementary factors related to causes of morbidity classified elsewhere

ACCIDENTS (V00-X58)

Transport accidents (V00-V99)

Note: This section is structured in 12 groups. Those relating to land transport accidents (V01-V89) reflect the victim's mode of transport and are subdivided to identify the victim's 'counterpart' or the type of event. The vehicle of which the injured person is an occupant is identified in the first two characters since it is seen as the most important factor to identify for prevention purposes. A transport accident is one in which the vehicle involved must be moving or running or in use for transport purposes at the time of the accident.

Use additional code to identify:

Airbag injury (W22.1)
Type of street or road (Y92.4-)
Use of cellular telephone and other electronic equipment at the time of the transport accident (Y93.c-)

Excludes 1: agricultural vehicles in stationary use or maintenance (W31.-)
   assault by crashing of motor vehicle (Y03.-)
   automobile or motor cycle in stationary use or maintenance- code to type of accident
   crashing of motor vehicle, undetermined intent (Y32)
   intentional self-harm by crashing of motor vehicle (X82)

Excludes 2: transport accidents due to cataclysm (X34-X38)

Definitions of Transport Vehicles:

A transport accident is any accident involving a device designed primarily for, or used at the time primarily for, conveying persons or good from one place to another.

A public highway [traffic way] or street is the entire width between property lines (or other boundary lines) of land open to the public as a matter of right or custom for purposes of moving persons or property from one place to another. A roadway is that part of the public highway designed, improved and customarily used for vehicular traffic.

A traffic accident is any vehicle accident occurring on the public highway [i.e. originating on, terminating on, or involving a vehicle partially on the highway]. A vehicle accident is assumed to have occurred on the public highway unless another place is specified, except in the case of accidents involving only off-road motor vehicles, which are classified as nontraffic accidents unless the contrary is stated.

A nontraffic accident is any vehicle accident that occurs entirely in any place other than a public highway.

A pedestrian is any person involved in an accident who was not at the time of the accident riding in or on a motor vehicle, railway train, streetcar or animal-drawn or other vehicle, or on a pedal cycle or animal. This includes, a person changing a tire or working on a parked car. It also includes the use of a pedestrian conveyance such as a baby carriage, ice-skates, roller skates, a skateboard, nonmotorized or motorized wheelchair, motorized mobility scooter, or nonmotorized scooter.

A driver is an occupant of a transport vehicle who is operating or intending to operate it.

A passenger is any occupant of a transport vehicle other than the driver, except a person traveling on the outside of the vehicle.

A person on the outside of a vehicle is any person being transported by a vehicle but not occupying the space normally reserved for the driver or passengers, or the space intended for the transport of property. This includes the body, bumper, fender, roof, running board or step of a vehicle.

A pedal cycle is any land transport vehicle operated solely by nonmotorized pedals including a bicycle or tricycle.

A pedal cyclist is any person riding a pedal cycle or in a sidecar or trailer attached to a pedal cycle.

A motorcycle is a two-wheeled motor vehicle with one or two riding saddles and sometimes with a third wheel for the support of a sidecar. The sidecar is considered part of the motorcycle.

A motorcycle rider is any person riding a motorcycle or in a sidecar or trailer attached to the motorcycle.

A three-wheeled motor vehicle is a motorized tricycle designed primarily for on-road use. This includes a motor- driven tricycle, a motorized rickshaw, or a three-wheeled motor car.

A car [automobile] is a four-wheeled motor vehicle designed primarily for carrying up to 7 persons. A trailer being towed by the car is considered part of the car.

A pick-up truck or van is a four or six-wheeled motor vehicle designed for carrying passengers as well as property or cargo weighing less than the local limit for classification as a heavy goods vehicle, and not requiring a special driver's license. This includes a minivan and a sport-utility vehicle (SUV).

A heavy transport vehicle is a motor vehicle designed primarily for carrying property, meeting local criteria for classification as a heavy goods vehicle in terms of weight and requiring a special driver's license.

A bus (coach) is a motor vehicle designed or adapted primarily for carrying more than 10 passengers, and requiring a special driver's license.
A railway train or railway vehicle is any device, with or without freight or passenger cars couple to it, designed for traffic on a railway track. This includes subterranean (subways) or elevated trains.

A streetcar, is a device designed and used primarily for transporting passengers within a municipality, running on rails, usually subject to normal traffic control signals, and operated principally on a right-of-way that forms part of the roadway. This includes a tram or trolley that runs on rails. A trailer being towed by a streetcar is considered part of the streetcar.

A special vehicle mainly used on industrial premises is a motor vehicle designed primarily for use within the buildings and premises of industrial or commercial establishments. This includes battery-powered trucks, forklifts, coal-cars in a coal mine, logging cars and trucks used in mines or quarries.

A special vehicle mainly used in agriculture is a motor vehicle designed specifically for use in farming and agriculture (horticulture), to work the land, tend and harvest crops and transport materials on the farm. This includes harvesters, farm machinery and tractor and trailers.

A special construction vehicle is a motor vehicle designed specifically for use on construction and demolition sites.

This includes bulldozers, diggers, earth levellers, dump trucks. backhoes, front-end loaders, pavers, and mechanical shovels.

A special all-terrain vehicle is a motor vehicle of special design to enable it to negotiate over rough or soft terrain , snow or sand. This includes snow mobiles, All-terrain vehicles (ATV), and dune buggies. It does not include passenger vehicle designated as Sport Utility Vehicles SUV).

A watercraft is any device designed for transporting passengers or goods on water. This includes motor or sail boats, ships, and hovercraft.

An aircraft is any device for transporting passengers or goods in the air. This includes hot-air balloons, gliders, helicopters and airplanes.

A military vehicle is any motorized vehicle operating on a public roadway owned by the military and being operated by a member of the military.

PEDESTRIAN INJURED IN TRANSPORT ACCIDENT (V00-V09)

Includes: person changing tire on transport vehicle
person examining engine of vehicle broken down in (on side of) road

Excludes 1: fall due to non-transport collision with other person (W03)
pedestrian on foot falling (slipping) on ice and snow (W00.-)
struck or bumped by another person (W51)

V00   Pedestrian Conveyance Accident
Use additional place of occurrence and activity external cause codes, if known (Y92.-, Y93.-)

Excludes 1: collision with another person without fall (W51)
fall due to person on foot colliding with another person on foot (W03)
fall from non-moving wheelchair, nonmotorized scooter and motorized mobility
scooter without collision (W05.-)
pedestrian (conveyance) collision with other land transport vehicle (V01-V09)
pedestrian on foot falling (slipping) on ice and snow (W00.-)

The appropriate 7th character is to be added to each code from category V00

A - initial encounter
D - subsequent encounter
S - sequela

V00.0   Pedestrian on foot injured in collision with pedestrian conveyance

V00.01   Pedestrian on foot injured in collision with roller-skater

V00.02   Pedestrian on foot injured in collision with skateboarder

V00.09   Pedestrian on foot injured in collision with other pedestrian conveyance

V00.1   Rolling-type pedestrian conveyance accident

Excludes 1: accident with baby stroller (V00.82-)
accident with wheelchair (powered) (V00.81-)
accident with motorized mobility scooter (V00.83-)

V00.11   In-line roller-skate accident

V00.111   Fall from in-line roller-skates

V00.112   In-line roller-skater colliding with stationary object

V00.118   Other in-line roller-skate accident

Excludes 1: roller-skater collision with other land transport vehicle (V01-V09 with 5th character 1)

V00.12   Non-in- line roller-skate accident

V00.121   Fall from non-in-line roller-skates

V00.122 Non-in-line roller-skater colliding with stationary object

V00.128 Other non-in-line roller-skating accident

> *Excludes 1*: roller-skater collision with other land transport vehicle (V01-V09 with 5th character 1)

V00.13 Skateboard accident

V00.131 Fall from skateboard

V00.132 Skateboarder colliding with stationary object

V00.138 Other skateboard accident

> *Excludes 1*: skateboarder collision with other land transport vehicle (V01-V09 with 5th character 2)

V00.14 Scooter (nonmotorized) accident

Excludes 1: motor scooter accident (V20-V29)

V00.141 Fall from scooter (nonmotorized)

V00.142 Scooter (nonmotorized) colliding with stationary object

V00.148 Other scooter (nonmotorized) accident

> *Excludes 1*: scooter (nonmotorized) collision with other land transport vehicle (V01-V09 with fifth character 9)

V00.15 Heelies accident
Rolling shoe
Wheeled shoe
Wheelies accident

V00.151 Fall from heelies

V00.152 Heelies colliding with stationary object

V00.158 Other heelies accident

V00.18 Accident on other rolling-type pedestrian conveyance

V00.181 Fall from other rolling-type pedestrian conveyance

V00.182 Pedestrian on other rolling-type pedestrian conveyance colliding with stationary object

V00.188 Other accident on other rolling-type pedestrian conveyance

V00.2 Gliding-type pedestrian conveyance accident

    V00.21   Ice-skates accident

        V00.211   Fall from ice-skates

        V00.212   Ice-skater colliding with stationary object

        V00.218   Other ice-skates accident

        Excludes 1: ice-skater collision with other land transport vehicle (V01-V09 with 5th digit 9)

    V00.22   Sled accident

        V00.221   Fall from sled

        V00.222   Sledder colliding with stationary object

        V00.228   Other sled accident

        Excludes 1: sled collision with other land transport vehicle (V01-V09 with 5th digit 9)

    V00.28   Other gliding-type pedestrian conveyance accident

        V00.281   Fall from other gliding-type pedestrian conveyance

        V00.282   Pedestrian on other gliding-type pedestrian conveyance colliding with stationary object

        V00.288   Other accident on other gliding-type pedestrian conveyance

        Excludes 1: gliding-type pedestrian conveyance collision with other land transport vehicle (V01-V09 with 5th digit 9)

V00.3 Flat-bottomed pedestrian conveyance accident

    V00.31   Snowboard accident

        V00.311   Fall from snowboard

        V00.312   Snowboarder colliding with stationary object

        V00.318   Other snowboard accident

        Excludes 1: snowboarder collision with other land transport vehicle (V01-V09 with 5th digit 9)

V00.32   Snow-ski accident

V00.321   Fall from snow-skis

V00.322   Snow-skier colliding with stationary object

FORWARD MAPPING SAMPLE (ICD-9-CM ➡ ICD-10-CM)			
ICD-9-CM CODE & DESCRIPTION		ICD-10-CM CODE & DESCRIPTION	
E88.00	Accidental fall on or from escalator	W10.0xxA	Fall (on)(from) escalator initial encounter
E88.01	Accidental fall on or from sidewalk curb	W10.1xxA	Fall (on)(from) sidewalk curb initial encounter
E88.09	Accidental fall on or from other stairs or steps	W10.8xxA	Fall (on) (from) other stairs and steps initial encounter
E88.10	Accidental fall from ladder	W11.xxxA	Fall on and from ladder initial encounter
E88.11	Accidental fall from scaffolding	W12.xxxA	Fall on and from scaffolding initial encounter
E88.2	Accidental fall from or out of building or other structure	W13.9xxA	Fall from out of or through building not otherwise specified
E88.30	Accident from diving or jumping into water (swimming pool)	W16.92xA	Jumping or diving into unspecified water causing other injury initial encounter
E88.31	Accidental fall into well	W17.0xxA	Fall into well initial encounter
E88.32	Accidental fall into storm drain or manhole	W17.1xxA	Fall into storm drain or manhole initial encounter
E88.39	Accidental fall into other hole or other opening in surface	W17.2xxA	Fall into hole initial encounter
E88.40	Accidental fall from playground equipment	W09.8xxA	Fall on or from other playground equipment initial encounter
E88.41	Accidental fall from cliff	W15.xxxA	Fall from cliff initial encounter
E88.42	Accidental fall from chair	W07.xxxA	Fall from chair initial encounter
E88.44	Accidental fall from bed	W06.xxxA	Fall from bed initial encounter
E88.45	Accidental fall from other furniture	W08.xxxA	Fall from other furniture initial encounter
E88.46	Accidental fall from commode	W18.11xA	Fall from or off toilet without subsequent striking against object initial encounter
E88.49	Other accidental fall from one level to another	W14.xxxA	Fall from tree initial encounter
E88.49	Other accidental fall from one level to another	W17.81xA	Fall down embankment (hill) initial encounter
E88.49	Other accidental fall from one level to another	W17.89xA	Other fall from one level to another initial encounter

E88.50	Accidental fall from (nonmotorized) scooter	V00.141A	Fall from scooter (nonmotorized) initial encounter
E88.51	Accidental fall from roller skates	V00.111A	Fall from in-line roller-skates initial encounter
E88.51	Accidental fall from roller skates	V00.151A	Fall from heelies initial encounter
E88.52	Accidental fall from skateboard	V00.131A	Fall from skateboard initial encounter
E88.53	Accidental fall from skis	V00.321A	Fall from snow-skis initial encounter
E88.54	Accidental fall from snowboard	V00.312A	Snowboarder colliding with stationary object initial encounter
E88.59	Accidental fall from other slipping tripping or stumbling	W18.49xA	Other slipping tripping and stumbling without falling initial encounter
E88.60	Accidental fall on same level from collision pushing or shoving by or with other person in sports	W03.xxxA	Other fall on same level due to collision with another person initial encounter
E88.69	Other and unspecified accidental falls on same level from collision pushing or shoving by or with other person	V00.388A	Other accident on other flat-bottomed pedestrian conveyance initial encounter
E88.7	Fracture cause unspecified	W19.xxxA	Unspecified fall initial encounter
E88.80	Accidental fall resulting in striking against sharp object	W01.110A	Fall on same level from slipping tripping and stumbling with subsequent striking against sharp glass initial encounter
E88.81	Accidental fall resulting in striking against other object	W01.198A	Fall on same level from slipping tripping and stumbling with subsequent striking against other object initial encounter
E88.88	Other accidental fall	W18.30xA	Fall on same level unspecified initial encounter
E88.89	Unspecified accidental fall	W19.xxxA	Unspecified fall initial encounter
E89.00	Explosion caused by conflagration in private dwelling	X00.8xxA	Other exposure to uncontrolled fire in building or structure initial encounter
E89.01	Fumes from combustion of polyvinylchloride (PVC) and similar material in conflagration in private dwelling	X08.8xxA	Exposure to other specified smoke fire and flames initial encounter
E89.02	Other smoke and fumes from conflagration in private dwelling	X00.1xxA	Exposure to smoke in uncontrolled fire in building or structure initial encounter

E89.03	Burning caused by conflagration in private dwelling	X00.0xxA	Exposure to flames in uncontrolled fire in building or structure initial encounter
E89.08	Other accident resulting from conflagration in private dwelling	X00.2xxA	Injury due to collapse of burning building or structure in uncontrolled fire initial encounter
E89.09	Unspecified accident resulting from conflagration in private dwelling	X00.8xxA	Other exposure to uncontrolled fire in building or structure initial encounter

BACKWARD MAPPING SAMPLE (ICD-10-CM ➜ ICD-9-CM)

ICD-10-CM CODE & DESCRIPTION		ICD-9-CM CODE & DESCRIPTION	
V40.0xxA	Car driver injured in collision with pedestrian or animal in nontraffic accident initial encounter	E82.20	Other motor vehicle nontraffic accident involving collision with moving object injuring driver of motor vehicle other than motorcycle
V40.0xxD	Car driver injured in collision with pedestrian or animal in nontraffic accident subsequent encounter	E82.20	Other motor vehicle nontraffic accident involving collision with moving object injuring driver of motor vehicle other than motorcycle
V40.0xxS	Car driver injured in collision with pedestrian or animal in nontraffic accident sequela	E92.90	Late effects of motor vehicle accident
V40.1xxA	Car passenger injured in collision with pedestrian or animal in nontraffic accident initial encounter	E82.21	Other motor vehicle nontraffic accident involving collision with moving object injuring passenger in motor vehicle other than motorcycle
V40.1xxD	Car passenger injured in collision with pedestrian or animal in nontraffic accident subsequent encounter	E82.21	Other motor vehicle nontraffic accident involving collision with moving object injuring passenger in motor vehicle other than motorcycle
V40.1xxS	Car passenger injured in collision with pedestrian or animal in nontraffic accident sequela	E92.90	Late effects of motor vehicle accident
V40.2xxA	Person on outside of car injured in collision with pedestrian or animal in nontraffic accident initial encounter	E82.28	Other motor vehicle nontraffic accident involving collision with moving object injuring other specified person
V40.2xxD	Person on outside of car injured in collision with pedestrian or animal in nontraffic accident subsequent encounter	E82.28	Other motor vehicle nontraffic accident involving collision with moving object injuring other specified person

V40.2xxS	Person on outside of car injured in collision with pedestrian or animal in nontraffic accident sequela	**E92.90**	Late effects of motor vehicle accident
V40.3xxA	Unspecified car occupant injured in collision with pedestrian or animal in nontraffic accident initial encounter	**E82.29**	Other motor vehicle nontraffic accident involving collision with moving object injuring unspecified person
V40.3xxD	Unspecified car occupant injured in collision with pedestrian or animal in nontraffic accident subsequent encounter	**E82.29**	Other motor vehicle nontraffic accident involving collision with moving object injuring unspecified person
V40.3xxS	Unspecified car occupant injured in collision with pedestrian or animal in nontraffic accident sequela	**E92.90**	Late effects of motor vehicle accident
V40.4xxA	Person boarding or alighting a car injured in collision with pedestrian or animal initial encounter	**E82.48**	Other motor vehicle nontraffic accident while boarding and alighting injuring other specified person
V40.4xxD	Person boarding or alighting a car injured in collision with pedestrian or animal subsequent encounter	**E82.48**	Other motor vehicle nontraffic accident while boarding and alighting injuring other specified person
V40.4xxS	Person boarding or alighting a car injured in collision with pedestrian or animal sequela	**E92.90**	Late effects of motor vehicle accident
V40.5xxA	Car driver injured in collision with pedestrian or animal in traffic accident initial encounter	**E81.40**	Motor vehicle traffic accident involving collision with pedestrian injuring driver of motor vehicle other than motorcycle
V40.5xxD	Car driver injured in collision with pedestrian or animal in traffic accident subsequent encounter	**E81.40**	Motor vehicle traffic accident involving collision with pedestrian injuring driver of motor vehicle other than motorcycle
V40.5xxS	Car driver injured in collision with pedestrian or animal in traffic accident sequela	**E92.90**	Late effects of motor vehicle accident
V40.6xxA	Car passenger injured in collision with pedestrian or animal in traffic accident initial encounter	**E81.41**	Motor vehicle traffic accident involving collision with pedestrian injuring passenger in motor vehicle other than motorcycle
V40.6xxD	Car passenger injured in collision with pedestrian or animal in traffic accident subsequent encounter	**E81.41**	Motor vehicle traffic accident involving collision with pedestrian injuring passenger in motor vehicle other than motorcycle

X00.0xxA	Exposure to flames in uncontrolled fire in building or structure initial encounter	E89.03	Burning caused by conflagration in private dwelling
X00.0xxD	Exposure to flames in uncontrolled fire in building or structure subsequent encounter	E89.03	Burning caused by conflagration in private dwelling
X00.0xxS	Exposure to flames in uncontrolled fire in building or structure sequela	E92.94	Late effects of accident caused by fire
X00.1xxA	Exposure to smoke in uncontrolled fire in building or structure initial encounter	E89.02	Other smoke and fumes from conflagration in private dwelling
X00.1xxD	Exposure to smoke in uncontrolled fire in building or structure subsequent encounter	E89.02	Other smoke and fumes from conflagration in private dwelling
X00.1xxS	Exposure to smoke in uncontrolled fire in building or structure sequela	E92.94	Late effects of accident caused by fire
X00.2xxA	Injury due to collapse of burning building or structure in uncontrolled fire initial encounter	E89.08	Other accident resulting from conflagration in private dwelling
X00.2xxD	Injury due to collapse of burning building or structure in uncontrolled fire subsequent encounter	E89.08	Other accident resulting from conflagration in private dwelling
X00.2xxS	Injury due to collapse of burning building or structure in uncontrolled fire sequela	E92.94	Late effects of accident caused by fire
X00.3xxA	Fall from burning building or structure in uncontrolled fire initial encounter	E89.08	Other accident resulting from conflagration in private dwelling
X00.3xxD	Fall from burning building or structure in uncontrolled fire subsequent encounter	E89.08	Other accident resulting from conflagration in private dwelling
X00.3xxS	Fall from burning building or structure in uncontrolled fire sequela	E92.94	Late effects of accident caused by fire
X00.4xxA	Hit by object from burning building or structure in uncontrolled fire initial encounter	E89.08	Other accident resulting from conflagration in private dwelling
X00.4xxD	Hit by object from burning building or structure in uncontrolled fire subsequent encounter	E89.08	Other accident resulting from conflagration in private dwelling

X00.4xxS	Hit by object from burning building or structure in uncontrolled fire sequela	E92.94	Late effects of accident caused by fire
X00.5xxA	Jump from burning building or structure in uncontrolled fire initial encounter	E89.08	Other accident resulting from conflagration in private dwelling
X00.5xxD	Jump from burning building or structure in uncontrolled fire subsequent encounter	E89.08	Other accident resulting from conflagration in private dwelling
X00.5xxS	Jump from burning building or structure in uncontrolled fire sequela	E92.94	Late effects of accident caused by fire
X00.8xxA	Other exposure to uncontrolled fire in building or structure initial encounter	E89.08	Other accident resulting from conflagration in private dwelling
X00.8xxD	Other exposure to uncontrolled fire in building or structure subsequent encounter	E89.08	Other accident resulting from conflagration in private dwelling
X00.8xxS	Other exposure to uncontrolled fire in building or structure sequela	E92.94	Late effects of accident caused by fire

CHAPTER 21: FACTORS INFLUENCING HEALTH STATUS AND CONTACT WITH HEALTH SERVICES (Z00-Z99)

GENERAL GUIDELINES

Note: The chapter specific guidelines provide additional information about the use of Z codes for specified encounters.

USE OF Z CODES IN ANY HEALTHCARE SETTING

Z codes are for use in any healthcare setting. Z codes may be used as either a first-listed (principal diagnosis code in the inpatient setting) or secondary code, depending on the circumstances of the encounter. Certain Z codes may only be used as first-listed or principal diagnosis.

Z CODES INDICATE A REASON FOR AN ENCOUNTER

Z codes are not procedure codes. A corresponding procedure code must accompany a Z code to describe any procedure performed.

CATEGORIES OF Z CODES

1) **Contact/Exposure**

   Category Z20 indicates contact with, and suspected exposure to, communicable diseases. These codes are for patients who do not show any sign or symptom of a disease but are suspected to have been exposed to it by close personal contact with an infected individual or are in an area where a disease is epidemic.

Category Z77, indicates contact with and suspected exposures hazardous to health.

Contact/exposure codes may be used as a first-listed code to explain an encounter for testing, or, more commonly, as a secondary code to identify a potential risk.

2) Inoculations and vaccinations

Code Z23 is for encounters for inoculations and vaccinations. It indicates that a patient is being seen to receive a prophylactic inoculation against a disease. Procedure codes are required to identify the actual administration of the injection and the type(s) of immunizations given. Code Z23 may be used as a secondary code if the inoculation is given as a routine part of preventive health care, such as a well-baby visit.

3) Status

Status codes indicate that a patient is either a carrier of a disease or has the sequelae or residual of a past disease or condition. This includes such things as the presence of prosthetic or mechanical devices resulting from past treatment. A status code is informative, because the status may affect the course of treatment and its outcome. A status code is distinct from a history code. The history code indicates that the patient no longer has the condition.

A status code should not be used with a diagnosis code from one of the body system chapters, if the diagnosis code includes the information provided by the status code. For example, code Z94.1, Heart transplant status, should not be used with a code from subcategory T86.2, Complications of heart transplant. The status code does not provide additional information. The complication code indicates that the patient is a heart transplant patient.

For encounters for weaning from a mechanical ventilator, assign a code from subcategory J96.1, Chronic respiratory failure, followed by code Z99.11, Dependence on respirator [ventilator] status.

The status Z codes/categories are:

Z14   Genetic carrier

     Genetic carrier status indicates that a person carries a gene, associated with a particular disease, which may be passed to offspring who may develop that disease. The person does not have the disease and is not at risk of developing the disease.

Z15   Genetic susceptibility to disease

     Genetic susceptibility indicates that a person has a gene that increases the risk of that person developing the disease.

     Codes from category Z15 should not be used as principal or first-listed codes. If the patient has the condition to which he/she is susceptible, and that condition is the reason for the encounter, the code for the current condition should be sequenced first. If the patient is being seen for follow-up after completed treatment for this condition, and the condition no longer exists, a follow-up code should be sequenced first, followed by the appropriate personal history and genetic susceptibility codes. If the purpose of the encounter is genetic counseling associated with procreative management, code Z31.5, Encounter for genetic counseling, should be assigned as the first-listed code, followed by a code from category Z15. Additional codes should be assigned for any applicable family or personal history.

Z16   Infection with drug-resistant microorganisms

This code indicates that a patient has an infection that is resistant to drug treatment. Sequence the infection code first.

Z17   Estrogen receptor status

Z18   Retained foreign body fragments

Z21   Asymptomatic HIV infection status

This code indicates that a patient has tested positive for HIV but has manifested no signs or symptoms of the disease.

Z22   Carrier of infectious disease

Carrier status indicates that a person harbors the specific organisms of a disease without manifest symptoms and is capable of transmitting the infection.

Z28.3   Underimmunization status

Z33.1   Pregnant state, incidental

This code is a secondary code only for use when the pregnancy is in no way complicating the reason for visit. Otherwise, a code from the obstetric chapter is required.

Z66   Do not resuscitate

This code may be used when it is documented by the provider that a patient is on do not resuscitate status at any time during the stay.

Z67   Blood type

Z68   Body mass index (BMI)

Z74.01 Bed confinement status

Z76.82 Awaiting organ transplant status

Z78   Other specified health status

Code Z78.1, Physical restraint status, may be used when it is documented by the provider that a patient has been put in restraints during the current encounter. Please note that this code should not be reported when it is documented by the provider that a patient is temporarily restrained during a procedure.

Z79   Long-term (current) drug therapy

Codes from this category indicate a patient's continuous use of a prescribed drug (including such things as aspirin therapy) for the long-term treatment of a condition or for prophylactic use. It is not for use for patients who have addictions to drugs. This subcategory is not for use of medications for detoxification or maintenance programs to prevent withdrawal symptoms in patients with drug dependence (e.g., methadone maintenance for opiate dependence). Assign the appropriate code for the drug dependence instead.

Assign a code from Z79 if the patient is receiving a medication for an extended period as a prophylactic measure (such as for the prevention of deep vein thrombosis) or as treatment of a chronic condition (such as arthritis) or a disease requiring a lengthy course of treatment (such as cancer). Do not assign a code from category Z79 for medication being administered for a brief period of time to treat an acute illness or injury (such as a course of antibiotics to treat acute bronchitis).

Z88   Allergy status to drugs, medicaments and biological substances

Except: Z88.9, Allergy status to unspecified drugs, medicaments and biological substances status

Z89   Acquired absence of limb

Z90   Acquired absence of organs, not elsewhere classified

Z91.0-   Allergy status, other than to drugs and biological substances

Z92.82   Status post administration of tPA (rtPA) in a different facility within the last 24 hours prior to admission to a current facility

Assign code Z92.82, Status post administration of tPA (rtPA) in a different facility within the last 24 hours prior to admission to current facility, as a secondary diagnosis when a patient is received by transfer into a facility and documentation indicates they were administered tissue plasminogen activator (tPA) within the last 24 hours prior to admission to the current facility.

This guideline applies even if the patient is still receiving the tPA at the time they are received into the current facility.

The appropriate code for the condition for which the tPA was administered (such as cerebrovascular disease or myocardial infarction) should be assigned first.

Code Z92.82 is only applicable to the receiving facility record and not to the transferring facility record.

Z93   Artificial opening status

Z94   Transplanted organ and tissue status

Z95   Presence of cardiac and vascular implants and grafts

Z96   Presence of other functional implants

Z97   Presence of other devices

Z98   Other postprocedural states
        Assign code Z98.85, Transplanted organ removal status, to indicate that a
        transplanted organ has been previously removed. This code should not be assigned
        for the encounter in which the transplanted organ is removed. The complication
        necessitating removal of the transplant organ should be assigned for that encounter.

        See section I.C19.g.3. for information on the coding of organ transplant
        complications.

Z99   Dependence on enabling machines and devices, not elsewhere classified

Note: Categories Z89-Z90 and Z93-Z99 are for use only if there are no complications or
malfunctions of the organ or tissue replaced, the amputation site or the equipment on which
the patient is dependent.

4) **History (of)**

There are two types of history Z codes, personal and family. Personal history codes explain a
patient's past medical condition that no longer exists and is not receiving any treatment, but
that has the potential for recurrence, and therefore may require continued monitoring.

Family history codes are for use when a patient has a family member(s) who has had a
particular disease that causes the patient to be at higher risk of also contracting the disease.

Personal history codes may be used in conjunction with follow- up codes and family history
codes may be used in conjunction with screening codes to explain the need for a test or
procedure. History codes are also acceptable on any medical record regardless of the reason
for visit. A history of an illness, even if no longer present, is important information that may
alter the type of treatment ordered.

The history Z code categories are:

Z80   Family history of primary malignant neoplasm

Z81   Family history of mental and behavioral disorders

Z82   Family history of certain disabilities and chronic diseases (leading to disablement)

Z83   Family history of other specific disorders

Z84   Family history of other conditions

Z85   Personal history of malignant neoplasm

Z86   Personal history of certain other diseases

Z87   Personal history of other diseases and conditions

Z91.4- Personal history of psychological trauma, not elsewhere classified

Z91.5   Personal history of self-harm

Z91.8- Other specified personal risk factors, not elsewhere classified

Z92   Personal history of medical treatment

       Except: Z92.0, Personal history of contraception
       Except: Z92.82, Status post administration of tPA (rtPA) in a different facility within the last 24 hours prior to admission to a current facility

5) Screening

Screening is the testing for disease or disease precursors in seemingly well individuals so that early detection and treatment can be provided for those who test positive for the disease (e.g., screening mammogram).

The testing of a person to rule out or confirm a suspected diagnosis because the patient has some sign or symptom is a diagnostic examination, not a screening. In these cases, the sign or symptom is used to explain the reason for the test.

A screening code may be a first-listed code if the reason for the visit is specifically the screening exam. It may also be used as an additional code if the screening is done during an office visit for other health problems. A screening code is not necessary if the screening is inherent to a routine examination, such as a pap smear done during a routine pelvic examination.

Should a condition be discovered during the screening then the code for the condition may be assigned as an additional diagnosis.
The Z code indicates that a screening exam is planned. A procedure code is required to confirm that the screening was performed.

The screening Z codes/categories:

Z11   Encounter for screening for infectious and parasitic diseases

Z12   Encounter for screening for malignant neoplasms

Z13   Encounter for screening for other diseases and disorders
       Except: Z13.9, Encounter for screening, unspecified

Z36   Encounter for antenatal screening for mother

6) Observation

There are two observation Z code categories. They are for use in very limited circumstances when a person is being observed for a suspected condition that is ruled out. The observation codes are not for use if an injury or illness or any signs or symptoms related to the suspected condition are present. In such cases the diagnosis/symptom code is used with the corresponding external cause code.

The observation codes are to be used as principal diagnosis only. Additional codes may be used in addition to the observation code but only if they are unrelated to the suspected condition being observed.

Codes from subcategory Z03.7, Encounter for suspected maternal and fetal conditions ruled out, may either be used as a first-listed or as an additional code assignment depending on the case. They are for use in very limited circumstances on a maternal record when an encounter is for a suspected maternal or fetal condition that is ruled out during that encounter (for example, a maternal or fetal condition may be suspected due to an abnormal test result). These codes should not be used when the condition is confirmed. In those cases, the confirmed condition should be coded. In addition, these codes are not for use if an illness or any signs or symptoms related to the suspected condition or problem are present. In such cases the diagnosis/symptom code is used.

Additional codes may be used in addition to the code from subcategory Z03.7, but only if they are unrelated to the suspected condition being evaluated.

Codes from subcategory Z03.7 may not be used for encounters for antenatal screening of mother.

For encounters for suspected fetal condition that are inconclusive following testing and evaluation, assign the appropriate code from category O35, O36, O40 or O41. The observation Z code categories:

Z03   Encounter for medical observation for suspected diseases and conditions ruled out

Z04   Encounter for examination and observation for other reasons

Except: Z04.9, Encounter for examination and observation for unspecified reason

7) Aftercare

Aftercare visit codes cover situations when the initial treatment of a disease has been performed and the patient requires continued care during the healing or recovery phase, or for the long-term consequences of the disease. The aftercare Z code should not be used if treatment is directed at a current, acute disease. The diagnosis code is to be used in these cases. Exceptions to this rule are codes Z51.0, Encounter for antineoplastic radiation therapy, and codes from subcategory Z51.1, Encounter for antineoplastic chemotherapy and immunotherapy. These codes are to be first-listed, followed by the diagnosis code when a patient's encounter is solely to receive radiation therapy, chemotherapy, or immunotherapy for the treatment of a neoplasm. If the reason for the encounter is more than one type of antineoplastic therapy, code Z51.0 and a code from subcategory Z51.1 may be assigned together, in which case one of these codes would be reported as a secondary diagnosis.

The aftercare Z codes should also not be used for aftercare for injuries. For aftercare of an injury, assign the acute injury code with the appropriate 7th character (for subsequent encounter).

The aftercare codes are generally first-listed to explain the specific reason for the encounter. An aftercare code may be used as an additional code when some type of aftercare is provided in addition to the reason for admission and no diagnosis code is applicable. An example of this would be the closure of a colostomy during an encounter for treatment of another condition.

Aftercare codes should be used in conjunction with other aftercare codes or diagnosis codes to provide better detail on the specifics of an aftercare encounter visit, unless otherwise directed by the classification. Should a patient receive multiple types of antineoplastic therapy during the same encounter, code Z51.0, Encounter for antineoplastic radiation therapy, and codes from subcategory Z51.1, Encounter for antineoplastic chemotherapy and immunotherapy, may be used together on a record. The sequencing of multiple aftercare codes depends on the circumstances of the encounter.

Certain aftercare Z code categories need a secondary diagnosis code to describe the resolving condition or sequelae. For others, the condition is included in the code title.

Additional Z code aftercare category terms include fitting and adjustment, and attention to artificial openings.

Status Z codes may be used with aftercare Z codes to indicate the nature of the aftercare. For example code Z95.1, Presence of aortocoronary bypass graft, may be used with code Z48.812, Encounter for surgical aftercare following surgery on the circulatory system, to indicate the surgery for which the aftercare is being performed. A status code should not be used when the aftercare code indicates the type of status, such as using Z43.0, Encounter for attention to tracheostomy, with Z93.0, Tracheostomy status.

The aftercare Z category/codes:

Z42   Encounter for plastic and reconstructive surgery following medical procedure or healed injury

Z43   Encounter for attention to artificial openings

Z44   Encounter for fitting and adjustment of external prosthetic device

Z45   Encounter for adjustment and management of implanted device

Z46   Encounter for fitting and adjustment of other devices

Z47   Orthopedic aftercare

Z48   Encounter for other postprocedural aftercare

Z49   Encounter for care involving renal dialysis

Z51   Encounter for other aftercare

8) Follow-up

The follow-up codes are used to explain continuing surveillance following completed treatment of a disease, condition, or injury. They imply that the condition has been fully treated and no longer exists. They should not be confused with aftercare codes, or injury codes with a 7th character for subsequent encounter, that explain ongoing care of a healing condition or its sequelae. Follow-up codes may be used in conjunction with history codes to provide the full picture of the healed condition and its treatment. The follow-up code is sequenced first, followed by the history code.

A follow-up code may be used to explain multiple visits. Should a condition be found to have recurred on the follow-up visit, then the diagnosis code for the condition should be assigned in place of the follow-up code.

The follow-up Z code categories:

Z08   Encounter for follow-up examination after completed treatment for malignant neoplasm

Z09   Encounter for follow-up examination after completed treatment for conditions other than malignant neoplasm

Z39   Encounter for maternal postpartum care and examination

9) Donor

Codes in category Z52, Donors of organs and tissues, are used for living individuals who are donating blood or other body tissue. These codes are only for individuals donating for others, not for self-donations. They are not used to identify cadaveric donations.

10) Counseling

Counseling Z codes are used when a patient or family member receives assistance in the aftermath of an illness or injury, or when support is required in coping with family or social problems. They are not used in conjunction with a diagnosis code when the counseling component of care is considered integral to standard treatment.

The counseling Z codes/categories: Z30.0- Encounter for general counseling and advice on contraception

Z31.5   Encounter for genetic counseling

Z31.6- Encounter for general counseling and advice on procreation

Z32.2   Encounter for childbirth instruction

Z32.3   Encounter for childcare instruction

Z69   Encounter for mental health services for victim and perpetrator of abuse

Z70   Counseling related to sexual attitude, behavior and orientation

Z71   Persons encountering health services for other counseling and medical advice, not elsewhere classified

Z76.81 Expectant mother prebirth pediatrician visit

11) Encounters for Obstetrical and Reproductive Services

Z codes for pregnancy are for use in those circumstances when none of the problems or complications included in the codes from the Obstetrics chapter exist (a routine prenatal visit or postpartum care). Codes in category Z34, Encounter for supervision of normal pregnancy, are always first-listed and are not to be used with any other code from the OB chapter.

The outcome of delivery, category Z37, should be included on all maternal delivery records. It is always a secondary code. Codes in category Z37 should not be used on the newborn record.

Z codes for family planning (contraceptive) or procreative management and counseling should be included on an obstetric record either during the pregnancy or the postpartum stage, if applicable.

Z codes/categories for obstetrical and reproductive services:

Z30   Encounter for contraceptive management

Z31   Encounter for procreative management

Z32.2   Encounter for childbirth instruction

Z32.3   Encounter for childcare instruction

Z33   Pregnant state

Z34   Encounter for supervision of normal pregnancy

Z36   Encounter for antenatal screening of mother

Z37   Outcome of delivery

Z39   Encounter for maternal postpartum care and examination

Z76.81 Expectant mother prebirth pediatrician visit

12) Newborns and Infants

Newborn Z codes/categories:

Z76.1   Encounter for health supervision and care of foundling

Z00.1- Encounter for routine child health examination

Z38   Liveborn infants according to place of birth and type of delivery

13) Routine and administrative examinations

The Z codes allow for the description of encounters for routine examinations, such as, a general check-up, or, examinations for administrative purposes, such as, a pre-employment physical. The codes are not to be used if the examination is for diagnosis of a suspected condition or for treatment purposes. In such cases the diagnosis code is used. During a routine exam, should a diagnosis or condition be discovered, it should be coded as an additional code. Pre-existing and chronic conditions and history codes may also be included as additional codes as long as the examination is for administrative purposes and not focused on any particular condition.

Some of the codes for routine health examinations distinguish between "with" and "without" abnormal findings. Code assignment depends on the information that is known at the time the encounter is being coded. For example, if no abnormal findings were found during the examination, but the encounter is being coded before test results are back, it is acceptable to assign the code for "without abnormal findings." When assigning a code for "with abnormal findings," additional code(s) should be assigned to identify the specific abnormal finding(s).

Pre-operative examination and pre-procedural laboratory examination Z codes are for use only in those situations when a patient is being cleared for a procedure or surgery and no treatment is given.

The Z codes/categories for routine and administrative examinations:

Z00   Encounter for general examination without complaint, suspected or reported diagnosis

Z01   Encounter for other special examination without complaint, suspected or reported diagnosis

Z02   Encounter for administrative examination
       Except: Z02.9, Encounter for administrative examinations, unspecified

Z32.0- Encounter for pregnancy test

14) Miscellaneous Z codes

The miscellaneous Z codes capture a number of other health care encounters that do not fall into one of the other categories. Certain of these codes identify the reason for the encounter; others are for use as additional codes that provide useful information on circumstances that may affect a patient's care and treatment.

Prophylactic Organ Removal

For encounters specifically for prophylactic removal of an organ (such as prophylactic removal of breasts due to a genetic susceptibility to cancer or a family history of cancer), the principal or first-listed code should be a code from category Z40, Encounter for prophylactic surgery, followed by the appropriate codes to identify the associated risk factor (such as genetic susceptibility or family history).

If the patient has a malignancy of one site and is having prophylactic removal at another site to prevent either a new primary malignancy or metastatic disease, a code for the malignancy should also be assigned in addition to a code from subcategory

Z40.0   Encounter for prophylactic surgery for risk factors related to malignant neoplasms.

A Z40.0 code should not be assigned if the patient is having organ removal for treatment of a malignancy, such as the removal of the testes for the treatment of prostate cancer.

Miscellaneous Z codes/categories:

Z28   Immunization not carried out
         Except: Z28.3, Underimmunization status

Z40   Encounter for prophylactic surgery

Z41   Encounter for procedures for purposes other than remedying health state
         Except: Z41.9, Encounter for procedure for purposes other than remedying health state, unspecified

Z53   Persons encountering health services for specific procedures and treatment, not carried out

Z55   Problems related to education and literacy

Z56   Problems related to employment and unemployment

Z57   Occupational exposure to risk factors

Z58   Problems related to physical environment

Z59   Problems related to housing and economic circumstances

Z60   Problems related to social environment

Z62   Problems related to upbringing

Z63   Other problems related to primary support group, including family circumstances

Z64   Problems related to certain psychosocial circumstances

Z65   Problems related to other psychosocial circumstances

Z72   Problems related to lifestyle

Z73   Problems related to life management difficulty

Z74   Problems related to care provider dependency
         Except: Z74.01, Bed confinement status

Z75   Problems related to medical facilities and other health care

Z76.0   Encounter for issue of repeat prescription

Z76.3   Healthy person accompanying sick person

Z76.4   Other boarder to healthcare facility

Z76.5   Malingerer [conscious simulation]

Z91.1-   Patient's noncompliance with medical treatment and regimen

Z91.89   Other specified personal risk factors, not elsewhere classified

15) Nonspecific Z codes

Certain Z codes are so non-specific, or potentially redundant with other codes in the classification, that there can be little justification for their use in the inpatient setting. Their use in the outpatient setting should be limited to those instances when there is no further documentation to permit more precise coding. Otherwise, any sign or symptom or any other reason for visit that is captured in another code should be used.

Nonspecific Z codes/categories:

Z02.9   Encounter for administrative examinations, unspecified

Z04.9   Encounter for examination and observation for unspecified reason

Z13.9   Encounter for screening, unspecified

Z41.9   Encounter for procedure for purposes other than remedying health state, unspecified

Z52.9   Donor of unspecified organ or tissue

Z86.59   Personal history of other mental and behavioral disorders

Z88.9   Allergy status to unspecified drugs, medicaments and biological substances status

Z92.0   Personal history of contraception

16) Z Codes That May Only be Principal/First-listed Diagnosis

The following Z codes/categories may only be reported as the principal/first-listed diagnosis, except when there are multiple encounters on the same day and the medical records for the encounters are combined:

Z00   Encounter for general examination without complaint, suspected or reported diagnosis

Z01   Encounter for other special examination without complaint, suspected or reported diagnosis

Z02   Encounter for administrative examination

Z03   Encounter for medical observation for suspected diseases and conditions ruled out

Z04   Encounter for examination and observation for other reasons

Z33.2   Encounter for elective termination of pregnancy

Z31.81 Encounter for male factor infertility in female patient

Z31.82 Encounter for Rh incompatibility status

Z31.83 Encounter for assisted reproductive fertility procedure cycle

Z31.84 Encounter for fertility preservation procedure

Z34   Encounter for supervision of normal pregnancy

Z39   Encounter for maternal postpartum care and examination

Z38   Liveborn infants according to place of birth and type of delivery

Z42   Encounter for plastic and reconstructive surgery following medical procedure or healed injury

Z51.0   Encounter for antineoplastic radiation therapy

Z51.1- Encounter for antineoplastic chemotherapy and immunotherapy

Z52   Donors of organs and tissues
        Except: Z52.9, Donor of unspecified organ or tissue

Z76.1   Encounter for health supervision and care of foundling

Z76.2   Encounter for health supervision and care of other healthy infant and child

Z99.12 Encounter for respirator [ventilator] dependence during power failure

SECTION II. SELECTION OF PRINCIPAL DIAGNOSIS

The circumstances of inpatient admission always govern the selection of principal diagnosis. The principal diagnosis is defined in the Uniform Hospital Discharge Data Set (UHDDS) as "that condition established after study to be chiefly responsible for occasioning the admission of the patient to the hospital for care."

The UHDDS definitions are used by hospitals to report inpatient data elements in a standardized manner. These data elements and their definitions can be found in the July 31, 1985, Federal Register (Vol. 50, No, 147), pp. 31038-40.

Since that time the application of the UHDDS definitions has been expanded to include all non-outpatient settings (acute care, short term, long term care and psychiatric hospitals; home health agencies; rehab facilities; nursing homes, etc).

In determining principal diagnosis the coding conventions in the ICD-10-CM, the Tabular List and Alphabetic Index take precedence over these official coding guidelines.

The importance of consistent, complete documentation in the medical record cannot be overemphasized. Without such documentation the application of all coding guidelines is a difficult, if not impossible, task.

CODES FOR SYMPTOMS, SIGNS, AND ILL-DEFINED CONDITIONS

Codes for symptoms, signs, and ill-defined conditions from Chapter 18 are not to be used as principal diagnosis when a related definitive diagnosis has been established.

TWO OR MORE INTERRELATED CONDITIONS, EACH POTENTIALLY MEETING THE DEFINITION FOR PRINCIPAL DIAGNOSIS.

When there are two or more interrelated conditions (such as diseases in the same ICD-10-CM chapter or manifestations characteristically associated with a certain disease) potentially meeting the definition of principal diagnosis, either condition may be sequenced first, unless the circumstances of the admission, the therapy provided, the Tabular List, or the Alphabetic Index indicate otherwise.

TWO OR MORE DIAGNOSES THAT EQUALLY MEET THE DEFINITION FOR PRINCIPAL DIAGNOSIS

In the unusual instance when two or more diagnoses equally meet the criteria for principal diagnosis as determined by the circumstances of admission, diagnostic workup and/or therapy provided, and the Alphabetic Index, Tabular List, or another coding guidelines does not provide sequencing direction, any one of the diagnoses may be sequenced first.

TWO OR MORE COMPARATIVE OR CONTRASTING CONDITIONS.

In those rare instances when two or more contrasting or comparative diagnoses are documented as "either/or" (or similar terminology), they are coded as if the diagnoses were confirmed and the diagnoses are sequenced according to the circumstances of the admission. If no further determination can be made as to which diagnosis should be principal, either diagnosis may be sequenced first.

A SYMPTOM(S) FOLLOWED BY CONTRASTING/COMPARATIVE DIAGNOSES

When a symptom(s) is followed by contrasting/comparative diagnoses, the symptom code is sequenced first. All the contrasting/comparative diagnoses should be coded as additional diagnoses.

ORIGINAL TREATMENT PLAN NOT CARRIED OUT

Sequence as the principal diagnosis the condition, which after study occasioned the admission to the hospital, even though treatment may not have been carried out due to unforeseen circumstances.

COMPLICATIONS OF SURGERY AND OTHER MEDICAL CARE

When the admission is for treatment of a complication resulting from surgery or other medical care, the complication code is sequenced as the principal diagnosis. If the complication is classified to the T80-T88 series and the code lacks the necessary specificity in describing the complication, an additional code for the specific complication should be assigned.

UNCERTAIN DIAGNOSIS

If the diagnosis documented at the time of discharge is qualified as "probable", "suspected", "likely", "questionable", "possible", or "still to be ruled out", or other similar terms indicating uncertainty, code the condition as if it existed or was established. The bases for these guidelines are the diagnostic workup, arrangements for further workup or observation, and initial therapeutic approach that correspond most closely with the established diagnosis.

Note: This guideline is applicable only to inpatient admissions to short-term, acute, long-term care and psychiatric hospitals.\

ADMISSION FROM OBSERVATION UNIT

1. **Admission Following Medical Observation**

    When a patient is admitted to an observation unit for a medical condition, which either worsens or does not improve, and is subsequently admitted as an inpatient of the same hospital for this same medical condition, the principal diagnosis would be the medical condition which led to the hospital admission.

2. **Admission Following Post-Operative Observation**

    When a patient is admitted to an observation unit to monitor a condition (or complication) that develops following outpatient surgery, and then is subsequently admitted as an inpatient of the same hospital, hospitals should apply the Uniform Hospital Discharge Data Set (UHDDS) definition of principal diagnosis as "that condition established after study to be chiefly responsible for occasioning the admission of the patient to the hospital for care."

ADMISSION FROM OUTPATIENT SURGERY

When a patient receives surgery in the hospital's outpatient surgery department and is subsequently admitted for continuing inpatient care at the same hospital, the following guidelines should be followed in selecting the principal diagnosis for the inpatient admission:

*   If the reason for the inpatient admission is a complication, assign the complication as the principal diagnosis.
*   If no complication, or other condition, is documented as the reason for the inpatient admission, assign the reason for the outpatient surgery as the principal diagnosis.

- If the reason for the inpatient admission is another condition unrelated to the surgery, assign the unrelated condition as the principal diagnosis.

SECTION III. REPORTING ADDITIONAL DIAGNOSES

GENERAL RULES FOR OTHER (ADDITIONAL) DIAGNOSES

For reporting purposes the definition for "other diagnoses" is interpreted as additional conditions that affect patient care in terms of requiring: clinical evaluation; or therapeutic treatment; or diagnostic procedures; or extended length of hospital stay; or increased nursing care and/or monitoring.

The UHDDS item 11-b defines Other Diagnoses as "all conditions that coexist at the time of admission, that develop subsequently, or that affect the treatment received and/or the length of stay. Diagnoses that relate to an earlier episode which have no bearing on the current hospital stay are to be excluded." UHDDS definitions apply to inpatients in acute care, short-term, long term care and psychiatric hospital setting. The UHDDS definitions are used by acute care short- term hospitals to report inpatient data elements in a standardized manner. These data elements and their definitions can be found in the July 31, 1985, Federal Register (Vol. 50, No, 147), pp. 31038-40.

Since that time the application of the UHDDS definitions has been expanded to include all non-outpatient settings (acute care, short term, long term care and psychiatric hospitals; home health agencies; rehab facilities; nursing homes, etc).

The following guidelines are to be applied in designating "other diagnoses" when neither the Alphabetic Index nor the Tabular List in ICD-10-CM provide direction. The listing of the diagnoses in the patient record is the responsibility of the attending provider.

PREVIOUS CONDITIONS

If the provider has included a diagnosis in the final diagnostic statement, such as the discharge summary or the face sheet, it should ordinarily be coded. Some providers include in the diagnostic statement resolved conditions or diagnoses and status-post procedures from previous admission that have no bearing on the current stay. Such conditions are not to be reported and are coded only if required by hospital policy.

However, history codes (categories Z80-Z87) may be used as secondary codes if the historical condition or family history has an impact on current care or influences treatment.

ABNORMAL FINDINGS

Abnormal findings (laboratory, x-ray, pathologic, and other diagnostic results) are not coded and reported unless the provider indicates their clinical significance. If the findings are outside the normal range and the attending provider has ordered other tests to evaluate the condition or prescribed treatment, it is appropriate to ask the provider whether the abnormal finding should be added.

Please note: This differs from the coding practices in the outpatient setting for coding encounters for diagnostic tests that have been interpreted by a provider.

UNCERTAIN DIAGNOSIS

If the diagnosis documented at the time of discharge is qualified as "probable", "suspected", "likely", "questionable", "possible", or "still to be ruled out" or other similar terms indicating uncertainty, code the condition as if it existed or was established. The bases for these guidelines are the diagnostic workup, arrangements for further workup or observation, and initial therapeutic approach that correspond most closely with the established diagnosis.

Note: This guideline is applicable only to inpatient admissions to short-term, acute, long-term care and psychiatric hospitals.

SECTION IV. DIAGNOSTIC CODING AND REPORTING GUIDELINES FOR OUTPATIENT SERVICES

These coding guidelines for outpatient diagnoses have been approved for use by hospitals/ providers in coding and reporting hospital-based outpatient services and provider-based office visits.

Information about the use of certain abbreviations, punctuation, symbols, and other conventions used in the ICD-10-CM Tabular List (code numbers and titles), can be found in Section IA of these guidelines, under "Conventions Used in the Tabular List." Information about the correct sequence to use in finding a code is also described in Section I.

The terms encounter and visit are often used interchangeably in describing outpatient service contacts and, therefore, appear together in these guidelines without distinguishing one from the other.

Though the conventions and general guidelines apply to all settings, coding guidelines for outpatient and provider reporting of diagnoses will vary in a number of instances from those for inpatient diagnoses, recognizing that:

The Uniform Hospital Discharge Data Set (UHDDS) definition of principal diagnosis applies only to inpatients in acute, short-term, long-term care and psychiatric hospitals.

Coding guidelines for inconclusive diagnoses (probable, suspected, rule out, etc.) were developed for inpatient reporting and do not apply to outpatients.

SELECTION OF FIRST-LISTED CONDITION

In the outpatient setting, the term first-listed diagnosis is used in lieu of principal diagnosis.

In determining the first-listed diagnosis the coding conventions of ICD-10-CM, as well as the general and disease specific guidelines take precedence over the outpatient guidelines.

Diagnoses often are not established at the time of the initial encounter/visit. It may take two or more visits before the diagnosis is confirmed.

The most critical rule involves beginning the search for the correct code assignment through the Alphabetic Index. Never begin searching initially in the Tabular List as this will lead to coding errors.

1) **Outpatient Surgery**

When a patient presents for outpatient surgery (same day surgery), code the reason for the surgery as the first-listed diagnosis (reason for the encounter), even if the surgery is not performed due to a contraindication.

2) **Observation Stay**

When a patient is admitted for observation for a medical condition, assign a code for the medical condition as the first-listed diagnosis.

When a patient presents for outpatient surgery and develops complications requiring admission to observation, code the reason for the surgery as the first reported diagnosis (reason for the encounter), followed by codes for the complications as secondary diagnoses.

CODES FROM A00.0 THROUGH T88.9, Z00-Z99

The appropriate code(s) from A00.0 through T88.9, Z00-Z99 must be used to identify diagnoses, symptoms, conditions, problems, complaints, or other reason(s) for the encounter/visit.

ACCURATE REPORTING OF ICD-10-CM DIAGNOSIS CODES

For accurate reporting of ICD-10-CM diagnosis codes, the documentation should describe the patient's condition, using terminology which includes specific diagnoses as well as symptoms, problems, or reasons for the encounter. There are ICD-10-CM codes to describe all of these.

CODES THAT DESCRIBE SYMPTOMS AND SIGNS

Codes that describe symptoms and signs, as opposed to diagnoses, are acceptable for reporting purposes when a diagnosis has not been established (confirmed) by the provider. Chapter 18 of ICD-10-CM, Symptoms, Signs, and Abnormal Clinical and Laboratory Findings Not Elsewhere Classified (codes R00-R99) contain many, but not all codes for symptoms.

ENCOUNTERS FOR CIRCUMSTANCES OTHER THAN A DISEASE OR INJURY

ICD-10-CM provides codes to deal with encounters for circumstances other than a disease or injury. The Factors Influencing Health Status and Contact with Health Services codes (Z00-Z99) are provided to deal with occasions when circumstances other than a disease or injury are recorded as diagnosis or problems.

LEVEL OF DETAIL IN CODING

1) **ICD-10-CM codes with 3, 4, 5, 6 or 7 characters**

ICD-10-CM is composed of codes with 3, 4, 5, 6 or 7 characters. Codes with three characters are included in ICD-10-CM as the heading of a category of codes that may be further subdivided by the use of fourth, fifth, sixth or seventh characters to provide greater specificity.

2) **Use of full number of characters required for a code**

A three-character code is to be used only if it is not further subdivided. A code is invalid if it has not been coded to the full number of characters required for that code, including the 7th character extension, if applicable.

ICD-10-CM CODE FOR THE DIAGNOSIS, CONDITION, PROBLEM, OR OTHER REASON FOR ENCOUNTER/VISIT

List first the ICD-10-CM code for the diagnosis, condition, problem, or other reason for encounter/visit shown in the medical record to be chiefly responsible for the services provided. List additional codes that describe any coexisting conditions. In some cases the first-listed diagnosis may be a symptom when a diagnosis has not been established (confirmed) by the physician.

UNCERTAIN DIAGNOSIS

Do not code diagnoses documented as "probable", "suspected," "questionable," "rule out," or "working diagnosis" or other similar terms indicating uncertainty. Rather, code the condition(s) to the highest degree of certainty for that encounter/visit, such as symptoms, signs, abnormal test results, or other reason for the visit.

Please note: This differs from the coding practices used by short-term, acute care, long-term care and psychiatric hospitals.

CHRONIC DISEASES

Chronic diseases treated on an ongoing basis may be coded and reported as many times as the patient receives treatment and care for the condition(s)

CODE ALL DOCUMENTED CONDITIONS THAT COEXIST

Code all documented conditions that coexist at the time of the encounter/visit, and require or affect patient care treatment or management. Do not code conditions that were previously treated and no longer exist. However, history codes (categories Z80- Z87) may be used as secondary codes if the historical condition or family history has an impact on current care or influences treatment.

PATIENTS RECEIVING DIAGNOSTIC SERVICES ONLY

For patients receiving diagnostic services only during an encounter/visit, sequence first the diagnosis, condition, problem, or other reason for encounter/visit shown in the medical record to be chiefly responsible for the outpatient services provided during the encounter/visit. Codes for other diagnoses (e.g., chronic conditions) may be sequenced as additional diagnoses.

For encounters for routine laboratory/radiology testing in the absence of any signs, symptoms, or associated diagnosis, assign Z01.89, Encounter for other specified special examinations. If routine testing is performed during the same encounter as a test to evaluate a sign, symptom, or diagnosis, it is appropriate to assign both the V code and the code describing the reason for the non-routine test.

For outpatient encounters for diagnostic tests that have been interpreted by a physician, and the final report is available at the time of coding, code any confirmed or definitive diagnosis(es) documented in the interpretation. Do not code related signs and symptoms as additional diagnoses.

NOTE: This differs from the coding practice in the hospital inpatient setting regarding abnormal findings on test results.

PATIENTS RECEIVING THERAPEUTIC SERVICES ONLY

For patients receiving therapeutic services only during an encounter/visit, sequence first the diagnosis, condition, problem, or other reason for encounter/visit shown in the medical record to be chiefly responsible for the outpatient services provided during the encounter/visit. Codes for other diagnoses (e.g., chronic conditions) may be sequenced as additional diagnoses.

The only exception to this rule is that when the primary reason for the admission/encounter is chemotherapy or radiation therapy, the appropriate Z code for the service is listed first, and the diagnosis or problem for which the service is being performed listed second.

PATIENTS RECEIVING PREOPERATIVE EVALUATIONS ONLY

For patients receiving preoperative evaluations only, sequence first a code from subcategory Z01.81, Encounter for pre-procedural examinations, to describe the pre-op consultations. Assign a code for the condition to describe the reason for the surgery as an additional diagnosis. Code also any findings related to the pre-op evaluation.

AMBULATORY SURGERY

For ambulatory surgery, code the diagnosis for which the surgery was performed. If the postoperative diagnosis is known to be different from the preoperative diagnosis at the time the diagnosis is confirmed, select the postoperative diagnosis for coding, since it is the most definitive.

ENCOUNTERS FOR GENERAL MEDICAL EXAMINATIONS WITH ABNORMAL FINDINGS

The subcategories for encounters for general medical examinations, Z00.0-, provide codes for with and without abnormal findings. Should a general medical examination result in an abnormal finding, the code for general medical examination with abnormal finding should be assigned as the first-listed diagnosis. A secondary code for the abnormal finding should also be coded.

SAMPLE ICD-10-CM CODES FROM THIS CHAPTER

Note: Z codes represent reasons for encounters. A corresponding procedure code must accompany a Z code if a procedure is performed. Categories Z00-Z99are provided for occasions when circumstances other than a disease, injury or external cause classifiable to categories A00-Y89 are recorded as 'diagnoses' or 'problems'. This can arise in two main ways:

(a) When a person who may or may not be sick encounters the health services for some specific purpose, such as to receive limited care or service for a current condition, to donate an organ or tissue, to receive prophylactic vaccination (immunization), or to discuss a problem which is in itself not a disease or injury.

(b) When some circumstance or problem is present which influences the person's health status but is not in itself a current illness or injury.

This chapter contains the following blocks:	
Z00-Z13	Persons encountering health services for examinations
Z14-Z15	Genetic carrier and genetic susceptibility to disease
Z16	Infection with drug resistant microorganisms
Z17	Estrogen receptor status
Z18	Retained foreign body fragments
Z20-Z28	Persons with potential health hazards related to communicable diseases
Z30-Z39	Persons encountering health services in circumstances related to reproduction
Z40-Z53	Encounters for other specific health care
Z55-Z65	Persons with potential health hazards related to socioeconomic and psychosocial circumstances
Z66	Do not resuscitate status
Z67	Blood type
Z68	Body mass index (BMI)
Z69-Z76	Persons encountering health services in other circumstances
Z77-Z99	Persons with potential health hazards related to family and personal history and certain conditions influencing health status

PERSONS ENCOUNTERING HEALTH SERVICES FOR EXAMINATIONS (Z00-Z13)

Note: Nonspecific abnormal findings disclosed at the time of these examinations are classified to categories R70-R94.

Excludes 1: examinations related to pregnancy and reproduction (Z30-Z36, Z39.-)

Z00   Encounter for general examination without complaint, suspected or reported diagnosis

Excludes 1: encounter for examination for administrative purposes (Z02.-)

Excludes 2: encounter for pre-procedural examinations (Z01.81-)
special screening examinations (Z11-Z13)

Z00.0 **Encounter for general adult medical examination**
Encounter for adult periodic examination (annual) (physical) and any associated laboratory and radiologic examinations

Excludes 1: encounter for examination of sign or symptom- code to sign or symptom
general health check-up of infant or child (Z00.12.-)

Z00.00   **Encounter for general adult medical examination without abnormal findings**
Encounter for adult health check-up NOS

Z00.01   **Encounter for general adult medical examination with abnormal findings**

Use additional code to identify abnormal findings

Z00.1 Encounter for newborn, infant and child health examinations

Z00.11 Newborn health examination
Health check for child under 29 days old
Use additional code to identify any abnormal findings

Excludes 1: health check for child over 28 days old (Z00.12-)

Z00.110 Health examination for newborn under 8days old
Health check for newborn under 8 days old

Z00.111 Health examination for newborn 8 to 28 days old
Health check for newborn 8 to 28 days old
Newborn weight check

Z00.12 Encounter for routine child health examination
Encounter for development testing of infant or child
Health check (routine) for child over 28 days old

Excludes 1: health check for child under 29 days old (Z0.11-)
health supervision of foundling or other healthy infant or
child (Z76.1-Z76.2)
newborn health examination (Z00.11-)

**Z00.121 Encounter for routine child health examination with
abnormal findings**
Use additional code to identify abnormal findings

**Z00.129 Encounter for routine child health examination without
abnormal findings**
Encounter for routine child health examination NOS

Z00.2 Encounter for examination for period of rapid growth in childhood

Z00.3 Encounter for examination for adolescent development state
Encounter for puberty development state

Z00.5 Encounter for examination of potential donor of organ and tissue

**Z00.6 Encounter for examination for normal comparison and control in clinical
research program**

Z00.7 Encounter for examination for period of delayed growth in childhood

**Z00.70 Encounter for examination for period of delayed growth in childhood
without abnormal findings**
**Z00.71 Encounter for examination for period of delayed growth in childhood
with abnormal findings**
Use additional code to identify abnormal findings

Z00.8   Encounter for other general examination
Encounter for health examination in population surveys

Z01   Encounter for other special examination without complaint, suspected or reported diagnosis

Includes: routine examination of specific system

Excludes 1: encounter for examination for administrative purposes (Z02.-)
encounter for examination for suspected conditions, proven not to exist (Z03.-)
encounter for laboratory and radiologic examinations as a component of general
medical examinations (Z00.0-)
encounter for laboratory, radiologic and imaging examinations for sign(s) and symptom(s) - code to the sign(s) or symptom(s)

Excludes 2: screening examinations (Z11-Z13)

Note: Codes from category Z01 represent the reason for the encounter. A separate procedure code is required to identify any examinations or procedures performed

Z01.0   Encounter for examination of eyes and vision

Excludes 1: examination for driving license (Z02.4)

Z01.00   Encounter for examination of eyes and vision without abnormal findings
Encounter for examination of eyes and vision NOS

Z01.01   Encounter for examination of eyes and vision with abnormal findings
Use additional code to identify abnormal findings

Z01.1   Encounter for examination of ears and hearing

Z01.10   Encounter for examination of ears and hearing without abnormal findings
Encounter for examination of ears and hearing NOS

Z01.11   Encounter for examination of ears and hearing with abnormal findings

Z01.110 Encounter for hearing examination following failed hearing screening

Z01.118 Encounter for examination of ears and hearing with other abnormal findings
Use additional code to identify abnormal findings

Z01.12   Encounter for hearing conservation and treatment

Z01.2   Encounter for dental examination and cleaning

Z01.20 **Encounter for dental examination and cleaning without abnormal findings**
Encounter for dental examination and cleaning NOS

FORWARD MAPPING SAMPLE (ICD-9-CM ➡ ICD-10-CM)

ICD-9-CM CODE & DESCRIPTION		ICDCD-10-CM CODE & DESCRIPTION	
V41.0	Problems with sight	Z97.3	Presence of spectacles and contact lenses
V41.1	Other eye problems	H57.9	Unspecified disorder of eye and adnexa
V41.2	Problems with hearing	Z97.4	Presence of external hearing-aid
V41.3	Other ear problems	H93.90	Unspecified disorder of ear unspecified ear
V41.4	Problems with voice production	R47.89	Other speech disturbances
V41.5	Problems with smell and taste	R43.9	Unspecified disturbances of smell and taste
V41.6	Problems with swallowing and mastication	R13.10	Dysphagia unspecified
V41.7	Problems with sexual function	F52.9	Unspecified sexual dysfunction not due to a substance or known physiological condition
V41.8	Other problems with special functions	R68.89	Other general symptoms and signs
V41.9	Unspecified problem with special functions	R69	Illness unspecified
V42.0	Kidney replaced by transplant	Z94.0	Kidney transplant status
V42.1	Heart replaced by transplant	Z94.1	Heart transplant status
V42.2	Heart valve replaced by transplant	Z95.3	Presence of xenogenic heart valve
V42.3	Skin replaced by transplant	Z94.5	Skin transplant status
V42.4	Bone replaced by transplant	Z94.6	Bone transplant status
V42.5	Cornea replaced by transplant	Z94.7	Corneal transplant status
V42.6	Lung replaced by transplant	Z94.2	Lung transplant status
V42.7	Liver replaced by transplant	Z94.4	Liver transplant status
V42.81	Bone marrow replaced by transplant	Z94.81	Bone marrow transplant status
V42.82	Peripheral stem cells replaced by transplant	Z94.84	Stem cells transplant status
V42.83	Pancreas replaced by transplant	Z94.83	Pancreas transplant status
V42.84	Organ or tissue replaced by transplant intestines	Z94.82	Intestine transplant status
V42.89	Other specified organ or tissue replaced by transplant	Z94.89	Other transplanted organ and tissue status
V42.9	Unspecified organ or tissue replaced by transplant	Z94.9	Transplanted organ and tissue status unspecified

V43.0	Eye globe replaced by other means	Z97.0	Presence of artificial eye
V43.1	Lens replaced by other means	Z96.1	Presence of intraocular lens
V43.21	Heart replaced by heart assist device	Z95.811	Presence of heart assist device
V43.22	Heart replaced by fully implantable artificial heart	Z95.812	Presence of fully implantable artificial heart
V43.3	Heart valve replaced by other means	Z95.2	Presence of prosthetic heart valve
V43.4	Blood vessel replaced by other means	Z95.828	Presence of other vascular implants and grafts
V43.5	Bladder replaced by other means	Z96.0	Presence of urogenital implants
V43.60	Unspecified joint replacement	Z96.60	Presence of unspecified orthopedic joint implant
V43.61	Shoulder joint replacement	Z96.619	Presence of unspecified artificial shoulder joint
V43.62	Elbow joint replacement	Z96.629	Presence of unspecified artificial elbow joint
V43.63	Wrist joint replacement	Z96.639	Presence of unspecified artificial wrist joint
V43.64	Hip joint replacement	Z96.649	Presence of unspecified artificial hip joint
V43.65	Knee joint replacement	Z96.659	Presence of unspecified artificial knee joint
V43.66	Ankle joint replacement	Z96.669	Presence of unspecified artificial ankle joint
V43.69	Other joint replacement	Z96.698	Presence of other orthopedic joint implants
V43.7	Limb replaced by other means	Z97.10	Presence of artificial limb (complete) (partial) unspecified

BACKWARD MAPPING SAMPLE (ICD-9-CM ➡ ICD-10-CM)			
ICD-10-CM CODE & DESCRIPTION		**ICD-9-CM CODE & DESCRIPTION**	
Z00.00	Encounter for general adult medical examination without abnormal findings	V70.0	Routine general medical examination at a health care facility
Z00.01	Encounter for general adult medical examination with abnormal findings	V70.0	Routine general medical examination at a health care facility
Z00.110	Health examination for newborn under 8 days old	V20.31	Health supervision for newborn under 8 days
Z00.111	Health examination for newborn 8 to 28 days old	V20.32	Health supervision for newborn 8 to 28 days old
Z00.121	Encounter for routine child health examination with abnormal findings	V20.2	Routine infant or child health check

Z00.129	Encounter for routine child health examination without abnormal findings	**V20.2**	Routine infant or child health check
Z00.2	Encounter for examination for period of rapid growth in childhood	**V21.0**	Period of rapid growth in childhood
Z00.3	Encounter for examination for adolescent development state	**V21.1**	Puberty
Z00.3	Encounter for examination for adolescent development state	**V21.2**	Other development of adolescence
Z00.5	Encounter for examination of potential donor of organ and tissue	**V70.8**	Other specified general medical examinations
Z00.6	Encounter for examination for normal comparison and control in clinical research program	**V70.7**	Examination of participant in clinical trial
Z00.70	Encounter for examination for period of delayed growth in childhood without abnormal findings	**V70.8**	Other specified general medical examinations
Z00.71	Encounter for examination for period of delayed growth in childhood with abnormal findings	**V70.8**	Other specified general medical examinations
Z00.8	Encounter for other general examination	**V70.6**	Health examination in population surveys
Z00.8	Encounter for other general examination	**V70.8**	Other specified general medical examinations
Z01.00	Encounter for examination of eyes and vision without abnormal findings	**V72.0**	Examination of eyes and vision
Z01.01	Encounter for examination of eyes and vision with abnormal findings	**V72.0**	Examination of eyes and vision
Z01.10	Encounter for examination of ears and hearing without abnormal findings	**V72.19**	Other examination of ears and hearing
Z01.110	Encounter for hearing examination following failed hearing screening	**V72.11**	Encounter for hearing examination following failed hearing screening
Z01.118	Encounter for examination of ears and hearing with other abnormal findings	**V72.19**	Other examination of ears and hearing
Z01.12	Encounter for hearing conservation and treatment	**V72.12**	Encounter for hearing conservation and treatment
Z01.20	Encounter for dental examination and cleaning without abnormal findings	**V72.2**	Dental examination
Z01.21	Encounter for dental examination and cleaning with abnormal findings	**V72.2**	Dental examination

Z01.30	Encounter for examination of blood pressure without abnormal findings	V72.85	Other specified examination
Z01.31	Encounter for examination of blood pressure with abnormal findings	V72.85	Other specified examination
Z01.411	Encounter for gynecological examination (general) (routine) with abnormal findings	V72.31	Routine gynecological examination
Z01.419	Encounter for gynecological examination (general) (routine) without abnormal findings	V72.31	Routine gynecological examination
Z01.42	Encounter for cervical smear to confirm findings of recent normal smear following initial abnormal smear	V72.32	Encounter for Papanicolaou cervical smear to confirm findings of recent normal smear following initial abnormal smear
Z01.810	Encounter for preprocedural cardiovascular examination	V72.81	Pre-operative cardiovascular examination
Z01.811	Encounter for preprocedural respiratory examination	V72.82	Pre-operative respiratory examination
Z01.812	Encounter for preprocedural laboratory examination	V72.63	Pre-procedural laboratory examination
Z01.818	Encounter for other preprocedural examination	V72.83	Other specified pre-operative examination
Z01.818	Encounter for other preprocedural examination	V72.84	Pre-operative examination, unspecified
Z01.82	Encounter for allergy testing	V72.85	Other specified examination
Z01.83	Encounter for blood typing	V72.86	Encounter for blood typing
Z01.84	Encounter for antibody response examination	V72.61	Antibody response examination
Z01.89	Encounter for other specified special examinations	V72.85	Other specified examination
Z02.0	Encounter for examination for admission to educational institution	V70.3	Other general medical examination for administrative purposes
Z02.1	Encounter for pre-employment examination	V70.5	Health examination of defined subpopulations
Z02.2	Encounter for examination for admission to residential institution	V70.3	Other general medical examination for administrative purposes

PRESENT ON ADMISSION REPORTING GUIDELINES

INTRODUCTION

These guidelines are to be used as a supplement to the *ICD-10-CM Official Guidelines for Coding and Reporting* to facilitate the assignment of the Present on Admission (POA) indicator for each diagnosis and external cause of injury code reported on claim forms (UB-04 and 837 Institutional).

These guidelines are not intended to replace any guidelines in the main body of the *ICD-10- CM Official Guidelines for Coding and Reporting*. The POA guidelines are not intended to provide guidance on when a condition should be coded, but rather, how to apply the POA indicator to the final set of diagnosis codes that have been assigned in accordance with Sections I, II, and III of the official coding guidelines. Subsequent to the assignment of the ICD-10-CM codes, the POA indicator should then be assigned to those conditions that have been coded.

As stated in the Introduction to the ICD-10-CM Official Guidelines for Coding and Reporting, a joint effort between the healthcare provider and the coder is essential to achieve complete and accurate documentation, code assignment, and reporting of diagnoses and procedures. The importance of consistent, complete documentation in the medical record cannot be overemphasized. Medical record documentation from any provider involved in the care and treatment of the patient may be used to support the determination of whether a condition was present on admission or not. In the context of the official coding guidelines, the term "provider" means a physician or any qualified healthcare practitioner who is legally accountable for establishing the patient's diagnosis.

These guidelines are not a substitute for the provider's clinical judgment as to the determination of whether a condition was/was not present on admission. The provider should be queried regarding issues related to the linking of signs/symptoms, timing of test results, and the timing of findings.

GENERAL REPORTING REQUIREMENTS

All claims involving inpatient admissions to general acute care hospitals or other facilities are subject to a law or regulation mandating collection of present on admission information.

Present on admission is defined as present at the time the order for inpatient admission occurs -- conditions that develop during an outpatient encounter, including emergency department, observation, or outpatient surgery, are considered as present on admission.

POA indicator is assigned to principal and secondary diagnoses (as defined in Section II of the Official Guidelines for Coding and Reporting) and the external cause of injury codes.

Issues related to inconsistent, missing, conflicting or unclear documentation must still be resolved by the provider.

If a condition would not be coded and reported based on UHDDS definitions and current official coding guidelines, then the POA indicator would not be reported.

Reporting Options

Y   =   Yes
N   =   No
U   =   Unknown
W   =   Clinically undetermined

Unreported/Not used (or "1" for Medicare usage) - (Exempt from POA reporting)

Reporting Definitions

Y   =   present at the time of inpatient admission

N   =   not present at the time of inpatient admission
U   =   documentation is insufficient to determine if condition is present on
        admission
W   =   provider is unable to clinically determine whether condition was
        present on admission or not

Timeframe for POA Identification and Documentation

There is no required timeframe as to when a provider (per the definition of "provider" used in these guidelines) must identify or document a condition to be present on admission. In some clinical situations, it may not be possible for a provider to make a definitive diagnosis (or a condition may not be recognized or reported by the patient) for a period of time after admission. In some cases it may be several days before the provider arrives at a definitive diagnosis. This does not mean that the condition was not present on admission. Determination of whether the condition was present on admission or not will be based on the applicable POA guideline as identified in this document, or on the provider's best clinical judgment.

If at the time of code assignment the documentation is unclear as to whether a condition was present on admission or not, it is appropriate to query the provider for clarification.

ASSIGNING THE POA INDICATOR

Condition is on the "Exempt from Reporting" list

Leave the "present on admission" field blank if the condition is on the list of ICD-10-CM codes for which this field is not applicable. This is the only circumstance in which the field may be left blank.

POA Explicitly Documented

Assign Y for any condition the provider explicitly documents as being present on admission.

Assign N for any condition the provider explicitly documents as not present at the time of admission.

Conditions diagnosed prior to inpatient admission

Assign "Y" for conditions that were diagnosed prior to admission (example: hypertension, diabetes mellitus, asthma)

Conditions diagnosed during the admission but clearly present before admission

Assign "Y" for conditions diagnosed during the admission that were clearly present but not diagnosed until after admission occurred.

Diagnoses subsequently confirmed after admission are considered present on admission if at the time of admission they are documented as suspected, possible, rule out, differential diagnosis, or constitute an underlying cause of a symptom that is present at the time of admission.

Condition develops during outpatient encounter prior to inpatient admission

Assign Y for any condition that develops during an outpatient encounter prior to a written order for inpatient admission.

Documentation does not indicate whether condition was present on admission

Assign "U" when the medical record documentation is unclear as to whether the condition was present on admission. "U" should not be routinely assigned and used only in very limited circumstances. Coders are encouraged to query the providers when the documentation is unclear.

Documentation states that it cannot be determined whether the condition was or was not present on admission

Assign "W" when the medical record documentation indicates that it cannot be clinically determined whether or not the condition was present on admission.

Chronic condition with acute exacerbation during the admission

If a single code identifies both the chronic condition and the acute exacerbation, see POA guidelines pertaining to combination codes.

If a single code only identifies the chronic condition and not the acute exacerbation (e.g., acute exacerbation of chronic leukemia), assign "Y." Conditions documented as possible, probable, suspected, or rule out at the time of discharge

If the final diagnosis contains a possible, probable, suspected, or rule out diagnosis, and this diagnosis was based on signs, symptoms or clinical findings suspected at the time of inpatient admission, assign "Y."

If the final diagnosis contains a possible, probable, suspected, or rule out diagnosis, and this diagnosis was based on signs, symptoms or clinical findings that were not present on admission, assign "N".

Conditions documented as impending or threatened at the time of discharge

If the final diagnosis contains an impending or threatened diagnosis, and this diagnosis is based on symptoms or clinical findings that were present on admission, assign "Y".
If the final diagnosis contains an impending or threatened diagnosis, and this diagnosis is based on symptoms or clinical findings that were not present on admission, assign "N".

Acute and Chronic Conditions

Assign "Y" for acute conditions that are present at time of admission and N for acute conditions that are not present at time of admission.

Assign "Y" for chronic conditions, even though the condition may not be diagnosed until after admission.

If a single code identifies both an acute and chronic condition, see the POA guidelines for combination codes.

Combination Codes

Assign "N" if any part of the combination code was not present on admission (e.g., COPD with acute exacerbation and the exacerbation was not present on admission; gastric ulcer that does not start bleeding until after admission; asthma patient develops status asthmaticus after admission)

Assign "Y" if all parts of the combination code were present on admission (e.g., patient with acute prostatitis admitted with hematuria)

If the final diagnosis includes comparative or contrasting diagnoses, and both were present, or suspected, at the time of admission, assign "Y".

For infection codes that include the causal organism, assign "Y" if the infection (or signs of the infection) was present on admission, even though the culture results may not be known until after admission (e.g., patient is admitted with pneumonia and the provider documents pseudomonas as the causal organism a few days later).

Same Diagnosis Code for Two or More Conditions

When the same ICD-10-CM diagnosis code applies to two or more conditions during the same encounter (e.g. two separate conditions classified to the same ICD-10-CM diagnosis code):
Assign "Y" if all conditions represented by the single ICD-10-CM code were present on admission (e.g. bilateral unspecified age-related cataracts).

Assign "N" if any of the conditions represented by the single ICD-10-CM code was not present on admission (e.g. traumatic secondary and recurrent hemorrhage and seroma is assigned to a single code T79.2, but only one of the conditions was present on admission).

Obstetrical Conditions

Whether or not the patient delivers during the current hospitalization does not affect assignment of the POA indicator. The determining factor for POA assignment is whether the pregnancy complication or obstetrical condition described by the code was present at the time of admission or not.

If the pregnancy complication or obstetrical condition was present on admission (e.g., patient admitted in preterm labor), assign "Y".

If the pregnancy complication or obstetrical condition was not present on admission (e.g., 2nd degree laceration during delivery, postpartum hemorrhage that occurred during current hospitalization, fetal distress develops after admission), assign "N".

If the obstetrical code includes more than one diagnosis and any of the diagnoses identified by the code were not present on admission assign "N". (e.g., Category O11, Pre-existing hypertension with pre-eclampsia)

Perinatal Conditions

Newborns are not considered to be admitted until after birth. Therefore, any condition present at birth or that developed in utero is considered present at admission and should be assigned "Y".

This includes conditions that occur during delivery (e.g., injury during delivery, meconium aspiration, exposure to streptococcus B in the vaginal canal).

Congenital conditions and anomalies

Assign "Y" for congenital conditions and anomalies (except for codes Q00- Q99 which are exempt). Congenital conditions are always considered present on admission.

External Cause of Injury Codes

Assign "Y" for any external cause code representing an external cause of morbidity that occurred prior to inpatient admission (e.g., patient fell out of bed at home, patient fell out of bed in emergency room prior to admission)

Assign "N" for any external cause code representing an external cause of morbidity that occurred during inpatient hospitalization (e.g., patient fell out of hospital bed during hospital stay, patient experienced an adverse reaction to a medication administered after inpatient admission) Categories and Codes Exempt from Diagnosis Present on Admission Requirement

Note: "Diagnosis present on admission" for these code categories are exempt because they represent circumstances regarding the healthcare encounter or factors influencing health status that do not represent a current disease or injury or are always present on admission.

B90-B94	Sequelae of infectious and parasitic diseases
E64	Sequelae of malnutrition and other nutritional deficiencies
I25.2	Old myocardial infarction
I69	Sequelae of cerebrovascular disease
O09	Supervision of high risk pregnancy
O66.5	Attempted application of vacuum extractor and forceps
O80	Encounter for full-term uncomplicated delivery
O94	Sequelae of complication of pregnancy childbirth and the puerperium
P00	Newborn (suspected to be) affected by maternal conditions that may be unrelated to present pregnancy
Q00-Q99	Congenital malformations deformations and chromosomal abnormalities
S00-T88.9	Injury poisoning and certain other consequences of external causes with 7th character representing subsequent encounter or sequela
V00.121	Fall from non-in-line roller-skates
V00.131	Fall from skateboard

V00.141	Fall from scooter (nonmotorized)
V00.311	Fall from snowboard
V00.321	Fall from snow-skis
V40-V49	Car occupant injured in transport accident
V80-V89	Other land transport accidents
V90-V94	Water transport accidents
V95-V97	Air and space transport accidents
W03	Other fall on same level due to collision with another person
W09	Fall on and from playground equipment
W15	Fall from cliff
W17.0	Fall into well
W17.1	Fall into storm drain or manhole
W18.01	Striking against sports equipment with subsequent fall
W20.8	Other cause of strike by thrown projected or falling object
W21	Striking against or struck by sports equipment
W30	Contact with agricultural machinery
W31	Contact with other and unspecified machinery
W32-W34	Accidental handgun discharge and malfunction
W35-W40	Exposure to inanimate mechanical forces
W52	Crushed pushed or stepped on by crowd or human stampede
W89	Exposure to man-made visible and ultraviolet light
X02	Exposure to controlled fire in building or structure
X03	Exposure to controlled fire not in building or structure
X04	Exposure to ignition of highly flammable material
X52	Prolonged stay in weightless environment
X71-X83	Intentional self-harm

Y21	Drowning and submersion undetermined intent
Y22	Handgun discharge undetermined intent
Y23	Rifle shotgun and larger firearm discharge undetermined intent
Y24	Other and unspecified firearm discharge undetermined intent
Y30	Falling jumping or pushed from a high place undetermined intent
Y35	Legal intervention
Y37	Military operations
Y36	Operations of war
Y38	Terrorism
Y92	Place of occurrence of the external cause
Y93	Activity code
Y99	External cause status
Z00	Encounter for general examination without complaint suspected or reported diagnosis
Z01	Encounter for other special examination without complaint suspected or reported diagnosis
Z02	Encounter for administrative examination
Z03	Encounter for medical observation for suspected diseases and conditions ruled out
Z08	Encounter for follow-up examination following completed treatment for malignant neoplasm
Z09	Encounter for follow-up examination after completed treatment for conditions other than malignant neoplasm
Z11	Encounter for screening for infectious and parasitic diseases
Z11.8	Encounter for screening for other infectious and parasitic diseases
Z12	Encounter for screening for malignant neoplasms
Z13	Encounter for screening for other diseases and disorders
Z13.4	Encounter for screening for certain developmental disorders in childhood
Z13.5	Encounter for screening for eye and ear disorders

Z13.6	Encounter for screening for cardiovascular disorders
Z13.83	Encounter for screening for respiratory disorder NEC
Z13.89	Encounter for screening for other disorder (inclusion term)
Z14	Genetic carrier
Z15	Genetic susceptibility to disease
Z17	Estrogen receptor status
Z18	Retained foreign body fragments
Z22	Carrier of infectious disease
Z23	Encounter for immunization
Z28	Immunization not carried out and underimmunization status
Z28.3	Underimmunization status
Z30	Encounter for contraceptive management
Z31	Encounter for procreative management
Z34	Encounter for supervision of normal pregnancy
Z36	Encounter for antenatal screening of mother
Z37	Outcome of delivery
Z38	Liveborn infants according to place of birth and type of delivery
Z39	Encounter for maternal postpartum care and examination
Z41	Encounter for procedures for purposes other than remedying health state
Z42	Encounter for plastic and reconstructive surgery following medical procedure or healed injury
Z43	Encounter for attention to artificial openings
Z44	Encounter for fitting and adjustment of external prosthetic device
Z45	Encounter for adjustment and management of implanted device
Z46	Encounter for fitting and adjustment of other devices
Z47.8	Encounter for other orthopedic aftercare

Z49	Encounter for care involving renal dialysis
Z51	Encounter for other aftercare
Z51.5	Encounter for palliative care
Z51.8	Encounter for other specified aftercare
Z52	Donors of organs and tissues
Z59	Problems related to housing and economic circumstances
Z63	Other problems related to primary support group including family circumstances
Z65	Problems related to other psychosocial circumstances
Z65.8	Other specified problems related to psychosocial circumstances
Z67.1- Z67.9	Blood type
Z68	Body mass index (BMI)
Z72	Problems related to lifestyle
Z74.01	Bed confinement status
Z76	Persons encountering health services in other circumstances
Z77.110- Z77.128	Environmental pollution and hazards in the physical environment
Z78	Other specified health status
Z79	Long term (current) drug therapy
Z80	Family history of primary malignant neoplasm
Z81	Family history of mental and behavioral disorders
Z82	Family history of certain disabilities and chronic diseases (leading to disablement)
Z83	Family history of other specific disorders
Z84	Family history of other conditions
Z85	Personal history of primary malignant neoplasm
Z86	Personal history of certain other diseases
Z87	Personal history of other diseases and conditions

Z87.828	Personal history of other (healed) physical injury and trauma
Z87.891	Personal history of nicotine dependence
Z88	Allergy status to drugs medicaments and biological substances
Z89	Acquired absence of limb
Z90.710	Acquired absence of both cervix and uterus
Z91.0	Allergy status other than to drugs and biological substances
Z91.4	Personal history of psychological trauma not elsewhere classified
Z91.5	Personal history of self-harm
Z91.8	Other specified risk factors not elsewhere classified
Z92	Personal history of medical treatment
Z93	Artificial opening status
Z94	Transplanted organ and tissue status
Z95	Presence of cardiac and vascular implants and grafts
Z97	Presence of other devices
Z98	Other postprocedural states
Z99	Dependence on enabling machines and devices not elsewhere classified

ICD-10-PCS OVERVIEW

The International Classification Of Diseases Tenth Revision Procedure Coding System (ICD-10-PCS) was created to accompany the World Health Organization's (WHO) ICD-10 diagnosis classification. The new procedure coding system was developed to replace ICD-9-CM procedure codes for reporting inpatient procedures.

Unlike the ICD-9-CM classification, ICD-10-PCS was designed to enable each code to have a standard structure and be very descriptive, and yet flexible enough to accommodate future needs. Information about the structure, organization, and application of ICD-10-PCS codes, along with reference material for coding with ICD-10-PCS, is provided in this manual.

WHAT IS ICD-10-PCS?

ICD-10-PCS is a procedure coding system that will be used to collect data, determine payment, and support the electronic health record for all inpatient procedures performed in the United States.

HISTORY OF ICD-10-PCS

The World Health Organization has maintained the International Classification of Diseases (ICD) for recording cause of death since 1893. It has updated the ICD periodically to reflect new discoveries in epidemiology and changes in medical understanding of disease.

The International Classification of Diseases Tenth Revision (ICD-10), published in 1992, is the latest revision of the ICD. The WHO authorized the National Center for Health Statistics (NCHS) to develop a clinical modification of ICD-10 for use in the United States. This version of ICD-10 is called ICD-10-CM. ICD-10-CM is intended to replace the previous U.S. clinical modification, ICD-9-CM, that has been in use since 1979. ICD-9-CM contains a procedure classification; ICD-10-CM does not.

The Centers for Medicare and Medicaid Services, the agency responsible for maintaining the inpatient procedure code set in the U.S., contracted with 3M Health Information Systems in 1993 to design and then develop a procedure classification system to replace Volume 3 of ICD-9-CM. ICD-10-PCS is the result.

ICD-10-PCS was initially released in 1998. It has been updated annually since that time.

ICD-9-CM VOLUME 3 COMPARED TO ICD-10-PCS

With ICD-10 implementation, the U.S. clinical modification of the ICD will not include a procedure classification based on the same principles of organization as the diagnosis classification. Instead, a separate procedure coding system has been developed to meet the rigorous and varied demands that are made of coded data in the healthcare industry. This represents a significant step toward building a health information infrastructure that functions optimally in the electronic age.

The following table highlights basic differences between ICD-9-CM Volume 3 and ICD-10-PCS.

ICD-9-CM VOLUME 3	ICD-10-PCS
Follows ICD structure (designed for diagnosis coding)	Designed/developed to meet healthcare needs for a procedure code system
Codes available as a fixed/finite set in list form	Codes constructed from flexible code components (values) using tables
Codes are numeric	Codes are alphanumeric
Codes are 3 through 4 digits long	All codes are seven characters long

ICD-10-PCS CODE STRUCTURE

Undergirding ICD-10-PCS is a logical, consistent structure that informs the system as a whole, down to the level of a single code. This means that the process of constructing codes in ICD-10-PCS is also logical and consistent: individual letters and numbers, called "values," are selected in sequence to occupy the seven spaces of the code, called "characters."

CHARACTERS

All codes in ICD-10-PCS are seven characters long. Each character in the seven-character code represents an aspect of the procedure, as shown in the following diagram of characters from the main section of ICD-10-PCS, called Medical and Surgical.

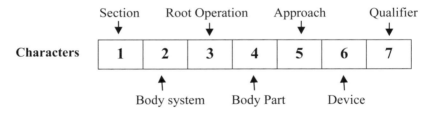

An ICD-10-PCS code is best understood as the result of a process rather than as an isolated, fixed quantity. The process consists of assigning values from among the valid choices for that part of the system, according to the rules governing the construction of codes.

VALUES

One of 34 possible values can be assigned to each character in a code: the numbers 0 through 9 and the alphabet (except I and O, because they are easily confused with the numbers 1 and 0). A finished code looks like the example below.

0	2	1	0	3	D	4

This code is derived by choosing a specific value for each of the seven characters. Based on details about the procedure performed, values for each character specifying the section, body system, root operation, body part, approach, device, and qualifier are assigned.

Because the definition of each character is a function of its physical position in the code, the same value placed in a different position in the code means something different. The value 0 in the first character means something different than 0 in the second character, or 0 in the third character, and so on.

CODE STRUCTURE: MEDICAL AND SURGICAL SECTION

The following pages define each character using the code 0LB50ZZ, "Excision of right lower arm and wrist tendon, open approach" as an example. This example comes from the Medical and Surgical section of ICD-10-PCS.

CHARACTER 1: SECTION

The first character in the code determines the broad procedure category, or section, where the code is found. In this example, the section is Medical and Surgical. 0 is the value that represents Medical and Surgical in the first character. The sample code looks like this so far:

Character 1 Section	Character 2 Body System	Character 3 Root Operation	Character 4 Body Part	Character 5 Approach	Character 6 Device	Character 7 Qualifier
Medical and Surgical						
0						

CHARACTER 2: BODY SYSTEM

The second character defines the body system—the general physiological system or anatomical region involved. Examples of body systems include Lower Arteries, Central Nervous System, and Respiratory System. In this example, the body system is Tendons, represented by the value L.

Character 1 Section	Character 2 Body System	Character 3 Root Operation	Character 4 Body Part	Character 5 Approach	Character 6 Device	Character 7 Qualifier
Medical and Surgical	Tendons					
0	L					

CHARACTER 3: ROOT OPERATION

The third character defines the root operation, or the objective of the procedure. Some examples of root operations are Bypass, Drainage, and Reattachment. In the sample code below, the root operation is Excision. When used in the third character of the code, the value B represents Excision.

Character 1 Section	Character 2 Body System	Character 3 Root Operation	Character 4 Body Part	Character 5 Approach	Character 6 Device	Character 7 Qualifier
Medical and Surgical	Tendons	Excision				
0	L	B				

CHARACTER 4: BODY PART

The fourth character defines the body part, or specific anatomical site where the procedure was performed. The body system (second character) provides only a general indication of the procedure site. The body part and body system values together provide a precise description of the procedure site.

Examples of body parts are Kidney, Tonsils, and Thymus. In this example, the body part value is 5, Lower Arm and Wrist, Right. when the second character is L, the value 5 when used in the fourth character of the code represents the right lower arm and wrist tendon.

Character 1 Section	Character 2 Body System	Character 3 Root Operation	Character 4 Body Part	Character 5 Approach	Character 6 Device	Character 7 Qualifier
Medical and Surgical	Tendons	Excision	Lower Arm and Wrist, Right			
0	L	B	5			

CHARACTER 5: APPROACH

The fifth character defines the approach, or the technique used to reach the procedure site. Seven different approach values are used in the Medical and Surgical section to define the approach. Examples of approaches include Open and Percutaneous Endoscopic.

In the sample code below, the approach is Open and is represented by the value 0.

Character 1 Section	Character 2 Body System	Character 3 Root Operation	Character 4 Body Part	Character 5 Approach	Character 6 Device	Character 7 Qualifier
Medical And Surgical	Tendons	Excision	Lower Arm And Wrist, Right	Open		
0	L	B	5	0		

CHARACTER 6: DEVICE

Depending on the procedure performed, there may or may not be a device left in place at the end of the procedure. The sixth character defines the device. Device values fall into four basic categories:

- Grafts and Prostheses
- Implants
- Simple or Mechanical Appliances
- Electronic Appliances

In this example, there is no device used in the procedure. The value Z is used to represent NO DEVICE, as shown below.

	Character 2 Body System	Character 3 Root Operation	Character 4 Body Part	Character 5 Approach	Character 6 Device	Character 7 Qualifier
Medical And Surgical	Tendons	Excision	Lower Arm And Wrist, Right	Open	No Device	
0	**L**	**B**	**5**	**0**	**Z**	

CHARACTER 7: QUALIFIER

The seventh character defines a qualifier for the code. A qualifier specifies an additional attribute of the procedure, if applicable.

Examples of qualifiers include Diagnostic and Stereotactic. Qualifier choices vary depending on the previous values selected. in this example, there is no specific qualifier applicable to this procedure, so the value is No Qualifier, represented by the letter Z.

	Character 2 Body System	Character 3 Root Operation	Character 4 Body Part	Character 5 Approach	Character 6 Device	Character 7 Qualifier
Medical And Surgical	Tendons	Excision	Lower Arm And Wrist, Right	Open	No Device	No Qualifier
0	**L**	**B**	**5**	**0**	**Z**	**Z**

0LB50ZZ is the complete specification of the procedure "Excision of right lower arm and wrist tendon, open approach."

ICD-10-PCS SYSTEM ORGANIZATION

ICD-10-PCS is composed of 16 sections, represented by the numbers 0 through 9 and the letters B through D and F.

- Medical and Surgical
- Obstetrics
- Placement
- Administration
- Measurement and Monitoring
- Extracorporeal Assistance and Performance
- Extracorporeal Therapies
- Osteopathic
- Other Procedures
- Chiropractic
- Imaging
- Nuclear Medicine
- Radiation Oncology
- Physical Rehabilitation and Diagnostic Audiology
- Mental Health
- Substance Abuse Treatment

MEDICAL AND SURGICAL SECTION

The first section, Medical and Surgical, contains the great majority of procedures typically reported in an inpatient setting. As shown in the previous section discussing ICD-10-PCS code structure, all procedure codes in the Medical and Surgical section begin with the section value 0.

	Character 2 Body System	Character 3 Root Operation	Character 4 Body Part	Character 5 Approach	Character 6 Device	Character 7 Qualifier
Medical and Surgical	Tendons	Excision	Lower arm and Wrist, right	Open	No device	No qualifier
0	**L**	**B**	**5**	**0**	**Z**	**Z**

Sections 1 through 9 of ICD-10-PCS comprise the Medical and Surgical-related sections. These sections include obstetrical procedures, administration of substances, measurement and monitoring of body functions, and extracorporeal therapies, as listed in the table below.

Section Value	Description
1	Obstetrics
2	Placement
3	Administration
4	Measurement and Monitoring
5	Extracorporeal Assistance and Performance
6	Extracorporeal Therapies
7	Osteopathic
8	Other Procedures
9	Chiropractic

In sections 1 and 2, all seven characters define the same aspects of the procedure as in the Medical and Surgical section.

Codes in sections 3 through 9 are structured for the most part like their counterparts in the Medical and Surgical section, with a few exceptions. For example, in sections 5 and 6, the fifth character is defined as duration instead of approach, as in this code for intra-aortic balloon pump (IABP):

Additional differences include these uses of the sixth character:

- Section 3 defines the sixth character as substance.
- Sections 4 and 5 define the sixth character as function.
- Sections 7 through 9 define the sixth character as method.

	Character 2 Body System	Character 3 Root Operation	Character 4 Body system	Character 5 Duration	Character 6 Function	Character 7 Qualifier
Extracorporeal Assist. And Performance	Physiological Systems	Assistance	Cardiac	Continuous	Output	Balloon Pump
5	A	0	2	2	1	0

ANCILLARY SECTIONS

Sections B through D and F through H comprise the ancillary sections of ICD-10-PCS. These six sections include imaging procedures, nuclear medicine, and substance abuse treatment, as listed in the following table.

Section Value	Description
B	Imaging
C	Nuclear Medicine
D	Radiation Oncology
F	Physical Rehabilitation and Diagnostic Audiology
G	Mental Health
H	Substance Abuse Treatment

The definitions of some characters in the ancillary sections differs from that seen in previous sections. In the Imaging section, the third character is defined as type, and the fifth and sixth characters define contrast and contrast/qualifier respectively, as in the CT scan example below.

	Character 2 Body System	Character 3 Type	Character 4 Body Part	Character 5 Contrast	Character 6 Qualifier	Character 7 Qualifier
Imaging	Central Nervous	Computerized Tomography	Brain	High Osmolar	Unenhanced and Enhanced	None
B	0	2	0	0	0	Z

Additional differences include:

- Section C defines the fifth character as radionuclide.
- Section D defines the fifth character as modality qualifier and the sixth character as isotope.
- Section F defines the fifth character as type qualifier and the sixth character as equipment.

TABLES

The complete ICD-10-PCS is presented in three parts: the Tables, the Index, and the List of Codes. The Tables are organized in a series, beginning with section 0, Medical and Surgical, and body system 0, Central Nervous, and proceeding in numerical order. Sections 0 through 9 are followed by sections B through D and F through H. The same convention is followed within each table for the second through the seventh characters—numeric values in order first, followed by alphabetical values in order.

The following examples use the Medical and Surgical section to describe the organization and format of the ICD-10-PCS Tables.

The Medical and Surgical section (first character 0) is organized by its 31 body system values. Each body system subdivision in the Medical and Surgical section contains tables that list the valid root operations for that body system. These are the root operation tables that form the system. These tables provide the valid choices of values available to construct a code.

The root operation tables consist of four columns and a varying number of rows, as in the following example of the root operation Bypass, in the Central Nervous body system.

0: MEDICAL AND SURGICAL (Section)
0: CENTRAL NERVOUS (Body system)
1: BYPASS: Altering the route of passage of the contents of a tubular body part (Root operation)

Body Part Character 4	Approach Character 5	Device Character 6	Qualifier Character 7
6 Cerebral Ventricle	0 Open	7 Autologous Tissue Substitute J Synthetic Substitute K Nonautologous Tissue Substitute	0 Nasopharynx 1 Mastoid Sinus 2 Atrium 3 Blood Vessel 4 Pleural Cavity 5 Intestine 6 Peritoneal Cavity 7 Urinary Tract 8 Bone Marrow B Cerebral Cisterns
U Spinal Canal	0 Open	7 Autologous Tissue Substitute J Synthetic Substitute K Nonautologous Tissue Substitute	4 Pleural Cavity 6 Peritoneal Cavity 7 Urinary Tract 9 Fallopian Tube

The values for characters 1 through 3 are provided at the top of each table. Four columns contain the applicable values for characters 4 through 7, given the values in characters 1 through 3.

A table may be separated into rows to specify the valid choices of values in characters 4 through 7. A built using values from more than one row of a table is not a valid code.

INDEX

The ICD-10-PCS Index can be used to access the Tables. The Index mirrors the structure of the Tables, so it follows a consistent pattern of organization and use of hierarchies.

The Index is organized as an alphabetic lookup. Two types of main terms are listed in the Index:

- Based on the value of the third character
- Common procedure terms

MAIN TERMS

For the medical and surgical and related sections, the root operation values are used as main terms in the index. in other sections, the values representing the general type of procedure performed, such as nuclear medicine or imaging type, are listed as main terms.

For the medical and surgical and related sections, values such as excision, bypass, and transplantation are included as main terms in the index. the applicable body system entries are listed beneath the main term, and refer to a specific table. for the ancillary sections, values such as fluoroscopy and positron emission tomography are listed as main terms.

In the example below, the index entry "bypass" refers to the medical and surgical section tables for all applicable body systems, including anatomical regions and central nervous system.

Bypass
    by Body System
        Anatomical Regions 0W1....
            Central Nervous System 001....

The body system listings may be followed by entries for specific body parts, as in the excerpt below. In the root operations CHANGE, INSERTION, REMOVAL, and REVISION, the device entries follow the body system listings.

    by Body Part
        Artery
            Aorta, Abdominal 0410...
            Aorta, Thoracic 021W...
            Axillary 031....
            Brachial 031....
            Common Carotid 031....

COMMON PROCEDURE TERMS

The second type of term listed in the Index uses procedure names, such as "appendectomy" or "fundoplication." These entries are listed as main terms, and refer to a table or tables from which a valid code can be constructed, as shown in the following example.

Cholecystectomy

- see Excision, Hepatobiliary System & Pancreas 0FB....
- see Resection, Hepatobiliary System & Pancreas 0FT....

LIST OF CODES

The ICD-10-PCS List of Codes is a resource that displays all valid codes in alphanumeric order. Each entry begins with the seven-character code, followed by the full text description.

The code descriptions are generated using rules that produce standardized, complete, and easy-to-read code descriptions.

ICD-10-PCS DESIGN

ICD-10-PCS is fundamentally different from ICD-9-CM in its structure, organization, and capabilities. It was designed and developed to adhere to recommendations made by the National Committee on Vital and Health Statistics (NCVHS). It also incorporates input from a wide range of organizations, individual physicians, healthcare professionals, and researchers.

Several structural attributes were recommended for a new procedure coding system. These attributes include

- Multiaxial structure
- Completeness
- Expandability

MULTIAXIAL STRUCTURE

The key attribute that provides the framework for all other structural attributes is multiaxial code structure. Multiaxial code structure makes it possible for the ICD-10-PCS to be complete, expandable, and to provide a high degree of flexibility and functionality.

As mentioned earlier, ICD-10-PCS codes are composed of seven characters. Each character represents a category of information that can be specified about the procedure performed. A character defines both the category of information and its physical position in the code.

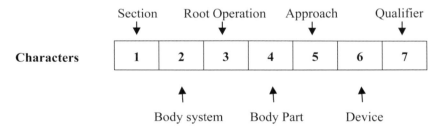

A character's position can be understood as a semi-independent axis of classification that allows different specific values to be inserted into that space, and whose physical position remains stable. Within a defined code range, a character retains the general meaning that it confers on any value in that position. For example, the fifth character retains the general meaning "approach" in sections 0 through 4 and 7 through 9 of the system. Any specific value in the fifth character will define a specific approach, such as Open.

Each group of values for a character contains all of the valid choices in relation to the other characters of the code, giving the system completeness. in the fifth character, for example, each significantly distinct approach is assigned its own approach value and all applicable approach values are included to represent the possible versions of a procedure.

Each group of values for a character can be added to as needed, giving the system expandability. if a significantly distinct approach is used to perform procedures, a new approach value can be added to the system.

Each group of values is confined to its own character, giving ICD-10-PCS a stable, predictable readability across a wide range of codes. In sections 0 through 4 and 7 through 9 of the system, for example, the fifth character always represents the approach.

ICD-10-PCS' multiaxial structure houses its capacity for completeness, expandability, and flexibility, giving it a high degree of functionality for multiple uses.

COMPLETENESS

Completeness is considered a key structural attribute for a new procedure coding system. The specific recommendation for completeness includes these characteristics:

- A unique code is available for each significantly different procedure.
- Each code retains its unique definition. Codes are not reused.

In Volume 3 of ICD-9-CM, procedures performed on many different body parts using different approaches or devices may be assigned to the same procedure code. In ICD-10-PCS, a unique code can be constructed for every significantly different procedure.

Within each section, a character defines a consistent component of a code, and contains all applicable values for that character. The values define individual expressions (open, percutaneous) of the character's general meaning (approach) that are then used to construct unique procedure codes.

Because all approaches by which a procedure is performed are assigned a separate approach value in the system, every procedure which uses a different approach will have its own unique code. This is true of the other characters as well. The same procedure performed on a different body part has its own unique code, the same procedure performed using a different device has its own unique code, and so on.

In the case of the coronary artery bypass graft (CABG), ICD-9-CM contains a total of nine codes to describe different versions of the procedure. These codes specify the version based on one aspect of the procedure, and the aspect defined is not consistent for all nine codes. Four of the codes specify the number of coronary arteries bypassed, four specify the source of the new blood flow, and one is an "unspecified" choice.

By contrast, ICD-10-PCS components can be combined to produce 34 unique codes defining all significantly different versions of the comparable CABG procedure. All 34 codes specify the same four aspects of the procedure: the number of coronary artery sites bypassed, the approach to the procedure site, the type of graft if used, and the origin of the bypass (source of the new blood flow). The differences are summarized in the table below.

ICD-9-CM VOLUME 3 CODE & DESCRIPTION		ICD-10-PCS CODE & DESCRIPTION	
36.11	Aortocoronary bypass of one coronary artery (1 of 4)	021009W	Bypass coronary artery, one site to aorta with autologous venous tissue, open approach(1 of 8)
36.15	Single internal mammary-coronary artery bypass (1 of 2)	02100Z8	Bypass coronary artery, one site to right internal mammary, open approach (1 of 16)

36.17	Abdominal-coronary artery bypass (1 of 2)	**02100AF**	Bypass coronary artery, one site to abdominal artery with autologous arterial tissue, open approach (1 of 10)
36.10	Aortocoronary bypass for heart revascularization, not otherwise specified (1 of 1)	**No Equivalent**	ICD-10-PCS codes all contain a minimum level of specificity

UNIQUE DEFINITIONS

Because ICD-10-PCS codes are constructed of individual values rather than lists of fixed codes and text descriptions, the unique, stable definition of a code in the system is retained. New values may be added to the system to represent a specific new approach or device or qualifier, but whole codes by design cannot be given new meanings and reused.

EXPANDABILITY

Expandability was also recommended as a key structural attribute. The specific recommendation for expandability includes these characteristics:

- Accommodate new procedures and technologies
- Add new codes without disrupting the existing structure

ICD-10-PCS is designed to be easily updated as new codes are required for new procedures and new techniques. Changes to ICD-10-PCS can all be made within the existing structure, because whole codes are not added. Instead, one of two possible changes is made to the system:

- A new value for a character is added as needed to the system.
- An existing value for a character is added to a table(s) in the system.

ICD-10-PCS UPDATE: PICVA

An example of how the updating of ICD-10-PCS works can be seen in the coronary artery bypass procedure called Percutaneous in-situ coronary venous arterialization (PICVA). This procedure is no more invasive than a percutaneous coronary angioplasty, but achieves the benefits of a bypass procedure by placing a specialized stent into the diseased coronary artery, through its wall into the adjacent coronary vein, and diverting blood flow through the stent into the artery past the blockage.

ICD-10-PCS was updated in 2004 to include an appropriate range of codes for the PICVA procedure (16 possible codes). This was accomplished simply by adding another row to the relevant table (see table 021, Bypass, Heart and Great Vessels) containing two approach values for the non-invasive approach, two device values for the possible types of stent, and a single qualifier.

0: MEDICAL AND SURGICAL 2: HEART AND GREAT VESSELS 1: BYPASS: Altering the route of passage of the contents of a tubular body part			
Body Part **Character 4**	**Approach** **Character 5**	**Device** **Character 6**	**Qualifier** **Character 7**
0 Coronary Artery, One Site **1** Coronary Artery, Two Sites **2** Coronary Artery, Three Sites **4** Coronary Artery, Four or More Sites	**3** Percutaneous **4** Percutaneous Endoscopic	**4** Drug-eluting Intraluminal Device **D** Intraluminal Device	**D** Coronary Vein

STRUCTURAL INTEGRITY

As shown in the previous example, ICD-10-PCS can be easily expanded without disrupting the structure of the system.

In the PICVA example, one new value—the qualifier value Coronary Vein—was added to the system to effect this change. All other values in the new row are existing values used to create unique, new codes.

This type of updating can be replicated anywhere in the system when a change is required. ICD-10-PCS allows unique new codes to be added to the system because values for the seven characters that make up a code can be combined as needed. The system can evolve as medical technology and clinical practice evolve, without disrupting the ICD-10-PCS structure.

ICD-10-PCS ADDITIONAL CHARACTERISTICS

ICD-10-PCS possesses several additional characteristics in response to government and industry recommendations. These characteristics are

- Standardized terminology within the coding system
- Standardized level of specificity
- No diagnostic information
- No explicit "not otherwise specified" (NOS) code options
- Limited use of "not elsewhere classified" (NEC) code options

STANDARDIZED TERMINOLOGY

Words commonly used in clinical vocabularies may have multiple meanings. This can cause confusion and result in inaccurate data. ICD-10-PCS is standardized and self-contained. Characters and values used in the system are defined in the system.

For example, the word "excision" is used to describe a wide variety of surgical procedures. In ICD-10-PCS, the word "excision" describes a single, precise surgical objective, defined as "Cutting out or off, without replacement, a portion of a body part."

NO EPONYMS OR COMMON PROCEDURE NAMES

The terminology used in ICD-10-PCS is standardized to provide precise and stable definitions of all procedures performed. This standardized terminology is used in all ICD-10-PCS code descriptions.

As a result, ICD-10-PCS code descriptions do not include eponyms or common procedure names. Two examples from ICD-9-CM are 22.61, "Excision of lesion of maxillary sinus with Caldwell-Luc approach," and 51.10, "Endoscopic retrograde cholangiopancreatography [ERCP]." In ICD-10-PCS, physicians' names are not included in a code description, nor are procedures identified by common terms or acronyms such as appendectomy or CABG. Instead, such procedures are coded to the root operation that accurately identifies the objective of the procedure.

The procedures described in the preceding paragraph by ICD-9-CM codes are coded in ICD-10-PCS according to the root operation that matches the objective of the procedure. Here the ICD-10-PCS equivalents would be Excision and Inspection respectively. By relying on the universal objectives defined in root operations rather than eponyms or specific procedure titles that change or become obsolete, ICD-10-PCS preserves the capacity to define past, present, and future procedures accurately using stable terminology in the form of characters and values.

NO COMBINATION CODES

With rare exceptions, ICD-10-PCS does not define multiple procedures with one code. This is to preserve standardized terminology and consistency across the system. Procedures that are typically performed together but are distinct procedures may be defined by a single "combination code" in ICD-9-CM. An example of a combination code in ICD-9-CM is 28.3, "Tonsillectomy with adenoidectomy."

A procedure that meets the reporting criteria for a separate procedure is coded separately in ICD-10-PCS. This allows the system to respond to changes in technology and medical practice with the maximum degree of stability and flexibility.

STANDARDIZED LEVEL OF SPECIFICITY

In ICD-9-CM, one code with its description and includes notes may encompass a vast number of procedure variations while another code defines a single specific procedure. ICD-10-PCS provides a standardized level of specificity for each code, so that each code represents a single procedure variation.

The ICD-9-CM code 39.31, "Suture of artery," does not specify the artery, whereas the code range 38.40 through 38.49, "Resection of artery with replacement," provides a fourth-digit subclassification for specifying the artery by anatomical region (thoracic, abdominal, etc.).

In ICD-10-PCS, the codes identifying all artery suture and artery replacement procedures possess the same degree of specificity. The ICD-9-CM examples above coded to their ICD-10-PCS equivalents would use the same artery body part values in all codes identifying the respective procedures.

In general, ICD-10-PCS code descriptions are much more specific than their ICD-9-CM counterparts, but sometimes an ICD-10-PCS code description is actually less specific. In most cases this is because the ICD-9-CM code contains diagnosis information. The standardized level of code specificity in ICD-10-PCS cannot always take account of these fluctuations in ICD-9-CM level of specificity. Instead, ICD-10-PCS provides a standardized level of specificity that can be predicted across the system.

DIAGNOSIS INFORMATION EXCLUDED

Another key feature of ICD-10-PCS is that information pertaining to a diagnosis is excluded from the code descriptions.

ICD-9-CM often contains information about the diagnosis in its procedure codes. Adding diagnosis information limits the flexibility and functionality of a procedure coding system. It has the effect of placing a code "off limits" because the diagnosis in the medical record does not match the diagnosis in the procedure code description. The code cannot be used even though the procedural part of the code description precisely matches the procedure performed.

Diagnosis information is not contained in any ICD-10-PCS code. The diagnosis codes, not the procedure codes, will specify the reason the procedure is performed.

NOS CODE OPTIONS RESTRICTED

ICD-9-CM often designates codes as "unspecified" or "not otherwise specified" codes. By contrast, the standardized level of specificity designed into ICD-10-PCS restricts the use of broadly applicable NOS or unspecified code options in the system. A minimal level of specificity is required to construct a valid code.

In ICD-10-PCS, each character defines information about the procedure and all seven characters must contain a specific value obtained from a single row of a table to build a valid code. Even values such as the sixth-character value Z, No Device and the seventh-character value Z, No Qualifier, provide important information about the procedure performed.

LIMITED NEC CODE OPTIONS

ICD-9-CM often designates codes as "not elsewhere classified" or "other specified" versions of a procedure throughout the code set. NEC options are also provided in ICD-10-PCS, but only for specific, limited use.

In the Medical and Surgical section, two significant "not elsewhere classified" options are the root operation value Q, Repair and the device value Y, Other Device.

The root operation Repair is a true NEC value. It is used only when the procedure performed is not one of the other root operations in the Medical and Surgical section.

Other Device, on the other hand, is intended to be used to temporarily define new devices that do not have a specific value assigned, until one can be added to the system. No categories of medical or surgical devices are permanently classified to Other Device.

ICD-10-PCS APPLICATIONS

ICD-10-PCS code structure results in qualities that optimize the performance of the system in electronic applications, and maximize the usefulness of the coded healthcare data. These qualities include

- Optimal search capability
- Consistent character definitions
- Consistent values wherever possible
- Code readability

Some have argued that, in the world of the electronic health record, the classification system as we know it is outmoded, that classification doesn't matter because a computer is able to find a code with equal ease whether the code has been generated at random or is part of a classification scheme. While this may be true from an IT perspective, assignment of randomly generated code numbers makes it impossible to aggregate data according to related ranges of codes. This is a critical capability for providers, payers, and researchers to make meaningful use of the data.

OPTIMAL SEARCH CAPABILITY

ICD-10-PCS is designed for maximum versatility in the ability to aggregate coded data. Values belonging to the same character as defined in a section or sections can be easily compared, since they occupy the same position in a code. This provides a high degree of flexibility and functionality for data mining.

For example, the body part value 6, Stomach, retains its meaning for all codes in the Medical and Surgical section that define procedures performed on the stomach. Because the body part value is dependent for its meaning on the body system in which it is found, the body system value D, Gastrointestinal, must also be included in the search.

A person wishing to examine data regarding all medical and surgical procedures performed on the stomach could do so simply by searching the code range below.

0D*6***

CONSISTENT CHARACTERS AND VALUES

In the previous example, the value 6 means Stomach only when the body system value is D, Gastrointestinal. In many other cases, values retain their meaning across a much broader range of codes. This provides consistency and readability.

For example, the value 0 in the fifth character defines the approach Open and the value 3 in the fifth character defines the approach Percutaneous across sections 0 through 4 and 7 through 9, where applicable. As a result, all open and percutaneous procedures represented by codes in sections 0-4 and 7-9 can be compared based on a single character—approach—by conducting a query on the code ranges below.

[0 through 4,7 through 9]***0** vs. [0 through 4,7through 9]***3**

Searches can be progressively refined by adding specific values. For example, one could search on a body system value or range of body system values, plus a body part value or range of body part values, plus a root operation value or range of root operation values.

To refine the search above, one could add the body system value for Gastrointestinal and the body part value for Stomach to limit the search to open vs. percutaneous procedures performed on the stomach:

0D*60** vs. 0D*63"

To refine the search even further and limit the comparison to open and percutaneous biopsies of the stomach, one could add the third-character value for the root operation Excision and the seventh-character qualifier Diagnostic, as below.

0DB60*X vs. 0DB63*X

Stability of characters and values across vast ranges of codes provides the maximum degree of functionality and flexibility for the collection and analysis of data. The search capabilities demonstrated above function equally well for all uses of healthcare data: investigating quality of care, resource utilization, risk management, conducting research, determining reimbursement, and many others.

Because the character definition is consistent, and only the individual values assigned to that character differ as needed, meaningful comparisons of data over time can be conducted across a virtually infinite range of procedures.

CODE READABILITY

ICD-10-PCS resembles a language in the sense that it is made up of semi-independent values combined by following the rules of the system, much the way a sentence is formed by combining words and following the rules of grammar and syntax. As with words in their context, the meaning of any single value is a combination of its position in the code and any preceding values on which it may be dependent.

For example, in the Medical and Surgical section, a body part value is always dependent for its meaning on the body system in which it is found. It cannot stand alone as a letter or a number and be meaningful. A fourth-character value of 6 by itself can mean 31 different things, but a fourth-character value of 6 in the context of a second-character value of D means one thing only—Stomach.

On the other hand, a root operation value is not dependent on any character but the section for its meaning, and identifies a single consistent objective wherever the third character is defined as root operation. For example, the third-character value T identifies the root operation Resection in both the Medical and Surgical and Obstetrics sections.

The approach value also identifies a single consistent approach wherever the fifth character is defined as approach. The fifth-character value 3 identifies the approach Percutaneous in the Medical and Surgical section, the Obstetrics section, the Administration section, and others.

The sixth-character device value or seventh-character qualifier value identifies the same device or qualifier in the context of the body system where it is found. Although there may be consistencies across body systems or within whole sections, this is not true in all cases.

Values in their designated context have a precise meaning, like words in a language. As seen in the code example which began this chapter, 0LB50ZZ represents the text description of the specific procedure "Excision of right lower arm and wrist tendon, open approach." Since ICD-10-PCS values in context have a single, precise meaning, a complete, valid code can be read and understood without its accompanying text description, much like one would read a sentence.

ICD-10-PCS PROCEDURES IN THE MEDICAL AND SURGICAL SECTION

This chapter provides reference material for the root operations in the Medical and Surgical section of ICD-10-PCS. The vast majority of codes reported in an inpatient setting are found in this section.

First, a table presents all root operations in the Medical and Surgical section, organized into logical groups. Following the table are definitions of each root operation, presented in the order shown in the table. Material on each root operation includes

- Definition, explanation, and examples of the root operation
- Coding notes as needed
- A representative procedure excerpt for each root operation, followed by the correct code for the procedure. The code is provided in table excerpt format, along with explanatory notes as needed.
- Coding exercises that provide example procedures and their corresponding ICD-10-PCS codes, with explanatory notes as needed

ROOT OPERATION GROUPS

The Medical and Surgical root operations are divided into groups that share similar attributes. These groups, and the root operations in each, are listed in the table below. Subsequent pages of this chapter provide a definition of each root operation in a group.

Root Operation	What Operation Does	Objective Of Procedure	Procedure Site	Example
Excision	Takes out some/all of a body part	Cutting out/off without replacement	Some of a body part	Breast lumpectomy
Resection	Takes out some/all of a body part	Cutting out/off without replacement	All of a body part	Total mastectomy
Detachment	Takes out some/all of a body part	Cutting out/off without replacement	Extremity only, any level	Amputation above elbow
Destruction	Takes out some/all of a body part	Eradicating without replacement	Some/all of a body part	Fulguration of endometrium
Extraction	Takes out some/all of a body part	Pulling out or off without replacement	Some/all of a body part	Suction D & C
Drainage	Takes out solids/fluids/ gases from a body part	Taking/letting out fluids/ gases	Within a body part	Incision and Drainage
Extirpation	Takes out solids/fluids/ gases from a body part	Taking/cutting out solid matter	Within a body part	Thrombectomy

Fragmentation	Takes out solids/fluids/ gases from a body part	Breaking solid matter into pieces	Within a body part	Lithotripsy
Division	Involves cutting or separation only	Cutting into/separating a body part	Within a body part	Neurotomy
Release	Involves cutting or separation only	Freeing a body part from constraint	Around a body part	Adhesiolysis
Transplantation	Puts in/puts back or move some/all of a body part	Putting in a living body part from a person/animal	Some/all of a body part	Kidney transplant
Reattachment	Puts in/puts back or move some/all of a body part	Putting back a detached body part	Some/all of a body part	Reattach severed finger
Transfer	Puts in/puts back or move some/all of a body part	Moving, to function for a similar body part	Some/all of a body part	Skin transfer flap
Reposition	Puts in/puts back or move some/all of a body part	Moving, to normal or other suitable location	Some/all of a body part	Move undescended testicle
Restriction	Alters the diameter/route of a tubular body part	Partially closing orifice/ lumen	Tubular body part	Gastroesophageal fundoplication
Occlusion	Alters the diameter/route of a tubular body part	Completely closing orifice/ lumen	Tubular body part	Fallopian tube ligation
Dilation	Alters the diameter/route of a tubular body part	Expanding orifice/lumen	Tubular body part	Percutaneous transluminal coronary angioplasty (PTCA)
Bypass	Alters the diameter/route of a tubular body part	Altering route of passage	Tubular body part	Coronary artery bypass graft (CABG)
Insertion	Always involve a device	Putting in non-biological device	In/on a body part	Central line insertion
Replacement	Always involve a device	Putting in device that replaces a body part	Some/all of a body part	Total hip replacement
Supplement	Always involve a device	Putting in device that reinforces or augments a body part	In/on a body part	Abdominal wall herniorrhaphy using mesh
Change	Always involve a device	Exchanging device w/out cutting/puncturing	In/on a body part	Drainage tube change
Removal	Always involve a device	Taking out device	In/on a body part	Central line removal

Revision	Always involve a device	Correcting a malfunctioning/displaced device	In/on a body part	Revision of pacemaker insertion
Inspection	Involves examination only	Visual/manual exploration	Some/all of a body part	Diagnostic cystoscopy
Map	Involves examination only	Locating electrical impulses/functional areas	Brain/cardiac conduction mechanism	Cardiac mapping
Repair	Includes other repairs	Restoring body part to its normal structure	Some/all of a body part	Suture laceration
Control	Includes other repairs	Stopping/attempting to stop postprocedural bleed	Anatomical region	Post-prostatectomy bleeding
Fusion	Includes other objectives	Rendering joint immobile	Joint	Spinal fusion
Alteration	Includes other objectives	Modifying body part for cosmetic purposes without affecting function	Some/all of a body part	Face lift
Creation	Includes other objectives	Making new structure for sex change operation	Perineum	Artificial vagina/penis

ROOT OPERATIONS THAT TAKE OUT SOME OR ALL OF A BODY PART

Five root operations represent procedures for taking out or otherwise eradicating some or all of a body part. These root operations are listed in the table below and described in detail in the pages that follow.

Root Operation	Objective of Procedure	Site of Procedure	Example
Excision	Cutting out/off without replacement	Some of a body part	Breast lumpectomy
Resection	Cutting out/off without replacement	All of a body part	Total mastectomy
Detachment	Cutting out/off without replacement	Extremity only, any level	Amputation above elbow
Destruction	Eradicating without replacement	Some/all of a body part	Fulguration of endometrium
Extraction	Pulling out or off without replacement	Some/all of a body part	Suction D&C

EXCISION—ROOT OPERATION B

Excision	Definition	Cutting out or off, without replacement, a portion of a body part
B	Explanation	The qualifier Diagnostic is used to identify excision procedures that are biopsies
	Examples	Partial nephrectomy, liver biopsy

Excision is coded when a portion of a body part is cut out or off using a sharp instrument. All root operations that employ cutting to accomplish the objective allow the use of any sharp instrument, including but not limited to

- Scalpel
- Wire
- Scissors
- Bone saw
- Electrocautery tip

> **CODING NOTE** **BONE MARROW AND ENDOMETRIAL BIOPSIES** are not coded to the root operation excision. They are coded to Extraction, with the qualifier Diagnostic.

Example: Excision of sebaceous cyst (right buttock)

...the patient was brought in the room and placed on the table in jack knife, prone position and a spinal block was used for anesthesia. She was prepped and draped in the usual sterile manner. A digital rectal examination was performed and we did not notice any communication between mass and rectum. The mass was palpated and a radial transverse incision was made over the mass.

Using blunt and sharp dissection the top of the mass was identified and shown to be a sebaceous cyst. The sebaceous cyst was freed from the surrounding tissue using blunt dissection. The entire cyst was removed. Hemostasis was obtained and the skin was closed using 5-0 Dexon interrupted sutures...

Character 1 Section	Character 2 Body System	Character 3 Root Operation	Character 4 Body Part	Character 5 Approach	Character 6 Device	Character 7 Qualifier
Medical and Surgical	Skin	Excision	Buttock	External	No Device	No Qualifier
0	**H**	**B**	**8**	**X**	**Z**	**Z**

RESECTION—ROOT OPERATION T

Resection	Definition	Cutting out or off, without replacement, all of a body part
T	Explanation	N/A
	Examples	Total nephrectomy, total lobectomy of lung

Resection is similar to Excision *(see page 2.9)*, except Resection includes all of a body part, or any subdivision of a body part that has its own body part value in ICD-10-PCS, while Excision includes only a portion of a body part.

CODING NOTE	**LYMPH NODES.** When an entire lymph node chain is cut out, the appropriate root operation is Resection. When a lymph node(s) is cut out, the root operation is Excision.

Example: Right hemicolectomy

...a vertical midline incision was used to enter the abdominal cavity. There was noted to be a mass in the region of the cecum. The mass was easily mobilized and it was felt that a right hemicolectomy was indicated. The right colon was mobilized by incising the white line of Toldt and reflecting colon medially. The loose tissue was taken down bluntly with a hand and adhesions were taken down sharply.

The colon was mobilized to the left end up to the level of the hepatic flexure. The mesentery was incised sharply with a knife and down to the level of the root of the mesentery. The mesentery of the right colon and the distal ileum was then taken down between Kelly's and tied with 2-0 silk, down to the level of the takeoff vessels.

After removing the right colon specimen off the field, a primary anastomosis was planned...

Character 1 Section	Character 2 Body System	Character 3 Root Operation	Character 4 Body Part	Character 5 Approach	Character 6 Device	Character 7 Qualifier
Medical and Surgical	Gastro-intestinal system	Resection	Large Intestine, Right	Open	No Device	No Qualifier
0	**D**	**T**	**F**	**0**	**Z**	**Z**

CODING NOTE	**ANASTOMOTIC.** Adjunct information about the anastomotic *technique* used to complete a colectomy procedure (e.g., side to end) is not specified in ICD-10-PCS. Only the specific Excision or Resection code is assigned.

DETACHMENT—ROOT OPERATION 6

Detachment represents a narrow range of procedures; it is used exclusively for amputation procedures.

Detachment 6	Definition	Cutting off all or part of the upper or lower extremities
	Explanation	The body part value is the site of the detachment, with a qualifier if applicable to further specify the level where the extremity was detached
	Examples	Below knee amputation, disarticulation of shoulder

Detachment procedure codes are found only in body systems X Anatomical Regions, Upper Extremities and Y Anatomical Regions, Lower Extremities, because amputations are performed on the extremities, across overlapping body layers, and so could not be coded to a specific musculoskeletal body system such as the bones or joints.

Detachment Qualifiers

The specific qualifiers used for Detachment are dependent on the body part value in the upper and lower extremities body systems. The table below defines the meaning of the qualifiers used in both the upper and lower extremities.

Body Part	Qualifier Value	Definition
Upper arm and upper leg	1	High: Amputation at the proximal portion of the shaft of the humerus or femur
	2	Mid: Amputation at the middle portion of the shaft of the humerus or femur
	3	Low: Amputation at the distal portion of the shaft of the humerus or femur
Hand and foot	0	Complete
	4	Complete 1st Ray
	5	Complete 2nd Ray
	6	Complete 3rd Ray
	7	Complete 4th Ray
	8	Complete 5th Ray
	9	Partial 1st Ray
	B	Partial 2nd Ray
	C	Partial 3rd Ray
	D	Partial 4th Ray
	F	Partial 5th Ray
		Complete: Amputation through the carpometacarpal joint of the hand, or through the tarsal-metatarsal joint of the foot Partial: Amputation anywhere along the shaft or head of the metacarpal bone of the hand, or of the metatarsal bone of the foot
Thumb, finger, or toe	0	Complete: Amputation at the metacarpophalangeal/metatarsal-phalangeal joint
	1	High: Amputation anywhere along the proximal phalanx
	2	Mid: Amputation through the proximal interphalangeal joint or anywhere along the middle phalanx

Character 1 Section	Character 2 Body System	Character 3 Root Operation	Character 4 Body Part	Character 5 Approach	Character 6 Device	Character 7 Qualifier
Medical and Surgical	Lower Extremities	Detachment	Foot, Left	Open	No Device	Partial 5th Ray
0	**Y**	**6**	**N**	**0**	**Z**	**f**

CODING NOTE	QUALIFIER VALUE. The surgeon uses the word "toe" to describe the amputation, but the operative report says he extends the amputation to the midshaft of the fifth metatarsal, which is the foot, so the qualifier is Partial 5th Ray.

ROOT OPERATIONS THAT TAKE OUT SOME OR ALL OF A BODY PART

DESTRUCTION—ROOT OPERATION 5

Destruction 5	Definition	Physical eradication of all or a portion of a body part by the direct use of energy, force or a destructive agent
	Explanation	None of the body part is physically taken out
	Examples	Fulguration of rectal polyp, cautery of skin lesion

Destruction "takes out" a body part in the sense that it obliterates the body part so it is no longer there. This root operation defines a broad range of common procedures, since it can be used anywhere in the body to treat a variety of conditions, including:

- Skin and genital warts
- Nasal and colon polyps
- Esophageal varices
- Endometrial implants
- Nerve lesions

Example: Radiofrequency coagulation of the trigeminal nerve

...The right cheek was infiltrated dermally with Xylocaine, and a small nick in the skin 2.5 cm lateral to the corner of the mouth was performed with an 18 gauge needle. The radiofrequency needle with 2 mm exposed tip was then introduced using the known anatomical landmarks and under lateral fluoroscopy guidance into the foramen ovale.

Confirmation of the placement of the needle was done by the patient grimacing to pain and by the lateral x-ray. The first treatment, 90 seconds in length, was administered with the tip of the needle 3 mm below the clival line at a temperature of 75 degrees C.

The needle was then advanced further to the mid clival line and another treatment of similar strength and duration was also administered. Finally the third and last treatment was administered with the tip of the needle about 3 cm above the line. The needle was removed. The patient tolerated the procedure well...

Character 1 Section	Character 2 Body System	Character 3 Root Operation	Character 4 Body Part	Character 5 Approach	Character 6 Device	Character 7 Qualifier
Medical And Surgical	Central Nervous	Destruction	Trigeminal Nerve	Percutaneous	No Device	No Qualifier
0	0	5	K	3	Z	Z

CODING NOTE	**APPROACH VALUE.** The small nick in the skin does not constitute an open approach. it was made to accommodate the radiofrequency needle. The needle was advanced all the way to the operative site, so the correct approach value is Percutaneous.

ROOT OPERATIONS THAT TAKE OUT SOME OR ALL OF A BODY PART

EXTRACTION—ROOT OPERATION D

Extraction **D**	Definition	Pulling or stripping out or off all or a portion of a body part by the use of force
	Explanation	The qualifier Diagnostic is used to identify extraction procedures that are biopsies
	Examples	Dilation and curettage, vein stripping

Extraction is coded when the method employed to take out the body part is pulling or stripping. Minor cutting, such as that used in vein stripping procedures, is included in Extraction if the objective of the procedure is nevertheless met by pulling or stripping. As with all applicable ICD-10-PCS codes, cutting used to reach the procedure site is specified in the approach value.

Example: Suction dilation & curettage

...after induction of general anesthesia the patient was placed in the dorsal lithotomy position and appropriately prepped and draped. Successive dilators were placed until the cervix was adequate for insertion of the suction cannula.

Suction cannula was placed and suction curettage performed with no residual endometrial lining. The tissue was sent to pathology to rule out endometrial cancer...

	Character 2 Body System	Character 3 Root Operation	Character 4 Body Part	Character 5 Approach	Character 6 Device	Character 7 Qualifier
Medical and Surgical	Female Reproductive	Extraction	Endometrium	Via Natural/ Artificial Opening	No Device	Diagnostic
0	**U**	**D**	**B**	**7**	**Z**	**X**

ROOT OPERATIONS THAT TAKE OUT SOLIDS/FLUIDS/GASES FROM A BODY PART

The table below lists the root operations that take out solids, fluids, or gases from a body part. Each is described in detail in the pages that follow.

Root Operation	Objective of Procedure	Site of Procedure	Example
Drainage	Taking/letting out fluids/gases	Within a body part	Incision and drainage
Extirpation	Taking/cutting out solid matter	Within a body part	Thrombectomy
Fragmentation	Breaking solid matter into pieces	Within a body part	Lithotripsy

DRAINAGE---ROOT OPERATION 9

Drainage 9	Definition	Taking or letting out fluids and/or gases from a body part
	Explanation	The qualifier Diagnostic is used to identify drainage procedures that are biopsies
	Examples	Thoracentesis, incision and drainage

The root operation Drainage is coded for both diagnostic and therapeutic drainage procedures. When drainage is accomplished by putting in a catheter, the device value Drainage Device is coded in the sixth character.

Example: *Urinary nephrostomy catheter placement*

...using fluoroscopy and sterile technique a needle was placed through the skin into a markedly dilated right renal collecting system. Guidewire was inserted and an 8 French locking catheter was positioned with the dilated right renal pelvis. It was attached to a bag and immediate drainage of urine was evident...

	Character 2 Body System	Character 3 Root Operation	Character 4 Body Part	Character 5 Approach	Character 6 Device	Character 7 Qualifier
Medical and Surgical	Urinary	Drainage	Kidney Pelvis, Right	Percutaneous	Drainage Device	No Qualifier
0	**T**	**9**	**3**	**3**	**0**	**Z**

ROOT OPERATIONS THAT TAKE OUT SOLIDS/FLUIDS/GASES FROM A BODY PART

EXTIRPATION—ROOT OPERATION C

Extirpation C	Definition	Taking or cutting out solid matter from a body part
	Explanation	The solid matter may be an abnormal byproduct of a biological function or a foreign body; it may be imbedded in a body part or in the lumen of a tubular body part. The solid matter may or may not have been previously broken into pieces.
	Examples	Thrombectomy, endarterectomy, choledocholithotomy

Extirpation represents a range of procedures where the body part itself is not the focus of the procedure. Instead, the objective is to remove solid material such as a foreign body, thrombus, or calculus from the body part.

Example: De-clotting of AV dialysis graft

...the right upper extremity was properly prepped and draped. Local anesthesia was used to explore the graft. A transverse incision in the previous site of the incision, 1 cm below the elbow crease, was performed. The venous limb of the graft was dissected free up to the venous anastomosis.

A small incision on the graft was performed. Then a 3 Fogarty catheter was passed on the venous side. The cephalic vein was found obstructed, not on the anastomotic site, but about 4 cm proximal to the anastomosis. A large number of clots were extracted. After the embolectomy a good back flow from the venous side was obtained.

Then the embolectomy was performed throughout the limb on the arterial side. More clots were extracted and a good arterial flow was obtained.

The procedure was concluded, closing the incision on the graft with 6-0prolene...

	Character 2 Body System	Character 3 Root Operation	Character 4 Body Part	Character 5 Approach	Character 6 Device	Character 7 Qualifier
Medical and Surgical	Upper Veins	Extirpation	Cephalic Vein, Right	Open	No Device	No Qualifier
0	**5**	**C**	**D**	**0**	**Z**	**Z**

CODING NOTE	**BODY PART VALUE.** Do not code separate body parts based on the words "venous side" and "arterial side" in the procedure report. They refer to the two ends of the cephalic vein used to create the fistula.

ROOT OPERATIONS THAT TAKE OUT SOLIDS/FLUIDS/GASES FROM A BODY PART

FRAGMENTATION—ROOT OPERATION F

Fragmentation	Definition	Breaking solid matter in a body part into pieces
F	Explanation	The Physical force (e.g., manual, ultrasonic) applied directly or indirectly is used to break the solid matter into pieces. The solid matter may be an abnormal byproduct of a biological function or a foreign body. The pieces of solid matter are not taken out.
	Examples	Extracorporeal shockwave lithotripsy, transurethral lithotripsy

Fragmentation is coded for procedures to break up, but not remove, solid material such as a calculus or foreign body. This root operation includes both direct and extracorporeal Fragmentation procedures.

Example: ESWL of left kidney

With the patient having been identified, under satisfactory IV sedation and using the MFL 1000 for extracorporeal shock wave lithotripsy, 1000 shocks were delivered to the stone in the lower pole of the left kidney, and 800 shocks were delivered to the stone in the upper pole of the same, with change in shape and density of the stone indicating fragmentation. The patient tolerated the procedure well...

Character 1 Section	Character 2 Body System	Character 3 Root Operation	Character 4 Body Part	Character 5 Approach	Character 6 Device	Character 7 Qualifier
Medical and Surgical	Urinary	Fragment.	Kidney Pelvis, Left	External	No Device	No Qualifier
0	**T**	**F**	**4**	**X**	**Z**	**Z**

ROOT OPERATIONS INVOLVING CUTTING OR SEPARATION ONLY

The table below lists the root operations that cut or separate a body part. Each is described in detail in the pages that follow.

Root Operation	Objective of Procedure	Site of Procedure	Example
Division	Cutting into/separating a body part	Within a body part	Neurotomy
Release	Freeing a body part from constraint	Around a body part	Adhesiolysis

DIVISION---ROOT OPERATION 8

Division 8	Definition	Cutting into a body part without draining fluids and/or gases from the body part in order to separate or transect a body part
	Explanation	All or a portion of the body part is separated into two or more portions
	Examples	Spinal cordotomy, osteotomy

The root operation Division is coded when the objective of the procedure is to cut into, transect, or otherwise separate all or a portion of a body part. When the objective is to cut or separate the area around a body part, the attachments to a body part, or between subdivisions of a body part that are causing abnormal constraint, then the root operation Release is coded instead.

Example: Anal sphincterotomy

Manual examination of the rectum and anus was done, and examination showed that the patient has an anterior anal fissure. For that reason, lateral sphincterotomy was done at the 3 o'clock position using the closed approach, dividing only the internal sphincter using the 11 blade...

	Character 2 Body System	Character 3 Root operation	Character 4 Body Part	Character 5 Approach	Character 6 Device	Character 7 Qualifier
Medical and Surgical	Gastro-intestinal System	Division	Anal Sphincter	Percutaneous	No Device	No Qualifier
0	**D**	**8**	**R**	**3**	**Z**	**Z**

CODING NOTE	**APPROACH VALUE.** This is coded to the Percutaneous approach, because the procedure report says that the sphincterotomy was done using the closed approach, dividing only the internal sphincter.

ROOT OPERATIONS INVOLVING CUTTING OR SEPARATION ONLY

RELEASE—ROOT OPERATION N

Release **N**	Definition	Freeing a body part from an abnormal physical constraint by cutting or by use of force
	Explanation	Some of the restraining tissue may be taken out but none of the body part is taken out
	Examples	Adhesiolysis, carpal tunnel release

The objective of procedures represented in the root operation Release is to free a body part from abnormal constraint. Release procedures are coded to the body part being freed. The procedure can be performed on the area around a body part, on the attachments to a body part, or between subdivisions of a body part that are causing the abnormal constraint.

Example: Release of median nerve

...the right arm was scrubbed with Betadine and prepped and draped in the usual sterile fashion. A well-padded tourniquet was fixed to the right proximal arm but not inflated until after draping. After draping, the right arm was exsanguinated with a combination of elevation and an Esmarch bandage, placing a sponge in the palm. The tourniquet was inflated to 250.

A transverse incision was made at the level of the proximal wrist crease between the palmaris longus and the flexor carpi ulnaris sharply through the skin with a knife, and subcutaneous tissue was dissected by blunt spreading.

The volar fascia was identified and a transverse incision was made sharply with a knife. The flat synovial retractor was pushed through the underneath of the transverse carpal ligament, removing synovium from beneath the ligament.

The entire carpal tunnel and the fat pad distally was visualized. The blade was inserted into the carpal tunnel, was elevated at the distal edge of the transverse carpal ligament, and was pulled proximally, spreading and cutting through the transverse carpal ligament.

It was visualized that the entire median nerve had been released, and that configuration of the end of the transverse carpal ligament was a rectangle, denoting that both the deep and the superficial fibers had been cut.

The wound was then copiously irrigated with saline...

Character 1 Section	Character 2 Body System	Character 3 Root Operation	Character 4 Body Part	Character 5 Approach	Character 6 Device	Character 7 Qualifier
Medical and Surgical	Peripheral Nervous	Release	Median Nerve	Open	No Device	No Qualifier
0	**1**	**N**	**5**	**0**	**Z**	**Z**

CODING NOTE	**BODY PART VALUE.** The body part value assigned is the structure released and not the structure cut to obtain the release, where the two differ. The transverse carpal ligament was cut to release the median nerve and not for its own sake.

ROOT OPERATIONS THAT PUT IN/PUT BACK OR MOVE SOME/ALL OF A BODY PART

The table below lists the root operations that put in, put back, or move some or all of a body part. Each is described in detail in the pages that follow.

Root Operation	Objective of Procedure	Site of Procedure	Example
Transplantation	Putting in a living body part from a person/animal	Some/all of a body part	Kidney transplant
Reattachment	Putting back a detached body part	Some/all of a body part	Reattach finger
Transfer	Moving a body part to function for a similar body part	Some/all of a body part	Skin transfer flap
Reposition	Moving a body part to normal or other suitable location	Some/all of a body part	Move undescended testicle

TRANSPLANTATION---ROOT OPERATION Y

Transplantation Y	Definition	Putting in or on all or a portion of a living body part taken from another individual or animal to physically take the place and/or function of all or a portion of a similar body part
	Explanation	The native body part may or may not be taken out, and the transplanted body part may take over all or a portion of its function
	Examples	Kidney transplant, heart transplant

A small number of procedures is represented in the root operation Transplantation and includes only the body parts currently being transplanted. Qualifier values specify the genetic compatibility of the body part transplanted.

Example: Right kidney transplant (syngeneic)

...the abdomen was sterilely prepped and draped in the usual fashion and incision in the right flank, the Gibson technique, performed. In doing so the right pelvis was entered and Book-Walter retractor appropriately positioned to provide exposure of the external iliac artery and vein.

The artery was placed on vessel loop retraction. We then proceeded with the kidney transplant, and the kidney which was trimmed on the back table was brought into the field. The right renal vein was cut short without reconstruction of the inferior vena cava, and single ureter was identified. Kidney was brought up in an ice chest and an end-to-end anastomosis was performed in the usual fashion with 5-0 Prolene between donor renal vein and external iliac vein on the right.

The long renal artery was brought into view, and end-to-side anastomosis performed in the usual fashion with 5-0 Prolene.

We then turned our attention to performing the neoureterocystostomy after appropriate positioning of the graft and evaluation of the vessels.

After the anastomosis was completed there was no evidence of leak. A Blake drain was brought out through a stab incision and the tip of the drain placed near the neoureterocystostomy and both wounds were closed. The infrainguinal wound was closed with running 3-0 Vicryl and the kidney transplant wound was closed with 1 PDS...

Character 1 Section	Character 2 Body System	Character 3 Root Operation	Character 4 Body Part	Character 5 Approach	Character 6 Device	Character 7 Qualifier
Medical and Surgical	Urinary	Transplant.	Kidney, Right	Open	No Device	Syngeneic
0	**T**	**Y**	**0**	**0**	**Z**	**1**

CODING NOTE	**BONE MARROW TRANSPLANT PROCEDURES** are coded in section 3 Transplant Administration to the root operation 2 Transfusion.

REATTACHMENT---ROOT OPERATION M

Reattachment	Definition	Putting back in or on all or a portion of a separated body part to its normal location or other suitable location
M	Explanation	Vascular circulation and nervous pathways may or may not be reestablished
	Examples	Reattachment of hand, reattachment of avulsed kidney

Procedures coded to Reattachment include putting back a body part that has been cut off or avulsed. Nerves and blood vessels may or may not be reconnected in a Reattachment procedure.

Example: Complex reattachment, left index finger

A sharp debridement of grossly contaminated tissue was carried out. It was noted that the extensor mechanism distal to the PIP joint had been lost. There were circumferential lacerations about the finger, save for a cutaneous bridge and ulnar vascular pedicle present at the PIP level.

Nonviable bony fragments were removed and then the distal portion of the PIP joint was reshaped with removal of cartilage using double- rongeurs. It was noted that the fractures through the proximal phalanx extended longitudinally. Stabilization was then carried out, with 0.062 K-wire brought down through the distal finger, out through the fingertip, and then back into the proximal phalanx centrally.

The A2 pulley was restored, using figure of eight interrupted sutures of 4 and 5-0 Vicryl, reapproximating the flexor tendons. The extensor mechanisms and tendons were repaired using 4 and 5-0 Vicryl, and anchored to the periosteum on the middle phalanx. A digital nerve was then carried out on the radial aspect of the digit at the PIP joint level using interrupted sutures of 9-0 Ethilon beneath the microscope.

At this point, the skin was trimmed, removing skin margins, and then multiple lacerations were closed with 5-0 Prolene...

Character 1 Section	Character 2 Body System	Character 3 Root Operation	Character 4 Body Part	Character 5 Approach	Character 6 Device	Character 7 Qualifier
Medical and Surgical	Upper Extremities	Reattachment	Index Finger, Left	Open	No Device	No Qualifier
0	**X**	**M**	**P**	**0**	**Z**	**Z**

TRANSFER---ROOT OPERATION X

Transfer	Definition	Moving, without taking out, all or a portion of a body part to another location to take over the function of all or a portion of a body part
X	Explanation	The body part transferred remains connected to its vascular and nervous supply
	Examples	Tendon transfer, skin pedicle flap transfer

The root operation Transfer is used to represent procedures where a body part is moved to another location without disrupting its vascular and nervous supply. In the body systems that classify the subcutaneous tissue, fascia and muscle body parts, qualifiers can be used to specify when more than one tissue layer was used in the transfer procedure, such as a musculocutaneous flap transfer.

Example: Fasciocutaneous flap from scalp to cheek

...development of the plane of dissection was completed into the superficial temporal fascia. Development of subgaleal dissection posteriorly was then completed, a distance of 7-8 cm, with hemo- stasis by electrocautery.

The flaps were advanced to the cheek defect and secured with 2-0 inverted PDS sutures and3-0 inverted Monocryl...

	Character 2 Body System	Character 3 Root Operation	Character 4 Body Part	Character 5 Approach	Character 6 Device	Character 7 Qualifier
Medical and Surgical	Subcut Tissue and Fascia	Transfer	Scalp	Open	No Device	Skin, Subcut And Fascia
0	**J**	**X**	**0**	**0**	**Z**	**C**

CODING NOTE	**BODY SYSTEM VALUE.** The body system value describes the deepest tissue layer in the flap. The qualifier can be used to describe the other tissue layers, if any, being transferred.

REPOSITION---ROOT OPERATION S

Reposition	Definition	Moving to its normal location or other suitable location all or a portion of a body part
S	Explanation	The body part is moved to a new location from an abnormal location, or from a normal location where it is not functioning correctly. The body part may or may not be cut out or off to be moved to the new location
	Examples	Reposition of undescended testicle, fracture reduction

Reposition represents procedures for moving a body part to a new location. The range of Reposition procedures includes moving a body part to its normal location, or moving a body part to a new location to enhance its ability to function.

Example: Reposition of undescended right testicle from pelvic region to scrotum

...Following satisfactory induction of general anesthesia, an incision was made in the inguinal region and dissection carried down to the pelvic cavity, where the right testis was located and mobilized.

The spermatic cord was located and freed from surrounding tissue, and its length judged to be sufficient.

A one centimeter incision was made in the scrotum and a pouch created in the usual fashion. The right testicle was mobilized down through the inguinal canal into the scrotum, and stitched in place.

Meticulous hemostasis was obtained, and the incisions closed in layers...

Character 1 Section	Character 2 Body System	Character 3 Root Operation	Character 4 Body Part	Character 5 Approach	Character 6 Device	Character 7 Qualifier
Medical and Surgical	Male Reproductive	Reposition	Testis, Right	Open	No Device	No Qualifier
0	**V**	**S**	**9**	**0**	**Z**	**Z**

ROOT OPERATIONS THAT ALTER THE DIAMETER/ROUTE OF A TUBULAR BODY PART

The table below lists the root operations that alter the diameter or route of a tubular body part. Tubular body parts are defined in ICD-10-PCS as those hollow body parts that provide a route of passage for solids, liquids, or gases. They include the cardiovascular system, and body parts such as those contained in the gastrointestinal tract, genitourinary tract, biliary tract, and respiratory tract. Each root operation is described in detail in the pages that follow.

Root Operation	Objective of Procedure	Site of Procedure	Example
Restriction	Partially closing orifice/ lumen	Tubular body part	Gastroesophageal fundoplication
Occlusion	Completely closing orifice/ lumen	Tubular body part	Fallopian tube ligation
Dilation	Expanding orifice/lumen	Tubular body part	Percutaneous transluminal coronary angioplasty (PTCA)
Bypass	Altering route of passage	Tubular body part	Coronary artery bypass graft (CABG)

ROOT OPERATIONS THAT ALTER THE DIAMETER/ROUTE OF A TUBULAR BODY PART

RESTRICTION—ROOT OPERATION V

Restriction	Definition	Partially closing an orifice or the lumen of a tubular body part
V	Explanation	The orifice can be a natural orifice or an artificially created orifice
	Examples	Esophagogastric fundoplication, cervical cerclage

The root operation Restriction is coded when the objective of the procedure is to narrow the diameter of a tubular body part or orifice. Restriction includes both intraluminal or extraluminal methods for narrowing the diameter.

Example: Laparoscopic gastroesophageal fundoplication

.. .Insufflation was accomplished through a 5 infraumbilical incision. Five separate 5 mm ports were placed under direct visualization other than the initial port. Laparoscopy revealed a large hiatal hernia. Electrocautery was used to free up adhesions from the hernia sac to the stomach.

Next, the fundus which had been mobilized was brought down into the stomach and it was felt there was enough mobilization to perform a fundoplication. A generous loose fundoplication was then performed by wrapping the fundus around the esophagus. Interrupted 0 Ethibond sutures were used to secure the stomach in this fashion.

There was generally good hemostasis throughout the case. All instruments were removed and ports closed.

Character 1 Section	Character 2 Body System	Character 3 Root Operation	Character 4 Body Part	Character 5 Approach	Character 6 Device	Character 7 Qualifier
Medical And Surgical	Gastro-intestinal System	Restriction	Esophago-gastric Junction	Percutaneous Endoscopic	No Device	No Qualifier
0	**D**	**V**	**4**	**4**	**Z**	**Z**

ROOT OPERATIONS THAT ALTER THE DIAMETER/ROUTE OF A TUBULAR BODY PART

OCCLUSION—ROOT OPERATION L

Occlusion	Definition	Completely closing an orifice or the lumen of a tubular body part
L	Explanation	The orifice can be a natural orifice or an artificially created orifice
	Examples	Fallopian tube ligation, ligation of inferior vena cava

The root operation Occlusion is coded when the objective of the procedure is to close off a tubular body part or orifice. Occlusion includes both intraluminal or extraluminal methods of closing off the body part. Division of the tubular body part prior to closing it is an integral part of the Occlusion procedure.

Example: Uterine artery embolization

... catheter was advanced over a 0.18 Terumo gold guidewire and advanced several centimeters super selectively into the left uterine artery. Contrast injection was performed here, confirming filling of the uterine artery and subsequent opacification of large vascular structures in the uterus compatible with uterine fibroids.

A syringe and a half of 500-700 micron biospheres was then instilled slowly through the catheter, and at the conclusion of this infusion there was cessation of flow through the uterine artery.

The catheter was then removed and hemostasis achieved...

Character 1 Section	Character 2 Body System	Character 3 Root Operation	Character 4 Body Part	Character 5 Approach	Character 6 Device	Character 7 Qualifier
Medical And Surgical	Lower Arteries	Occlusion	Internal Iliac Artery, Left	Percutaneous	Intraluminal Device	Uterine Artery, Left
0	4	L	F	3	D	U

ROOT OPERATIONS THAT ALTER THE DIAMETER/ROUTE OF A TUBULAR BODY PART

DILATION—ROOT OPERATION 7

Dilation 7	Definition	Expanding an orifice or the lumen of a tubular body part
	Explanation	The orifice can be a natural orifice or an artificially created orifice. Accomplished by stretching a tubular body part using intraluminal pressure or by cutting part of the orifice or wall of the tubular body part
	Examples	Percutaneous transluminal angioplasty, pyloromyotomy

The root operation Dilation is coded when the objective of the procedure is to enlarge the diameter of a tubular body part or orifice. Dilation includes both intraluminal or extraluminal methods of enlarging the diameter. A device placed to maintain the new diameter is an integral part of the Dilation procedure, and is coded to a sixth-character device value in the Dilation procedure code.

Example: PTCA of left anterior descending

...under 1% Lidocaine local anesthesia, the right femoral artery was entered by the Seldinger technique and a 7French sheath was placed. A Judkins left guiding catheter was advanced to the left coronary ostium and using a .014 Entree wire and a 2.5 x 30 mm Panther balloon, it was easily placed across the lesion in the left anterior descending.

The balloon was inflated times two for five minutes for up to 9 atmospheres. Angiography demonstrated an excellent result...

Character 1 Section	Character 2 Body System	Character 3 Root Operation	Character 4 Body Part	Character 5 Approach	Character 6 Device	Character 7 Qualifier
Medical and Surgical	Heart and Great Vessels	Dilation	Coronary Art., One Site	Percutaneous	No Device	No Qualifier
0	**2**	**7**	**0**	**3**	**Z**	**Z**

ROOT OPERATIONS THAT ALTER THE DIAMETER/ROUTE OF A TUBULAR BODY PART

BYPASS—ROOT OPERATION 1

Bypass 1	Definition	Altering the route of passage of the contents of a tubular body part
	Explanation	Rerouting contents of a body part to a downstream area of the normal route, to a similar route and body part, or to an abnormal route and dissimilar body part. Includes one or more anastomoses, with or without the use of a device
	Examples	Coronary artery bypass, colostomy formation

Example: Aorto-bifemoral bypass graft

...the patient was prepped and draped, and groin incisions were opened. The common femoral vein and its branches were isolated and Teflon tapes were placed around the vessels.

The aorta and iliacs were mobilized. Bleeding points were controlled with electrocautery and Liga clips. Tapes were placed around the vessel, the vessel measured, and the aorta was found to be 12 mm. A 12 x 7 bifurcated microvelour graft was then preclotted with the patient's own blood.

An end-to-end anastomosis was made on the aorta and the graft using a running suture of 2-0 Prolene. The limbs were taken down through tunnels noting that the ureters were anterior, and at this point an end-to-side anastomosis was made between the graft and the femoral arteries with running suture of 4-0 Prolene.

The inguinal incisions were closed.

Bypass is coded when the objective of the procedure is to reroute the contents of a tubular body part. The range of Bypass procedures includes normal routes such as those made in coronary artery bypass procedures, and abnormal routes such as those made in colostomy formation procedures.

Character 1 Section	Character 2 Body System	Character 3 Root Operation	Character 4 Body Part	Character 5 Approach	Character 6 Device	Character 7 Qualifier
Medical And Surgical	Lower Arteries	Bypass	Abdominal Aorta	Open	Synthetic Substitute	Bilat Femoral Arteries
0	**4**	**1**	**0**	**0**	**J**	**K**

ROOT OPERATIONS THAT ALWAYS INVOLVE A DEVICE

The table below lists the root operations that always involve a device. Each is described in detail in the pages that follow.

Root Operation	Objective of Procedure	Site of Procedure	Example
Insertion	Putting in non-biological device	In/on a body part	Central line insertion
Replacement	Putting in device that replaces a body part	Some/all of a body part	Total hip replacement
Supplement	Putting in device that reinforces or augments a body part	In/on a body part	Abdominal wall herniorrhaphy using mesh
Change	Exchanging device w/out cutting/ puncturing	In/on a body part	Drainage tube change
Removal	Taking out device	In/on a body part	Central line removal
Revision	Correcting a malfunctioning/ displaced device	In/on a body part	Revision of pacemaker insertion

INSERTION---ROOT OPERATION H

Insertion	Definition	Putting in a non-biological device that monitors, assists, performs or prevents a physiological function but does not physically take the place of a body part
H	Explanation	N/A
	Examples	Insertion of radioactive implant, insertion of central venous catheter

The root operation Insertion represents those procedures where the sole objective is to put in a device without doing anything else to a body part. Procedures typical of those coded to Insertion include putting in a vascular catheter, a pacemaker lead, or a tissue expander.

Example: Port-a-cath placement

...the right chest and neck were prepped and draped in the usual manner and 10 cc's of 1% Lidocaine were injected in the right infraclavicular area.

The right subclavian vein was then punctured and a wire was passed through the needle into the superior vena cava. This was documented by fluoroscopy. Introducer kit was introduced into the subclavian vein and the Port-a-cath was placed through the introducer and by fluoroscopy was placed down to the superior vena cava.

The pocket was then made over the right pectoralis major muscle, superior to the breast, and the Port-a-cath reservoir was placed into this pocket and tacked down with 0 Prolene sutures.

The catheter was then tunneled through a subcutaneous tunnel to this receptacle. Hemostasis was achieved and the subcutaneous tissue closed.

Character 1 Section	Character 2 Body System	Character 3 Root Operation	Character 4 Body Part	Character 5 Approach	Character 6 Device	Character 7 Qualifier
Medical and Surgical	Heart and Gr. Vessels	Insertion	Superior Vena Cava	Percutaneous	Vascular Access Device	No Qualifier
0	**2**	**H**	**V**	**3**	**X**	**Z**

Character 1 Section	Character 2 Body System	Character 3 Root Operation	Character 4 Body Part	Character 5 Approach	Character 6 Device	Character 7 Qualifier
Medical and Surgical	Subcut Tissue and Fascia	Insertion	Chest	Open	Reservoir	No Qualifier
0	**J**	**H**	**6**	**0**	**W**	**Z**

REPLACEMENT---ROOT OPERATION R

Replacement **R**	Definition	Putting in or on biological or synthetic material that physically takes the place and/or function of all or a portion of a body part
	Explanation	The body part may have been taken out or replaced, or may be taken out, physically eradicated, or rendered nonfunctional during the Replacement procedure. A Removal procedure is coded for taking out the device used in a previous replacement procedure.
	Examples	Total hip replacement, bone graft, free skin graft

The objective of procedures coded to the root operation Replacement is to put in a device that takes the place of some or all of a body part. Replacement encompasses a wide range of procedures, from joint replacements to grafts of all kinds.

> ## *Example: Prosthetic lens implantation*
>
> *...a superior peritomy was made on the left eye and adequate hemostasis was achieved using eraser cautery. A posterior one-half thickness groove was placed posterior to the blue line. This was beveled forward toward clear cornea.*
>
> *The anterior chamber was entered at the 11:30position with a blade. The eye was filled with viscoelastic substance. A can-opener type capsulotomy was performed with a cystotome. Hydrodissection was carried out and the lens was rocked gently with a cystotome to loosen it from the cortex.*
>
> *The wound was then opened with corneal scleral scissors. The lens was prolapsed in the anterior chamber and removed. The anterior chamber was then temporarily closed with 8-0 Vicryl sutures and cortical clean-up was performed.*
>
> *One of the sutures was removed and a posterior chamber intraocular lens (Alcon model MZ50BD) was inspected, rinsed, and placed into a capsular bag. Miochol was then instilled into the anterior chamber. The conjunctiva was pulled over the incision and cauterized into place...*

Character 1 Section	Character 2 Body System	Character 3 Root Operation	Character 4 Body Part	Character 5 Approach	Character 6 Device	Character 7 Qualifier
Medical And Surgical	Eye	Replacement	Lens, Left	Percutaneous	Synthetic Substitute	No Qualifier
0	**8**	**R**	**K**	**3**	**J**	**Z**

SUPPLEMENT---ROOT OPERATION U

Supplement **U**	Definition	Putting in or on biologic or synthetic material that physically reinforces and/or augments the function a portion of a body part
	Explanation	The biological material is non-living, or is living and from the same individual. The body part may have been previously replaced, and the Supplement procedure is performed to physically reinforce and/or augment the function of the replaced body part.
	Examples	Herniorrhaphy using mesh, free nerve graft, mitral valve ring annuloplasty, put a new acetabular liner in a previous hip replacement

The objective of procedures coded to the root operation Supplement is to put in a device that reinforces or augments the functions of some or all of a body part. The body part may have been taken out during a previous procedure, but is not taken out as part of the Supplement procedure. Supplement includes a wide range of procedures, from hernia repairs using mesh reinforcement to heart valve annuloplasties and grafts such as nerve grafts that supplement but do not physically take the place of the existing body part.

Example: Posterior colporrhaphy with Gynemesh

...attention was then turned to the posterior wall. Two Allis clamps were placed at the mucocutaneous junction in the region of the fourchette, and another clamp was placed at the apex of the rectocele.

The tissue between the distal clamps and the fourchette was excised, and carefully measured so that the introitus would be a 3-finger introitus The posterior vaginal mucosa was then incised in the midline by sharp and blunt dissection. The mucosa was then dissected to the level at the Allis clamp at the apex of the rectocele, and dissected with blunt and sharp dissection from the underlying tissue. The rectocele was then imbricated using mattress sutures of 2-0 Vicryl, and the area of the levator ani reinforced with Gynemesh.

Two sutures of 2-0 Vicryl were taken in the levator ani muscle, the excess posterior vaginal mucosa excised, and then closed with interrupted sutures of 2-0 Vicryl.

The perineal muscles were then approximated in the midline in layers, using 2-0 Vicryl, after which the perineal skin was approximated using interrupted sutures of 2-0 Vicryl...

Character 1 Section	Character 2 Body System	Character 3 Root Operation	Character 4 Body Part	Character 5 Approach	Character 6 Device	Character 7 Qualifier
Medical and Surgical	Female Reproductive	Supplement	Vagina	Open	Synthetic Substitute	No Qualifier
0	**U**	**U**	**G**	**0**	**J**	**Z**

CHANGE---ROOT OPERATION 2

Change **2**	Definition	Taking out or off a device from a body part and putting back an identical or similar device in or on the same body part without cutting or puncturing the skin or a mucous membrane
	Explanation	All Change procedures are coded using the approach External
	Examples	Urinary catheter change, gastrostomy tube change

The root operation Change represents only those procedures where a similar device is exchanged without making a new incision or puncture. Typical Change procedures include exchange of drainage devices and feeding devices.

> **CODING NOTE** **CHANGE.** In the root operation Change, general body part values are used when the specific body part value is not in the table

Example: Percutaneous endoscopic gastrostomy (PEG) tube exchange

Character 1 Section	Character 2 Body System	Character 3 Root Operation	Character 4 Body Part	Character 5 Approach	Character 6 Device	Character 7 Qualifier
Medical and Surgical	Gastro-intestinal System	Change	Upper Intestinal Tract	External	Feeding Device	No Qualifier
0	**D**	**2**	**0**	**X**	**U**	**Z**

ROOT OPERATIONS THAT ALWAYS INVOLVE A DEVICE

REMOVAL—ROOT OPERATION P

Removal **P**	Definition	Taking out or off a device from a body part
	Explanation	If a device is taken out and a similar device put in without cutting or puncturing the skin or mucous membrane, the procedure is coded to the root operation Change. Otherwise, the procedure for taking out a device is coded to the root operation Removal.
	Examples	Drainage tube removal, cardiac pacemaker removal

Removal represents a much broader range of procedures than those for removing the devices contained in the root operation Insertion. A procedure to remove a device is coded to Removal if it is not an integral part of another root operation, and regardless of the approach or the original root operation by which the device was put in.

CODING NOTE	**REMOVAL.** In the root operation Removal, general body part values are used when the specific body part value is not in the table.

Example: Removal of right forearm external fixator

...the right upper extremity was prepped and draped in a sterile fashion. A tourniquet was placed at 250 mm of pressure.

The external fixator was removed using the appropriate wrench. The four pins in the ulna were then removed manually, as well as with the drill. The wounds were irrigated with antibiotic solution and a sterile dressing applied...

Character 1 Section	Character 2 Body System	Character 3 Root Operation	Character 4 Body Part	Character 5 Approach	Character 6 Device	Character 7 Qualifier
Medical and Surgical	Upper Bones	Removal	Ulna, Right	External	External Fixation	No Qualifier
0	**P**	**P**	**K**	**X**	**5**	**Z**

ROOT OPERATIONS THAT ALWAYS INVOLVE A DEVICE

REVISION—ROOT OPERATION W

Revision **W**	Definition	Correcting, to the extent possible, a malfunctioning or displaced device
	Explanation	Revision can include correcting a malfunctioning device by taking out and/or putting in part of the device
	Examples	Adjustment of pacemaker lead, adjustment of hip prosthesis

Revision is coded when the objective of the procedure is to correct the position or function of a previously placed device, without taking the entire device out and putting a whole new device in its place. A complete re-do of a procedure is coded to the root operation performed.

CODING NOTE	**REVISION.** In the root operation Revision, general body part values are used when the specific body part value is not in the table.

Example: Revision of artificial anal sphincter

...Proceeding through a suprapubic incision, this was then extended after injecting local anesthetic, thereby exposing the underlying tubing, which was then delivered through the suprapubic region.

Meticulous hemostasis was achieved using electrocautery. At that point the pump device was then repositioned in the left lower quadrant abdominal wall region. The tubing was reinserted using dilators, and the skin reapproximated using 2-0 Vicryl sutures. Sterile dressing was then applied...

Character 1 Section	Character 2 Body System	Character 3 Root Operation	Character 4 Body Part	Character 5 Approach	Character 6 Device	Character 7 Qualifier
Medical and Surgical	Gastrointestinal System	Revision	Anus	Open	Artificial Sphincter	No Qualifier
0	**D**	**W**	**Q**	**0**	**L**	**Z**

ROOT OPERATIONS INVOLVING EXAMINATION ONLY

The table below lists the root operations that involve examination of a body part. Each is described in detail in the pages that follow.

Root operation	Objective of Procedure	Site of Procedure	Example
Inspection	Visual/manual exploration	Some/all of a body part	Diagnostic cystoscopy
Map	Location electrical impulses/ functional areas	Brain/cardiac conduction mechanism	Cardiac mapping

ROOT OPERATIONS INVOLVING EXAMINATION ONLY

INSPECTION—ROOT OPERATION J

Inspection	Definition	Visually and/or Manually Exploring A Body Part
J	Explanation	Visual Exploration May Be Performed With Or Without Optical Instrumentation. Manual Exploration May Be Performed Directly Or Through Intervening Body Layers
	Examples	Diagnostic Arthroscopy, Exploratory Laparotomy

The root operation Inspection represents procedures where the sole objective is to examine a body part. Procedures that are discontinued without any other root operation being performed are also coded to Inspection.

Example: Diagnostic colposcopy with examination of cervix

...Colposcopy was done which revealed pseudo-white areas at 2 o'clock and 6o'clock on the cervix, with abnormal cells and irregular white borders noted on both...

Character 1 Section	Character 2 Body System	Character 3 Root Operation	Character 4 Body Part	Character 5 Approach	Character 6 Device	Character 7 Qualifier
Medical And Surgical	Female Reproductive	Inspection	Uterus And Cervix	Via Natural/ Artificial Opening Endo	No Device	No Qualifier
0	U	J	D	8	Z	Z

MAP---ROOT OPERATION K

Map K	Definition	Locating the route of passage of electrical impulses and/or locating functional areas in a body part
	Explanation	Applicable only to the cardiac conduction mechanism and the central nervous system
	Examples	Cardiac mapping, cortical mapping

Mapping represents a very narrow range of procedures. Procedures include only cardiac mapping and cortical mapping.

Example: Cardiac mapping

. ..under sterile technique arterial sheath was placed in the right femoral artery. The electrical catheter was advanced up the aorta and into the left atrium under fluoroscopic guidance and mapping commenced. After adequate recordings were obtained the catheter was withdrawn and hemostasis achieved with manual pressure on the right femoral artery...

Character 1 Section	Character 2 Body System	Character 3 Root Operation	Character 4 Body Part	Character 5 Approach	Character 6 Device	Character 7 Qualifier
Medical and Surgical	Heart & Great Vessels	Map	Conduction Mechanism	Percutaneous	No Device	No Qualifier
0	2	K	8	3	Z	Z

ROOT OPERATIONS THAT DEFINE OTHER REPAIRS

The table below lists the root operations that define other repairs. CONTROL describes the effort to locate and stop postprocedural hemorrhage. Repair is described in detail in the pages that follow.

Root Operation	Objective of Procedure	Site of Procedure	Example
Control	Stopping/attempting to stop postprocedural bleed	Anatomical region	Post-prostatectomy bleeding control
Repair	Restoring body part to its normal structure	Some/all of a body part	Suture laceration

CONTROL---ROOT OPERATION 3

Control 3	Definition	Stopping, or attempting to stop, postprocedural bleeding
	Explanation	The site of the bleeding is coded as an anatomical region and not to a specific body part
	Examples	Control of post-prostatectomy hemorrhage, control of post-tonsillectomy hemorrhage

CONTROL is used to represent a small range of procedures performed to treat postprocedural bleeding. If performing Bypass, Detachment, Excision, Extraction, Reposition, Replacement, or Resection is required to stop the bleeding, then Control is not coded separately.

CODING NOTE **CONTROL** includes irrigation or evacuation of hematoma done at the operative site. Both irrigation and evacuation may be necessary to clear the operative field and effectively stop the bleeding.

Example: Re-opening of laparotomy site with ligation of arterial bleeder

Character 1 Section	Character 2 Body System	Character 3 Root Operation	Character 4 Body Part	Character 5 Approach	Character 6 Device	Character 7 Qualifier
Medical and Surgical	Anatomical Regions, Gen.	Control	Peritoneal Cavity	Open	No Device	No Qualifier
0	W	3	g	0	Z	Z

ROOT OPERATIONS THAT DEFINE OTHER REPAIRS

REPAIR—ROOT OPERATION Q

Repair Q	Definition	Restoring, to the extent possible, a body part to its normal anatomic structure and function
	Explanation	Used only when the method to accomplish the repair is not one of the other root operations
	Examples	Herniorrhaphy, suture of laceration

The root operation Repair represents a broad range of procedures for restoring the anatomic structure of a body part such as suture of lacerations. Repair also functions as the "not elsewhere classified (NEC)" root operation, to be used when the procedure performed does not meet the definition of one of the other root operations. Fixation devices are included for procedures to repair the bones and joints.

Example: Left open inguinal herniorrhaphy

...an incision in the left groin extending on the skin from the internal to the external inguinal ring was made. The external oblique aponeurosis was exposed.

The hernia sac was then ligated at the internal ring with non-dissolving sutures. A hernia repair was then performed. The internal oblique fascia was sutured in interrupted stitches to the ilio-pubic fascia. The spermatic cord was then returned to its anatomical position.

The external oblique aponeurosis was then repaired in interrupted sutures. Complete hemostasis was obtained, and the skin closed...

Character 1 Section	Character 2 Body System	Character 3 Root Operation	Character 4 Body Part	Character 5 Approach	Character 6 Device	Character 7 Qualifier
Medical and Surgical	Lower Extremities	Repair	Inguinal Region, Left	Open	No Device	No Qualifier
0	**Y**	**Q**	**6**	**0**	**Z**	**Z**

ROOT OPERATIONS THAT DEFINE OTHER OBJECTIVES

The last three root operations in the Medical and Surgical section, Fusion, Alteration, and Creation, describe procedures performed for three distinct reasons. Beyond that they have little in common. A Fusion procedure puts a dysfunctional joint out of service rather than restoring function to the joint. Alteration encompasses a whole range of procedures that share only the fact that they are done to improve the way the patient looks. Creation represents only two very specific sex change operations.

Root operation	Objective of procedure	Site of procedure	Example
Fusion	Rendering joint immobile	Joint	Spinal fusion
Alteration	Modifying body part for cosmetic purposes without affecting function	Some/all of a body part	Face lift
Creation	Making new structure for sex change operation	Perineum	Artificial vagina/penis

FUSION---ROOT OPERATION G

Fusion **G**	Definition	Joining together portions of an articular body part rendering the articular body part immobile
	Explanation	The body part is joined together by fixation device, bone graft, or other means
	Examples	Spinal fusion, ankle arthrodesis

A limited range of procedures is represented in the root operation Fusion, because fusion procedures are by definition only performed on the joints. Qualifier values are used to specify whether a vertebral joint fusion uses an anterior or posterior approach, and whether the anterior or posterior column of the spine is fused.

Example: Anterior cervical fusion C-2 through C-4 with bone bank graft

...after skull tong traction was applied, incision was made in the left neck, and Gardner retractors placed to separate the intervertebral muscles at the C-2 through C-4 levels.

Using the drill, a trough was incised on the anterior surface of the C-2 vertebra, and the C-2/C-3 space evacuated with a rongeur, and the accompanying cartilage removed. This procedure was then repeated at the C-3/C-4 level.

Bone bank patella strut graft was trimmed with a saw and fashioned to fit the C-2/C-3 interspace. After adequate adjustments in the size and shape had been made, the graft was tapped securely into place. The procedure was repeated for the C-3/C-4 level.

X-rays revealed good alignment and final position. Traction was gradually decreased to maintain position. Retractors were removed and the fascia was reapproximated with 0 Vicryl...

Character 1 Section	Character 2 Body System	Character 3 Root Operation	Character 4 Body part	Character 5 Approach	Character 6 Device	Character 7 Qualifier
Medical and Surgical	Upper Joints	Fusion	Cervical Joint, 2 or More	OPEN	Nonautologous Tissue Substance	Ant Approach Ant Column
0	**R**	**G**	**2**	**0**	**K**	**0**

ALTERATION---ROOT OPERATION 0

Alteration **0**	Definition	Modifying the natural anatomic structure of a body part without affecting the function of the body part
	Explanation	Principal purpose is to improve appearance
	Examples	Face lift, breast augmentation

Alteration is coded for all procedures performed solely to improve appearance. All methods, approaches, and devices used for the objective of improving appearance are coded here.

CODING NOTE	ALTERATION. Because some surgical procedures can be performed for either medical or cosmetic purposes, coding for Alteration requires diagnostic confirmation that the surgery is in fact performed to improve appearance.

Example: Cosmetic blepharoplasty

...attention was turned to the redundant upper eyelid skin. The ellipse of skin as marked preoperatively was excised bilaterally.

The medial and lateral fat compartments were open bilaterally. The medial compartment had severe fatty excess and periorbital fat herniation. This was resected. The lateral fat compartment was opened and the lateral fat tailored as well.

Subdermal closure was performed with interrupted 3-0 sutures bilaterally. The skin was closed.

Character 1 Section	Character 2 Body System	Character 3 Root Operation	Character 4 Body Part	Character 5 Approach	Character 6 Device	Character 7 Qualifier
Medical And Surgical	Eye	Alteration	Upper Eyelid, Left	Open	No Device	No Qualifier
0	8	0	P	0	Z	Z

Character 1 Section	Character 2 Body System	Character 3 Root Operation	Character 4 Body Part	Character 5 Approach	Character 6 Device	Character 7 Qualifier
Medical And Surgical	Eye	Alteration	Upper Eyelid, Right	Open	No Device	No Qualifier
0	8	0	N	0	Z	Z

CREATION---ROOT OPERATION 4

Creation 4	Definition	Making a new genital structure that does not physically take the place of a body part
	Explanation	Used only for sex change operations
	Examples	Creation of vagina in a male, creation of penis in a female

Creation is used to represent a very narrow range of procedures. Only the procedures performed for sex change operations are included here.

CODING NOTE	**HARVESTING.** If a separate procedure is performed to harvest autograft tissue, *autograft tissue* it is coded to the appropriate root operation in addition to the primary procedure.

Example: Creating a vagina in a male patient using autograft

Character 1 Section	Character 2 Body System	Character 3 Root Operation	Character 4 Body Part	Character 5 Approach	Character 6 Device	Character 7 Qualifier
Medical and Surgical	Anatomical Regions, Gen.	Creation	Perineum, Male	Open	Autologous Tissue Subst.	Vagina
0	**W**	**4**	**M**	**0**	**7**	**0**

ICD-10-PCS PROCEDURES IN THE MEDICAL AND SURGICAL-RELATED SECTIONS

This chapter provides reference material for procedure codes in sections 1 through 9 of ICD-10-PCS. These nine sections define procedures related to the Medical and Surgical section. Codes in these sections contain characters not previously defined, such as substance, function, and method.

First, a table is provided, listing the sections in order. Following the table, reference material is provided for each section, and includes

- General description of the section
- A table listing each root operation in the section, with its corresponding definition
- Coding notes as needed
- Representative examples of procedures coded in that section, in table excerpt format, with explanatory notes as needed
- Coding exercises that provide example procedures and their corresponding ICD-10-PCS codes, with explanatory notes as needed

LIST OF MEDICAL AND SURGICAL-RELATED SECTIONS OF ICD-10-PCS

Nine additional sections of ICD-10-PCS include procedures related to the Medical and Surgical section, such as obstetrical procedures, administration of substances, and extracorporeal procedures.

Section Value	Description
1	Obstetrics
2	Placement
3	Administration
4	Measurement and Monitoring
5	Extracorporeal Assistance and Performance
6	Extracorporeal Therapies
7	Osteopathic
8	Other Procedures
9	Chiropractic

OBSTETRICS—SECTION 1

The Obstetrics section follows the same conventions established in the Medical and Surgical section, with all seven characters retaining the same meaning, as shown in this example of a low forceps extraction.

	Character 2 Body System	Character 3 Root Operation	Character 4 Body Part	Character 5 Approach	Character 6 Device	Character 7 Qualifier
Obstetrics	Pregnancy	Extraction	Products of Conception	Via Nat./Artificial Opening	No Device	Low Forceps
1	**0**	**D**	**0**	**7**	**Z**	**3**

ROOT OPERATIONS

There are twelve root operations in the Obstetrics section. Ten of these are also found in the Medical and Surgical section.

The two root operations unique to Obstetrics are defined below.

Value	Description	Definition
A	Abortion	Artificially terminating a pregnancy
E	Delivery	Assisting the passage of the products of conception from the genital canal

CODING NOTE	**ABORTION** is subdivided according to whether an additional device such as a laminaria or abortifacient is used, or whether the abortion was performed by mechanical means. If either a laminaria or abortifacient is used, then the approach is Via Natural or Artificial Opening. All other abortion procedures are those done by mechanical means (the products of conception are physically removed using instrumentation), and the device value is Z, No Device.

Example: Transvaginal abortion using vacuum aspiration technique

	Character 2 Body System	Character 3 Root Operation	Character 4 Body Part	Character 5 Approach	Character 6 Device	Character 7 Qualifier
Obstetrics	Pregnancy	Abortion	Products Of Conception	Via Nat/Artificial Opening	No Device	Vacuum
1	**0**	**A**	**0**	**7**	**Z**	**6**

CODING NOTE	**DELIVERY** applies only to manually-assisted, vaginal delivery and is defined as assisting the passage of the products of conception from the genital canal. Cesarean deliveries are coded in this section to the root operation Extraction.

Example: Manually-assisted delivery

	Character 2 Body System	Character 3 Root Operation	Character 4 Body Part	Character 5 Approach	Character 6 Device	Character 7 Qualifier
Obstetrics	Pregnancy	Delivery	Products Of Conception	External	No Device	No Qualifier
1	**0**	**E**	**0**	**X**	**Z**	**Z**

OTHER OBSTETRICS CODING EXAMPLES

Procedure	Code
Abortion by dilation and evacuation following laminaria insertion	10A07ZW
Manually assisted spontaneous abortion	10E0XZZ Since the pregnancy was not artificially terminated, this is coded to DELIVERY, because it captures the procedure objective. The fact that it was an abortion will be identified in the diagnosis code.
Abortion by abortifacient insertion	10A07ZX
Bimanual pregnancy examination	10J07ZZ
Extraperitoneal c-section, low transverse incision	10D00Z2
Fetal spinal tap, percutaneous	10903ZA
Fetal kidney transplant, laparoscopic	10Y04ZS
Open in utero repair of congenital diaphragmatic hernia	10Q00ZK Diaphragm is classified to the RESPIRATORY body system in the MEDICAL AND SURGICAL section.
Laparoscopy with total excision of tubal pregnancy	10T24ZZ
Transvaginal removal of fetal monitoring electrode	10P073Z

PLACEMENT—SECTION 2

The Placement section follows the same conventions established in the Medical and Surgical section, with all seven characters retaining the same meaning, as in the example of cast change on the right forearm below.

	Character 2 Body System	Character 3 Root Operation	Character 4 Body Part	Character 5 Approach	Character 6 Device	Character 7 Qualifier
Placement	Anatomical Regions	Change	Lower Arm, Right	External	Cast	No Qualifier
2	W	0	C	X	2	Z

ROOT OPERATIONS

The root operations in the Placement section include only those procedures performed without making an incision or a puncture.

Value	Description	Definition
0	Change	Taking out or off a device from a body region and putting back an identical or similar device in or on the same body region without cutting or puncturing the skin or a mucous membrane
1	Compression	Putting pressure on a body region
2	Dressing	Putting material on a body region for protection
3	Immobilization	Limiting or preventing motion of a body region
4	Packing	Putting material in a body region
5	Removal	Taking out or off a device from a body region
6	Traction	Exerting a pulling force on a body region in a distal direction

Example: Change of vaginal packing

Character 1 Section	Character 2 Body System	Character 3 Root Operation	Character 4 Body Part	Character 5 Approach	Character 6 Device	Character 7
Placement	Anatomical Orifices	Change	Female Genital Tract	External	Packing Material	No Qualifier
2	Y	0	4	X	5	Z

Example: Placement of pressure dressing on abdominal wall

	Character 2 Body System	Character 3 Root operation	Character 4 Body Region	Character 5 Approach	Character 6 Device	Character 7 Qualifier
Placement	Anatomical Regions	Compression	Abdominal Wall	External	Pressure Dressing	No Qualifier
2	W	1	3	X	6	Z

Example: Application of sterile dressing to head wound

Character 1 Section	Character 2 Body System	Character 3 Root operation	Character 4 Body Region	Character 5 Approach	Character 6 Device	Character 7 Qualifier
Placement	Anatomical Regions	Dressing	Head	External	Bandage	No Qualifier
2	W	2	0	X	4	Z

CODING NOTE	**IMMOBILIZATION:** The procedures to fit a device, such as splints and braces, as described in F0DZ6EZ and F0DZ7EZ, apply only to the rehabilitation setting. splints and braces placed in other inpatient settings are coded to Immobilization, table 2X3 in the Placement section.

Example: Placement of splint on left finger

	Character 2 Body System	Character 3 Root operation	Character 4 Body Region	Character 5 Approach	Character 6 Device	Character 7 Qualifier
Placement	Anatomical Regions	Immobilization	Finger, Left	External	Splint	No Qualifier
2	W	3	K	X	1	Z

Example: Placement of nasal packing

Character 1 Section	Character 2 Body System	Character 3 Root operation	Character 4 Body Region	Character 5 Approach	Character 6 Device	Character 7 Qualifier
Placement	Anatomical Orifices	Packing	Nasal	External	Packing Material	No Qualifier
2	Y	4	1	X	5	Z

Example: Removal of stereotactic head frame

Character 1 Section	Character 2 Body System	Character 3 Root operation	Character 4 Body Region	Character 5 Approach	Character 6 Device	Character 7 Qualifier
Placement	Anatomical Regions	Removal	Head	External	Stereotactic Apparatus	No Qualifier
2	W	5	0	X	8	Z

	CODING NOTE	TRACTION in this section includes only the task performed using a mechanical traction apparatus. Manual traction performed by a physical therapist is coded to Manual Therapy Techniques in section F, Physical Rehabilitation and Diagnostic Audiology.

Example: Lumbar traction using motorized split-traction table

	Character 2 Body System	Character 3 Root Operation	Character 4 Body Part	Character 5 Approach	Character 6 Device	Character 7 Qualifier
Placement	Anatomical Regions	Traction	Back	External	Traction Apparatus	No Qualifier
2	**W**	**6**	**5**	**X**	**0**	**Z**

OTHER PLACEMENT CODING EXAMPLES

Procedure	Code
Placement of packing material, right ear	2Y42X5Z
Mechanical traction of entire left leg	2W6MX0Z
Removal of splint, right shoulder	2W5AX1Z
Placement of neck brace	2W32X3Z
Change of vaginal packing	2Y04X5Z
Packing of wound, chest wall	2W44X5Z
Sterile dressing placement to left groin region	2W27X4Z
Removal of packing material from pharynx	2Y50X5Z
Placement of intermittent pneumatic compression device, covering entire right arm	2W18X7Z
Exchange of pressure dressing to left thigh	2W0PX6Z

ADMINISTRATION—SECTION 3

The Administration section includes infusions, injections, and transfusions, as well as other related procedures, such as irrigation and tattooing. All codes in this section define procedures where a diagnostic or therapeutic substance is given to the patient, as in the platelet transfusion example below.

	Character 2 Body System	Character 3 Root Operation	Character 4 Body System	Character 5 Approach	Character 6 Substance	Character 7 Qualifier
Administration	Circulatory	Transfusion	Central Vein	Percutaneous	Platelets	Non-auto logous
3	0	2	4	3	R	1

ROOT OPERATIONS

Root operations in this section are classified according to the broad category of substance administered. If the substance given is a blood product or a cleansing substance, then the procedure is coded to Transfusion and Irrigation respectively. All the other substances administered, such as anti-neoplastic substances, are coded to the root operation Introduction.

Value	Description	Definition
0	Introduction	Putting in or on a therapeutic, diagnostic, nutritional, physiological, or prophylactic substance except blood or blood products
1	Irrigation	Putting in or on a cleansing substance
2	Transfusion	Putting in blood or blood products'

Example: Nerve block injection to median nerve

Character 1 Section	Character 2 Body System	Character 3 Root operation	Character 4 Body System	Character 5 Approach	Character 6 Substance	Character 7 Qualifier
Administration	Phys. Sys. & Anat. Regions	Introduction	Peripheral Nerves	Percutaneous	Regional Anesthetic	No Qualifier
3	E	0	T	3	C	Z

Example: Flushing of eye

Character 1 Section	Character 2 Body System	Character 3 Root operation	Character 4 Body System	Character 5 Approach	Character 6 Substance	Character 7 Qualifier
Administration	Phys. Sys. & Anat. Regions	Irrigation	Eye	External	Irrigating Substance	No Qualifier
3	E	1	C	X	8	Z

Example: Transfusion of cell saver red cells into central venous line

Character 1 Section	Character 2 Body System	Character 3 Root operation	Character 4 Body System	Character 5 Approach	Character 6 Substance	Character 7 Qualifier
Administration	Circulatory	Transfusion	Central Vein	Percutaneous	Red Blood Cells	Autologous
3	**0**	**2**	**4**	**3**	**N**	**0**

OTHER ADMINISTRATION CODING EXAMPLES

Procedure	Code
Peritoneal dialysis via indwelling catheter	3E1M39Z
Transvaginal artificial insemination	3E0P7LZ
Infusion of total parenteral nutrition via central venous catheter	3E0436Z
Esophagogastroscopy with Botox injection into esophageal sphincter	3E0G8GC Botulinum toxin is a paralyzing agent with temporary effects; it does not sclerose or destroy the nerve.
Percutaneous irrigation of knee joint	3E1U38Z
Epidural injection of mixed steroid and local anesthetic for pain control	3E0S33Z This is coded to the substance value ANTI-INFLAMMATORY. The anesthetic is only added to lessen the pain of the injection.
Chemical pleurodesis using injection of tetracycline	3E0L3TZ
Transfusion of antihemophilic factor, (nonautologous) via arterial central line	30263V1
Transabdominal in-vitro fertilization, implantation of donor ovum	3E0P3Q1
Autologous bone marrow transplant via central venous line	30243G0
Implantation of anti-microbial envelope with cardiac defibrillator placement, open	3E0102A

MEASUREMENT AND MONITORING—SECTION 4

There are two root operations in this section, and they differ in only one respect: Measurement defines one procedure and Monitoring defines a series of procedures.

ROOT OPERATIONS

Measurement describes a single level taken, while Monitoring describes a series of levels obtained at intervals. For example,

- A single temperature reading is considered Measurement.
- Temperature taken every half hour for 8 hours is considered Monitoring. Instead of defining a device, the sixth character defines the physiological or physical function being tested.

Value	Description	Definition
0	Measurement	Determining the level of a physiological or physical function at a point in time
1	Monitoring	Determining the level of a physiological or physical function repetitively over a period of time

Example: External electrocardiogram (EKG), single reading

Character 1 Section	Character 2 Body System	Character 3 Root Operation	Character 4 Body System	Character 5 Approach	Character 6 Function	Character 7 Qualifier
Measurement & Monitoring	Physiological Systems	Measurement	Cardiac	External	Electrical Activity	No Qualifier
4	A	0	2	X	4	Z

Example: Urinary pressure monitoring

Character 1 Section	Character 2 Body System	Character 3 Root operation	Character 4 Body System	Character 5 Approach	Character 6 Device	Character 7 Qualifier
Measurement & Monitoring	Physiological Systems	Monitoring	Urinary	Via Nat./Artificial Opening	Pressure	No Qualifier
4	A	1	D	7	B	Z

OTHER MEASURING AND MONITORING CODING EXAMPLES

Procedure	Code
Cardiac stress test, single measurement	4A02XM4
EGD with biliary flow measurement	4A0C85Z
Right and left heart cardiac catheterization with bilateral sampling and pressure measurements	4A023N8
Peripheral venous pulse, external, single measurement	4A04XJ1
Holter monitoring	4A12X45

Respiratory rate, external, single measurement	4A09XCZ
Fetal heart rate monitoring, transvaginal	4A1H7CZ
Visual mobility test, single measurement	4A07X7Z
Pulmonary artery wedge pressure monitoring from Swan-Ganz catheter	4A133B3
Olfactory acuity test, single measurement	4A08X0Z

EXTRACORPOREAL ASSISTANCE AND PERFORMANCE— SECTION 5

This section includes procedures performed in a critical care setting, such as mechanical ventilation and cardioversion. It also includes other procedures, such as hemodialysis and hyperbaric oxygen treatment. These procedures all use equipment to support a physiological function in some way, whether it is breathing, circulating the blood, or restoring the natural rhythm of the heart.

The fifth and sixth characters in this section define duration and function respectively. These characters describe the duration of the procedure and the body function being acted upon, rather than the approach and device used.

Root operations

Assistance and Performance are two variations of the same kinds of procedures, varying only in the degree of control exercised over the physiological function.

Value	Description	Definition
0	Assistance	Taking over a portion of a physiological function by extracorporeal means
1	Performance	Completely taking over a physiological function by extracorporeal means
2	Restoration	Returning, or attempting to return, a physiological function to its original state by extracorporeal means

CODING NOTE	ASSISTANCE defines procedures that support a physiological function but do not take complete control of it, such as intra-aortic balloon pump to support cardiac output and hyperbaric oxygen treatment.

Example: Hyperbaric oxygenation of wound

Character 1 Section	Character 2 Body System	Character 3 Root Operation	Character 4 Body System	Character 5 Duration	Character 6 Function	Character 7 Qualifier
Extracorporeal Assistance & Performance	Physiological Systems	Assistance	Circulatory	Intermittent	Oxygenation	Hyperbaric

5	A	0	5	1	2	

CODING NOTE   **PERFORMANCE** defines procedures where complete control is exercised over a physiological function, such as total mechanical ventilation, cardiac pacing, and cardiopulmonary bypass.

Example: Cardiopulmonary bypass in conjunction with CABG

Character 1 Section	Character 2 Body System	Character 3 Root Operation	Character 4 Body System	Character 5 Duration	Character 6 Function	Character 7 Qualifier
Extracorporeal Assistance & Performance	Physiological Systems	Performance	Cardiac	Continuous	Output	No Qualifier
5	A	1	2	2	1	Z

Character 1 Section	Character 2 Body System	Character 3 Root Operation	Character 4 Body System	Character 5 Duration	Character 6 Function	Character 7 Qualifier
Extracorporeal Assistance & Performance	Physiological Systems	Performance	Respiratory	Less Than 24 Consecutive Hrs	Ventilation	No Qualifier
5	A	1	9	3	5	Z

CODING NOTE   **RESTORATION** defines only external cardioversion and defibrillation procedures. Failed cardio-version procedures are also included in the definition of Restoration, and are coded the same as successful procedures.

Example: Attempted cardiac defibrillation, unsuccessful

Character 1 Section	Character 2 Body System	Character 3 Root Operation	Character 4 Body System	Character 5 Duration	Character 6 Function	Character 7 Qualifier
Extracorporeal Assist. And Performance	Physiological Systems	Restoration	Cardiac	Single	Rhythm	No Qualifier
5	A	2	2	0	4	Z

OTHER EXTRACORPOREAL ASSISTANCE AND PERFORMANCE CODING EXAMPLES

Procedure	Code
Intermittent mechanical ventilation, 16 hours	5A1935Z
Liver dialysis, single encounter	5A1C00Z

Cardiac countershock with successful conversion to sinus rhythm	5A2204Z
IPPB (intermittent positive pressure breathing) for mobilization of secretions, 22 hours	5A09358
Renal dialysis, series of encounters	5A1D60Z
IABP (intra-aortic balloon pump) continuous	5A02210 The procedure to insert the balloon pump is coded to the root operation INSERTION in the MEDICAL AND SURGICAL section.
Intra-operative cardiac pacing, continuous	5A1223Z
ECMO (extracorporeal membrane oxygenation), continuous	5A15223
Controlled mechanical ventilation (CMV), 45 hours	5A1945Z The endotracheal tube associated with the mechanical ventilation procedure is considered a component of the equipment used in performing the procedure and is not coded separately.
Pulsatile compression boot with intermittent inflation	5A02115 This is coded to the function value CARDIAC OUTPUT, because the purpose of such compression devices is to return blood to the heart faster

EXTRACORPOREAL THERAPIES—SECTION 6

Section 6, Extracorporeal Therapies, describes other extracorporeal procedures that are not defined by Assistance and Performance in section 5 *(see page 3 16)*. Examples are bili-lite phototherapy, apheresis, and whole body hypothermia.

The second character contains a single general body system choice, Physiological Systems, as in the phototherapy example below. The sixth character is defined as a qualifier, but contains no specific qualifier values. The seventh-character qualifier identifies various blood components separated out in pheresis procedures.

Character 1 Section	Character 2 Body System	Character 3 Root Operation	Character 4 Body System	Character 5 Duration	Character 6 Function	Character 7 Qualifier
Extracorporeal Therapies	Physiological Systems	Phototherapy	Skin	Single	No Qualifier	No Qualifier

6	A	6	0	0	Z	Z

ROOT OPERATIONS

The meaning of each root operation is consistent with the term as used in the medical community. Decompression and Hyperthermia have a more specialized meaning. All are defined in the table below.

Value	Description	Definition
0	Atmospheric Control	Extracorporeal control of atmospheric pressure and composition
1	Decompression	Extracorporeal elimination of undissolved gas from body fluids
2	Electromagnetic Therapy	Extracorporeal treatment by electromagnetic rays
3	Hyperthermia	Extracorporeal raising of body temperature
4	Hypothermia	Extracorporeal lowering of body temperature
5	Pheresis	Extracorporeal separation of blood products
6	Phototherapy	Extracorporeal treatment by light rays
7	ultrasound Therapy	Extracorporeal treatment by ultrasound
8	Ultraviolet Light Therapy	Extracorporeal treatment by ultraviolet light
9	Shock Wave Therapy	Extracorporeal treatment by shock waves

CODING NOTE **DECOMPRESSION** describes a single type of procedure—treatment for decompression sickness (the bends) in a hyperbaric chamber.

Example: Hyperbaric decompression treatment, single

Character 1 Body System	Character 2 Root	Character 3 Body System	Character 4 Duration	Character 5 Qualifier	Character 6 Qualifier	Character 7 Qualifier
Extracorporeal Therapies	Physiological Systems	Decomp-ression	Circulatory	Single	No Qualifier	No Qualifier
6	A	1	5	0	Z	Z

CODING NOTE **HYPERTHERMIA** is used both to treat temperature imbalance, and as an adjunct radiation treatment for cancer. When performed to treat temperature imbalance, the procedure is coded to this section. When performed for cancer treatment, whole-body hyperthermia is classified as a modality qualifier in section D, Radiation Oncology.

Example: Whole body hypothermia treatment for temperature imbalance, series

	Character 2 Body System	Character 3 Root Operation	Character 4 Body System	Character 5 Duration	Character 6 Qualifier	Character 7 Qualifier
Extracorporeal Therapies	Physiological Systems	Hypothermia	None	Multiple	No Qualifier	No Qualifier
6	A	4	Z	1	Z	Z

CODING NOTE	PHERESIS is used in medical practice for two main purposes: to treat diseases where too much of a blood component is produced, such as leukemia, or to remove a blood product such as platelets from a donor, for transfusion into a patient who needs them.

Example: Therapeutic leukapheresis, single treatment

Character 1 Section	Character 2 Body System	Character 3 Root Operation	Character 4 Body System	Character 5 Duration	Character 6 Qualifier	Character 7 Qualifier
Extracorporeal Therapies	Physiological Systems	Pheresis	Circulatory	Single	No Qualifier	Leukocytes
6	A	5	5	0	Z	1

Example: Phototherapy of circulatory system, series treatment

Character 1 Section	Character 2 Body System	Character 3 Root Operation	Character 4 Body System	Character 5 Duration	Character 6 Qualifier	Character 7 Qualifier
Extracorporeal Therapies	Physiological Systems	Phototherapy	Circulatory	Multiple	No Qualifier	No Qualifier
6	A	6	5	1	Z	Z

Example: Ultraviolet Light Phototherapy, Series Treatment

Character 1 Section	Character 2 Body System	Character 3 Root Operation	Character 4 Body System	Character 5 Duration	Character 6 Qualifier	Character 7 Qualifier
Extracorporeal Therapies	Physiological Systems	UV Light Phototherapy	Skin	Multiple	No Qualifier	No Qualifier
6	A	8	0	1	Z	Z

OTHER EXTRACORPOREAL THERAPIES CODING EXAMPLES

Procedure	Code
Donor thrombocytapheresis, single encounter	6A550Z2
Bili-lite UV phototherapy, series treatment	6A801ZZ
Whole body hypothermia, single treatment	6A4Z0ZZ
Circulatory phototherapy, single encounter	6A650ZZ
Shock wave therapy of plantar fascia, single treatment	6A930ZZ
Antigen-free air conditioning, series treatment	6A0Z1ZZ
TMS (transcranial magnetic stimulation), series treatment	6A221ZZ
Therapeutic ultrasound of peripheral vessels, single treatment	6A750ZZ
Plasmapheresis, series treatment	6A551Z3
Extracorporeal electromagnetic stimulation (EMS) for urinary incontinence, single treatment	6A210ZZ

OSTEOPATHIC—SECTION 7

Section 7, Osteopathic, is one of the smallest sections in ICD-10-PCS. There is a single body system, Anatomical Regions, and a single root operation, Treatment.

The sixth-character methods such as Lymphatic Pump and Fascial Release are not explicitly defined in ICD-10-PCS, and rely on the standard definitions as used in this specialty.

Value	Description	Definition
0	Treatment	Manual treatment to eliminate or alleviate somatic dysfunction and related disorders

Example: Fascial release of abdomen, osteopathic treatment

	Character 2 Body System	Character 3 Operation	Character 4 Body Region	Character 5 Approach	Character 6 Method	Character 7 Qualifier
Osteopathic	Anatomical Regions	Treatment	Abdomen	External	Fascial Release	No Qualifier
7	W	0	9	X	1	Z

Example: General osteopathic mobilization of legs

Character 1 Section	Character 2 Body System	Character 3 Operation	Character 4 Body Region	Character 5 Approach	Character 6 Method	Character 7
Osteopathic	Anatomical Regions	Treatment	Lower Extremities	External	General Mobilization	No Qualifier
7	W	0	6	X	2	Z

OTHER OSTEOPATHIC CODING EXAMPLES

PROCEDURES	CODE
Isotonic muscle energy treatment of right leg	7W06X8Z
Low velocity-high amplitude osteopathic treatment of head	7W00X5Z
Lymphatic pump osteopathic treatment of left axilla	7W07X6Z
Indirect osteopathic treatment of sacrum	7W04X4Z
Articulatory osteopathic treatment of cervical region	7W01X0Z

OTHER PROCEDURES—SECTION 8

The Other Procedures section contains codes for procedures not included in the other medical and surgical-related sections A single root operation, Other Procedures, is defined below.

Value	Description	Definition
0	Other Procedures	Methodologies which attempt to remediate or cure a disorder or disease

There are relatively few procedure codes in this section, for nontraditional, whole body therapies including acupuncture and meditation. There is also a code for the fertilization portion of an in-vitro fertilization procedure.

Example: Acupuncture

	Character 2 Body System	Character 3 Root Operation	Character 4 Body Region	Character 5 Approach	Character 6 Method	Character 7 Qualifier
Other Procedures	Phys. Sys. & Anat. Regions	Other Procedures	Integumentary Sys. & Breast	Percutaneous	Acupuncture	No Qualifier
8	E	0	H	3	0	Z

Example: Yoga therapy

Character 1 Section	Character 2 Body System	Character 3 Root Operation	Character 4 Body Region	Character 5 Approach	Character 6 Method	Character 7 Qualifier
Other Procedures	Phys. Sys. & Anat. Regions	Other Procedures	None	External	Other Method	Yoga Therapy
8	**E**	**0**	**Z**	**X**	**Y**	**4**

OTHER PROCEDURES CODING EXAMPLES

Procedure	Code
Near infrared spectroscopy of leg vessels	8E023DZ
CT computer assisted sinus surgery	8E09XBG The primary procedure is coded separately.
Suture removal, abdominal wall	8E0WXY8
Isolation after infectious disease exposure	8E0ZXY6
Robotic assisted open prostatectomy	8E0W0CZ The primary procedure is coded separately.

CHIROPRACTIC—SECTION 9

The Chiropractic section consists of a single body system, Anatomical Regions, and a single root operation, Manipulation, defined below.

Value	Description	Definition
B	Manipulation	Manual procedure that involves a directed thrust to move a joint past the physiological range of motion, without exceeding the anatomical limit

Example: Chiropractic treatment of cervical spine, short lever specific contact

	Character 2 Body System	Character 3 Root Operation	Character 4 Body Region	Character 5 Approach	Character 6 Method	Character 7 Qualifier
Chiropractic	Anatomical Regions	Manipulation	Cervical	External	Short Lever Sp. Contact	No Qualifier
9	**W**	**B**	**1**	**X**	**H**	**Z**

Example: Non-manual chiropractic manipulation of pelvis

Character 1 Section	Character 2 Body System	Character 3 Root Operation	Character 4 Body Region	Character 5 Approach	Character 6 Method	Character 7 Qualifier
Chiropractic	Anatomical Regions	Manipulation	Pelvis	External	Non-Manual	No Qualifier
9	**W**	**B**	**5**	**X**	**B**	**Z**

OTHER CHIROPRACTIC CODING EXAMPLES

Procedure	Code
Chiropractic treatment of lumbar region using long lever specific contact	9WB3XGZ
Chiropractic manipulation of abdominal region, indirect visceral	9WB9XCZ
Chiropractic extra-articular treatment of hip region	9WB6XDZ
Chiropractic treatment of sacrum using long and short lever specific contact	9WB4XJZ
Mechanically-assisted chiropractic manipulation of head	9WB0XKZ

PROCEDURES IN THE ANCILLARY SECTIONS

This section provides reference material for procedure codes in the six ancillary sections of ICD-10-PCS (B through D, F through H). Codes in these sections contain characters not previously defined, such as contrast, modality qualifier and equipment.

First, a table is provided, listing the sections in order. Following the table, reference material is provided for each section, and includes

- General description of the section
- A table listing each root type in the section, with its corresponding definition (sections B, C and F only)
- Coding notes as needed
- Representative examples of procedures coded in that section, in table excerpt format, with explanatory notes as needed
- Coding exercises that provide example procedures and their corresponding ICD-10-PCS codes, with explanatory notes as needed

LIST OF ANCILLARY SECTIONS IN ICD-10-PCS

Six ancillary sections of ICD-10-PCS include procedures such as imaging, radiation oncology, and rehabilitation.

Section Value	Description
B	Imaging
C	Nuclear Medicine

D	Radiation Oncology
F	Physical Rehabilitation and Diagnostic Audiology
G	Mental Health
H	Substance Abuse Treatment

IMAGING—SECTION B

Imaging follows the same conventions established in the Medical and Surgical section (*see chapter* 2), for the section, body system, and body part characters. However, the third and fourth characters introduce definitions not used in previous sections.

- Third character defines procedure by root type, instead of root operation.
- Fifth character defines contrast if used.
- Sixth character is a qualifier that specifies an image taken without contrast followed by one with contrast.
- Seventh character is a qualifier that is not specified in this section.

ROOT TYPES

The Imaging root types are defined in the following table.

Value	Description	Definition
0	Plain Radiography	Planar display of an image developed from the capture of external ionizing radiation on photographic or photoconductive plate
1	Fluoroscopy	Single plane or bi-plane real time display of an image developed from the capture of external ionizing radiation on a fluorescent screen. The image may also be stored by either digital or analog means
2	Computerized Tomography (CT scan)	Computer reformatted digital display of multiplanar images developed from the capture of multiple exposures of external ionizing radiation
3	Magnetic Resonance Imaging (MRI)	Computer reformatted digital display of multiplanar images developed from the capture of radio-frequency signals emitted by nuclei in a body site excited within a magnetic field
4	Ultrasonography	Real time display of images of anatomy or flow information developed from the capture of reflected and attenuated high frequency sound waves

Example: X-ray of right clavicle, limited study

Character 1 Section	Character 2 Body System	Character 3 Root Type	Character 4 Body Part	Character 5 Contrast	Character 6 Qualifier	Character 7 Qualifier
Imaging	Veins	Fluoroscopy	Dialysis Shunt/Fistula	Other Contrast	None	None

| B | 5 | 1 | W | Y | Z | Z |

Example: CT of brain without contrast followed by high osmolar contrast

Character 1 Section	Character 2 Body System	Character 3 Root Type	Character 4 Body Part	Character 5 Contrast	Character 6 Qualifier	Character 7 Qualifier
Imaging	Central Nervous	Computerized Tomography	Brain	High Osmolar	Unenhanced and Enhanced	None
B	**0**	**2**	**0**	**0**	**0**	**Z**

Example: MRI of liver using Gadoteridol

Character 1 Section	Character 2 Body System	Character 3 Root Type	Character 4 Body Part	Character 5 Contrast	Character 6 Qualifier	Character 7 Qualifier
Imaging	Hepatobiliary & Pancreas	Magnetic Resonance Imaging	Liver	Other Contrast	None	None
B	**F**	**3**	**5**	**Y**	**Z**	**Z**

Example: Ultrasound of prostate gland

Character 1 Section	Character 2 Body System	Character 3 Root Type	Character 4 Body Part	Character 5 Contrast	Character 6 Qualifier	Character 7 Qualifier
Imaging	Male Reproductive	Ultra-sonography	Prostate and Seminal Vesicles	None	None	None
B	**V**	**4**	**9**	**Z**	**Z**	**Z**

Example: X-ray of right clavicle, limited study

	Character 2 Body System	Character 3 Root Type	Character 4 Body Part	Character 5 Contrast	Character 6 Qualifier	Character 7 Qualifier
Imaging	Non-axial Upper Bones	Plain Radiography	Clavicle, Right	None	None	None
B	**P**	**0**	**4**	**Z**	**Z**	**Z**

OTHER IMAGING CODING EXAMPLES

Procedure	Code
Non-contrast CT of abdomen and pelvis	BW21ZZZ
Intravascular ultrasound, left subclavian artery	B342ZZ3

Fluoroscopic guidance for insertion of central venous catheter in SVC, low osmolar contrast	B5181ZA
Endoluminal ultrasound of gallbladder and bile ducts	BF43ZZZ
Left ventriculography using low osmolar contrast	B2151ZZ
Esophageal videofluoroscopy study with oral barium contrast	BD11YZZ
Portable X-ray study of right radius/ulna shaft, standard series	BP0JZZZ
Routine fetal ultrasound, second trimester twin gestation	BY4DZZZ
CT scan of bilateral lungs, high osmolar contrast with densitometry	BB240ZZ
Fluoroscopic guidance for percutaneous transluminal angioplasty (PTA) of left common femoral artery, low osmolar contrast	B41G1ZZ

NUCLEAR MEDICINE—SECTION C

Nuclear Medicine is organized like the Imaging section *(see page 4.5)*. The only significant difference is that the fifth character defines the radionuclide instead of the contrast material used in the procedure, as described below.

- The fifth character specifies the radionuclide, the radiation source used in the procedure. Choices are applicable for the root procedure type.
- The sixth and seventh characters are qualifiers, and are not specified in this section.

ROOT TYPES

The third character classifies the procedure by root type instead of by root operation.

Value	Description	Definition
1	Planar Nuclear Medicine Imaging	Introduction of radioactive materials into the body for single plane display of images developed from the capture of radioactive emissions
2	Tomographic (Tomo) Nuclear Medicine Imaging	Introduction of radioactive materials into the body for three-dimensional display of images developed from the capture of radioactive emissions
3	Positron Emission Tomography (PET)	Introduction of radioactive materials into the body for three-dimensional display of images developed from the simultaneous capture, 180 degrees apart, of radioactive emissions
4	Nonimaging Nuclear Medicine Uptake	Introduction of radioactive materials into the body for measurements of organ function, from the detection of radioactive emissions
5	Nonimaging Nuclear Medicine Probe	Introduction of radioactive materials into the body for the study of distribution and fate of certain substances by the detection of radioactive emissions from an external source

6	Nonimaging Nuclear medicine Assay	Introduction of radioactive materials into the body for the study of body fluids and blood elements, by the detection of radioactive emissions
7	Systemic Nuclear Medicine Therapy	Introduction of unsealed radioactive materials into the body for treatment

Example: Adenosine sestamibi (technetium) planar scan of heart muscle at rest

	Character 2 Body System	Character 3 Root Type	Character 4 Body Part	Character 5 Radionuclide	Character 6 Qualifier.	Character 7 Qualifier
Nuclear Medicine	Heart	Planar Nuclear Imaging	Myocardium	Technetium 99m	None	None
C	2	1	G	1	Z	Z

Example: Technetium tomo scan of liver

Character 1 Section	Character 2 Body System	Character 3 Root Type	Character 4 Body Part	Character 5 Radionuclide	Character 6 Qualifier	Character 7 Qualifier
Nuclear Medicine	Hepatobiliary And Pancreas	Tomo Nuclear Imaging	Liver	Technetium 99M	None	None
C	F	2	5	1	Z	Z

OTHER NUCLEAR MEDICINE CODING EXAMPLES

Procedure	Code
Tomo scan of right and left heart, unspecified radiopharmaceutical, qualitative gated rest	C226YZZ
Technetium pentetate assay of kidneys, ureters, and bladder	CT631ZZ
Uniplanar scan of spine using technetium oxidronate, with first pass study	CP151ZZ
Thallous chloride tomographic scan of bilateral breasts	CH22SZZ
PET scan of myocardium using rubidium	C23GQZZ
Gallium citrate scan of head and neck, single plane imaging	CW1BLZZ
Xenon gas non-imaging probe of brain	C050VZZ
Upper GI scan, radiopharmaceutical unspecified, for gastric emptying	CD15YZZ
Carbon 11 PET scan of brain with quantification	C030BZZ
Iodinated albumin nuclear medicine assay, blood plasma volume study	C763HZZ

RADIATION ONCOLOGY—SECTION D

Radiation Oncology contains the radiation procedures performed for cancer treatment. Character meanings are described below.

- Third character defines root type, which is the basic modality.
- Fifth character further specifies treatment modality.
- Sixth character defines the radioactive isotope used, if applicable.
- Seventh character is a qualifier, and is not specified in this section.

ROOT TYPE

The third character defines the treatment modality as root type.

Examples are Brachytherapy and Stereotactic Radiosurgery. Four different root types are used in this section, as listed in the table below.

Value	Description
0	Beam Radiation
1	Brachytherapy
2	Stereotactic Radiosurgery
Y	Other Radiation

Example: LDR Brachytherapy of cervix using Iridium 192

Character 1 Section	Character 2 Body System	Character 3 Root Type	Character 4 Body part	Character 5 Modal. Qualifier	Character 6 isotope	Character 7 Qualifier
Radiation Oncology	Female Reproductive	Brachytherapy	Cervix	LDR Brachy-therapy	Iridium 192	None
D	**U**	**1**	**1**	**B**	**8**	**Z**

Example: Intraoperative radiation therapy (IORT) of bladder

Character 1 Section	Character 2 Body Sys	Character 3 Root Type	Character 4 Body part	Character 5 Modal. Qualifier	Character 6 isotope	Character 7 Qualifier
Radiation Oncology	Urinary System	Other Radiation	Bladder	IORT	None	None
D	**T**	**Y**	**2**	**C**	**Z**	**Z**

OTHER RADIATION ONCOLOGY CODING EXAMPLES

Procedure	Code
Plaque radiation of left eye, single port	D8Y0FZZ

8 MeV photon beam radiation to brain	D0011ZZ
IORT of colon, 3 ports	DDY5CZZ
HDR Brachytherapy of prostate using Palladium 103	DV109BZ
Electron radiation treatment of right breast, custom device	DM013ZZ
Hyperthermia oncology treatment of pelvic region	DWY68ZZ
Contact radiation of tongue	D9Y57ZZ
Heavy particle radiation treatment of pancreas, four risk sites	DF034ZZ
LDR brachytherapy to spinal cord using iodine	D016B9Z
Whole body Phosphorus 32 administration with risk to hematopoietic system	DWY5GFZ

PHYSICAL REHABILITATION AND DIAGNOSTIC AUDIOLOGY— SECTION F

Physical Rehabilitation and Diagnostic Audiology contains character definitions unlike the other sections in ICD-10-PCS. The following table defines the special character definitions:

Value	Description	Definition
0	Speech Assessment	Measurement of speech and related functions
1	Motor and/or Nerve Function Assessment	Measurement of motor, nerve, and related functions
2	Activities of Daily Living Assessment	Measurement of functional level for activities of daily living
3	Hearing Assessment	Measurement of hearing and related functions
4	Hearing Aid Assessment	Measurement of the appropriateness and/or effectiveness of a hearing device
5	Vestibular Assessment	Measurement of the vestibular system and related functions
6	Speech Treatment	Application of techniques to improve, augment, or compensate for speech and related functional impairment
7	Motor Treatment	Exercise or activities to increase or facilitate motor function
8	Activities of Daily Living Treatment	Exercise or activities to facilitate functional competence for activities of daily living
9	Hearing Treatment	Application of techniques to improve, augment, or compensate for hearing and related functional impairment
b	Hearing Aid Treatment	Application of techniques to improve the communication abilities of individuals with cochlear implant

C	Vestibular Treatment	Application of techniques to improve, augment, or compensate for vestibular and related functional impairment
D	Device Fitting	Fitting of a device designed to facilitate or support achievement of a higher level of function
F	Caregiver Training	Training in activities to support patient's optimal level of function

- Second character is a section qualifier that specifies whether the procedure is a rehabilitation or diagnostic audiology procedure.
- Third character defines the general procedure root type.
- Fourth character defines the body system and body region combined, where applicable
- Fifth character further specifies the procedure type.
- Sixth character specifies the equipment used, if any.

ROOT TYPES

This section uses the third character to classify procedures into 14 root types. They are defined in the table below.

CODING NOTE	**TREATMENT** procedures include swallowing dysfunction exercises, bathing and showering techniques, wound management, gait training, and a host of activities typically associated with rehabilitation.

Example: Wound care treatment of left calf ulcer using pulsatile lavage

	Character 2 Section Qualifier	Character 3 Root Type	Character 4 Body System & Region	Character 5 Type Qualifier	Character 6 Equipment	Character 7 Qualifier
Rehabilitation & Diagnostic Audiology	Rehabilitation	Activities Of Daily Living Treatment	Musculo-skeletal Lower Extremity	Wound Management	Physical Agents	None
F	**0**	**8**	**L**	**5**	**B**	**Z**

CODING NOTE	**ASSESSMENTS** are further classified into more than 100 different tests or methods. The majority of these focus on the faculties of hearing and speech, but others focus on various aspects of body function, and on the patient's quality of life, such as muscle performance, neuromotor development, and reintegration skills.

Example: Articulation and phonology assessment using spectrograph

Character 1 Section	Character 2 Section Qualifier	Character 3 Root Type	Character 4 Body System & Region	Character 5 Type Qualifier	Character 6 Equipment	Character 7 Qualifier
Rehabilitation & Diagnostic Audiology	Rehabilitation	Speech Assessment	None	Articulation/ Phonology	Speech Analysis	None

F	0	0	Z	9	Q	Z

CODING NOTE	**DEVICE FITTING**. The fifth character used in Device Fitting describes the device being fitted rather than the method used to fit the device. Detailed descriptions of the devices are provided in the reference materials, the table specific to Device Fitting.

Example: Individual fitting of moveable brace, right knee

	Character 2 Section Qualifier	Character 3 Root Type	Character 4 Body System & Region	Character 5 Type Qualifier	Character 6 Equipment	Character 7 Qualifier
Rehabilitation & Diagnostic Audiology	Rehabilitation	Device Fitting	None	Dynamic Orthosis	Orthosis	None
F	**0**	**D**	**Z**	**6**	**E**	**Z**

CODING NOTE	**CAREGIVER TRAINING** is divided into eighteen different broad subjects taught to help a caregiver provide proper patient care.

Example: Caregiver training in feeding, no special equipment used

Character 1 Section	Character 2 Section Qualifier	Character 3 Root Type	Character 4 Body System & Region	Character 5 Type Qualifier	Character 6 Equipment	Character 7 Qualifier
Rehabilitation & Diagnostic Audiology	Rehabilitation	Caregiver Training	None	Feeding and Eating	None	None
F	**0**	**F**	**Z**	**2**	**Z**	**Z**

OTHER PHYSICAL REHABILITATION AND DIAGNOSTIC AUDIOLOGY CODING EXAMPLES

Procedure	Code
Bekesy assessment using audiometer	F13Z31Z
Individual fitting of left eye prosthesis	F0DZ8UZ
Physical therapy for range of motion and mobility, patient right hip, no special equipment	F07L0ZZ
Bedside swallow assessment using assessment kit	F00ZHYZ
Caregiver training in airway clearance techniques	F0FZ8ZZ
Application of short arm cast in rehabilitation setting	F0DZ7EZ Inhibitory cast is listed in the equipment reference table under E, ORTHOSIS.
Verbal assessment of patient's pain level	F02ZFZZ

Caregiver training in communication skills using manual communication board	F0FZJMZ Manual communication board is listed in the equipment reference table under M, AUGMENTATIVE/ALTERNATIVE COMMUNICATION.
Group musculoskeletal balance training exercises, whole body, no special equipment	F07M6ZZ Balance training is included in the MOTOR TREATMENT reference table under THERAPEUTIC EXERCISE.
Individual therapy for auditory processing using tape recorder	F09Z2KZ Tape recorder is listed in the equipment reference table under AUDIOVISUAL EQUIPMENT.

MENTAL HEALTH—SECTION G

Mental Health contains specific values in the third and fourth characters to describe mental health procedures. The remaining characters function as placeholders only. Character meanings are described below.

- Third character describes the mental health procedure root type.
- Fourth character further specifies the procedure type as needed.
- Second, fifth, sixth, and seventh characters do not convey specific information about the procedure. The value Z functions as a placeholder in these characters.

ROOT TYPE

The third character describes the mental health root type. There are 11 root type values in this section, as listed in the table below.

Value	Description
1	Psychological Tests
2	Crisis Intervention
5	Individual Psychotherapy
6	Counseling
7	Family Psychotherapy
B	Electroconvulsive Therapy
C	Biofeedback
F	Hypnosis
G	Narcosynthesis
H	Group Therapy
J	Light Therapy

Example: Galvanic skin response (GSR) biofeedback

Character 1 Section	Character 2 Body System	Character 3 Root Type	Character 4 Type Qualifier	Character 5 Qualifier	Character 6 Qualifier	Character 7 Qualifier
Mental Health	None	Biofeedback	Other Biofeedback	None	None	None
G	Z	C	9	Z	Z	Z

Procedure	Code
Cognitive-behavioral psychotherapy, individual	GZ58ZZZ
Narcosynthesis	GZGZZZZ
Light therapy	GZJZZZZ
ECT (Electroconvulsive therapy), unilateral, multiple seizure	GZB1ZZZ
Crisis intervention	GZ2ZZZZ
Neuropsychological testing	GZ13ZZZ
Hypnosis	GZFZZZZ
Developmental testing	GZ10ZZZ
Vocational counseling	GZ61ZZZ
Family psychotherapy	GZ72ZZZ

SUBSTANCE ABUSE TREATMENT—SECTION H

Substance Abuse Treatment is structured like a smaller version of the Mental Health section. Character meanings are described below.

- Third character describes the root type.
- Fourth character is a qualifier that further classifies the root type
- Second, fifth, sixth, and seventh characters do not convey specific information about the procedure. The value Z functions as a placeholder in these characters.

ROOT TYPES

There are seven different root type values classified in this section, as listed in the following table.

Value	Description
2	Detoxification Services
3	Individual Counseling
4	Group Counseling
5	Individual Psychotherapy
6	Family Counseling

8	Medication Management
9	Pharmacotherapy

Example: Pharmacotherapy treatment with Antabuse for alcohol addiction

Character 1 Section	Character 2 Body System	Character 3 Root Type	Character 4 Type Qualifier	Character 5 Qualifier	Character 6 Qualifier	Character 7 Qualifier
Substance Abuse Treatment	None	Pharmaco-therapy	Antabuse	None	None	None
H	Z	9	3	Z	Z	Z

OTHER SUBSTANCE ABUSE CODING EXAMPLES

Procedure	Code
Naltrexone treatment for drug dependency	HZ94ZZZ
Substance abuse treatment family counseling	HZ63ZZZ
Medication monitoring of patient on methadone maintenance	HZ81ZZZ
Individual interpersonal psychotherapy for drug abuse	HZ54ZZZ
Patient in for alcohol detoxification treatment	HZ2ZZZZ
Group motivational counseling	HZ47ZZZ
Individual 12-step psychotherapy for substance abuse	HZ53ZZZ
Post-test infectious disease counseling for IV drug abuser	HZ3CZZZ
Psychodynamic psychotherapy for drug dependent patient	HZ5CZZZ
Group cognitive-behavioral counseling for substance abuse	HZ42ZZZ

ICD-10-PCS ROOT OPERATIONS AND APPROACHES

This section contains reference tables listing the root operations and approaches used in the Medical and Surgical section. The first table includes the definition of each root operation, with explanation and examples. The second table includes the definition of each approach.

The root operations are listed by name in alphabetical order. The approaches are listed by approach value, in numeric order followed by alphabetical order. For the full ICD-10-PCS definitions, please refer to the Definitions portion of the ICD-10 Procedure Coding System.

ROOT OPERATIONS		
Alteration	Definition	Modifying the anatomic structure of a body part without affecting the function of the body part
	Explanation	Principal purpose is to improve appearance
	Examples	Face lift, breast augmentation
Bypass	Definition	Altering the route of passage of the contents of a tubular body part
	Explanation	Rerouting contents of a body part to a downstream area of the normal route, to a similar route and body part, or to an abnormal route and dissimilar body part. Includes one or more anastomoses, with or without the use of a device
	Examples	Coronary artery bypass, colostomy formation
Change	Definition	Taking out or off a device from a body part and putting back an identical or similar device in or on the same body part without cutting or puncturing the skin or a mucous membrane
	Explanation	All CHANGE procedures are coded using the approach EXTERNAL
	Examples	Urinary catheter change, gastrostomy tube change
Control	Definition	Stopping, or attempting to stop, postprocedural bleeding
	Explanation	The site of the bleeding is coded as an anatomical region and not to a specific body part
	Examples	Control of post-prostatectomy hemorrhage, control of post-tonsillectomy hemorrhage
Creation	Definition	Making a new genital structure that does not take over the function of a body part
	Explanation	Used only for sex change operations
	Examples	Creation of vagina in a male, creation of penis in a female
Destruction	Definition	Physical eradication of all or a portion of a body part by the direct use of energy, force or a destructive agent
	Explanation	None of the body part is physically taken out
	Examples	Fulguration of rectal polyp, cautery of skin lesion

Detachment	Definition	Cutting off all or a portion of the upper or lower extremities
	Explanation	The body part value is the site of the detachment, with a qualifier if applicable to further specify the level where the extremity was detached
	Examples	Below knee amputation, disarticulation of shoulder
Dilation	Definition	Expanding an orifice or the lumen of a tubular body part
	Explanation	The orifice can be a natural orifice or an artificially created orifice. Accomplished by stretching a tubular body part using intraluminal pressure or by cutting part of the orifice or wall of the tubular body part
	Examples	Percutaneous transluminal angioplasty, pyloromyotomy
Division	Definition	Cutting into a body part without draining fluids and/or gases from the body part in order to separate or transect a body part
	Explanation	All or a portion of the body part is separated into two or more portions
	Examples	Spinal cordotomy, osteotomy
Drainage	Definition	Taking or letting out fluids and/or gases from a body part
	Explanation	The qualifier DIAGNOSTIC is used to identify drainage procedures that are biopsies
	Examples	Thoracentesis, incision and drainage
Excision	Definition	Cutting out or off, without replacement, a portion of a body part
	Explanation	The qualifier DIAGNOSTIC is used to identify excision procedures that are biopsies
	Examples	Partial nephrectomy, liver biopsy
Extirpation	Definition	Taking or cutting out solid matter from a body part
	Explanation	The solid matter may be an abnormal byproduct of a biological function or a foreign body; it may be imbedded in a body part or in the lumen of a tubular body part. The solid matter may or may not have been previously broken into pieces
	Examples	Thrombectomy, choledocholithotomy
Extraction	Definition	Pulling or stripping out or off all or a portion of a body part by the use of force
	Explanation	The qualifier DIAGNOSTIC is used to identify extraction procedures that are biopsies
	Examples	Dilation and curettage, vein stripping

Fragmentation	Definition	Breaking solid matter in a body part into pieces
	Explanation	Physical force (e.g., manual, ultrasonic) applied directly or indirectly is used to break the solid matter into pieces. The solid matter may be an abnormal byproduct of a biological function or a foreign body. The pieces of solid matter are not taken out
	Examples	Extracorporeal shockwave lithotripsy, transurethral lithotripsy
Fusion	Definition	Joining together portions of an articular body part rendering the articular body part immobile
	Explanation	The body part is joined together by fixation device, bone graft, or other means
	Examples	Spinal fusion, ankle arthrodesis
Insertion	Definition	Putting in a nonbiological device that monitors, assists, performs or prevents a physiological function but does not physically take the place of a body part
	Explanation	N/A
	Examples	Insertion of radioactive implant, insertion of central venous catheter
Inspection	Definition	Visually and/or manually exploring a body part
	Explanation	Visual exploration may be performed with or without optical instrumentation. Manual exploration may be performed directly or through intervening body layers
	Examples	Diagnostic arthroscopy, exploratory laparotomy
Map	Definition	Locating the route of passage of electrical impulses and/or locating functional areas in a body part
	Explanation	Applicable only to the cardiac conduction mechanism and the central nervous system
	Examples	Cardiac mapping, cortical mapping
Occlusion	Definition	Completely closing an orifice or the lumen of a tubular body part
	Explanation	The orifice can be a natural orifice or an artificially created orifice
	Examples	Fallopian tube ligation, ligation of inferior vena cava
Reattachment	Definition	Putting back in or on all or a portion of a separated body part to its normal location or other suitable location
	Explanation	Vascular circulation and nervous pathways may or may not be reestablished
	Examples	Reattachment of hand, reattachment of avulsed kidney

Release	Definition	Freeing a body part from an abnormal physical constraint by cutting or by use of force
	Explanation	Some of the restraining tissue may be taken out but none of the body part is taken out
	Examples	Adhesiolysis, carpal tunnel release
Removal	Definition	Taking out or off a device from a body part
	Explanation	If a device is taken out and a similar device put in without cutting or puncturing the skin or mucous membrane, the procedure is coded to the root operation CHANGE. Otherwise, the procedure for taking out a device is coded to the root operation REMOVAL
	Examples	Drainage tube removal, cardiac pacemaker removal
Repair	Definition	Restoring, to the extent possible, a body part to its normal anatomic structure and function
	Explanation	Used only when the method to accomplish the repair is not one of the other root operations
	Examples	Colostomy takedown, suture of laceration
Replacement	Definition	Putting in or on biological or synthetic material that physically takes the place and/or function of all or a portion of a body part
	Explanation	The body part may have been taken out or replaced, or may be taken out, physically eradicated, or rendered nonfunctional during the Replacement procedure. A Removal procedure is coded for taking out the device used in a previous replacement procedure
	Examples	Total hip replacement, bone graft, free skin graft
Reposition	Definition	Moving to its normal location, or other suitable location, all or a portion of a body part
	Explanation	The body part is moved to a new location from an abnormal location, or from a normal location where it is not functioning correctly. The body part may or may not be cut out or off to be moved to the new location
	Examples	Reposition of undescended testicle, fracture reduction
Resection	Definition	Cutting out or off, without replacement, all of a body part
	Explanation	N/A
	Examples	Total nephrectomy, total lobectomy of lung
Restriction	Definition	Partially closing an orifice or the lumen of a tubular body part
	Explanation	The orifice can be a natural orifice or an artificially created orifice
	Examples	Esophagogastric fundoplication, cervical cerclage

Revision	Definition	Correcting, to the extent possible, a portion of a malfunctioning device or the position of a displaced device
	Explanation	Revision can include correcting a malfunctioning or displaced device by taking out or putting in components of the device such as a screw or pin
	Examples	Adjustment of position of pacemaker lead, recementing of hip prosthesis
Supplement	Definition	Putting in or on biological or synthetic material that physically reinforces and/or augments the function of a portion of a body part
	Explanation	The biological material is non-living, or is living and from the same individual. The body part may have been previously replaced, and the Supplement procedure is performed to physically reinforce and/or augment the function of the replaced body part
	Examples	Herniorrhaphy using mesh, free nerve graft, mitral valve ring annuloplasty, put a new acetabular liner in a previous hip replacement
Transfer	Definition	Moving, without taking out, all or a portion of a body part to another location to take over the function of all or a portion of a body part
	Explanation	The body part transferred remains connected to its vascular and nervous supply
	Examples	Tendon transfer, skin pedicle flap transfer
Transplantation	Definition	Putting in or on all or a portion of a living body part taken from another individual or animal to physically take the place and/or function of all or a portion of a similar body part
	Explanation	The native body part may or may not be taken out, and the transplanted body part may take over all or a portion of its function
	Examples	Kidney transplant, heart transplant

APPROACHES	
Open	Cutting through the skin or mucous membrane and any other body layers necessary to expose the site of the procedure
Percutaneous	Entry, by puncture or minor incision, of instrumentation through the skin or mucous membrane and any other body layers necessary to reach the site of the procedure
Percutaneous Endoscopic	Entry, by puncture or minor incision, of instrumentation through the skin or mucous membrane and any other body layers necessary to reach and visualize the site of the procedure
Via Natural or Artificial Opening	Entry of instrumentation through a natural or artificial external opening to reach the site of the procedure

Via Natural or Artificial Opening Endoscopic	Entry of instrumentation through a natural or artificial external opening to reach and visualize the site of the procedure
Via Natural or Artificial Opening With Percutaneous Endoscopic Assistance	Entry of instrumentation through a natural or artificial external opening and entry, by puncture or minor incision, of instrumentation through the skin or mucous membrane and any other body layers necessary to aid in the performance of the procedure
External	Procedures performed directly on the skin or mucous membrane and procedures performed indirectly by the application of external force through the skin or mucous membrane

ICD-10-PCS CODING GUIDELINES

This section lists the ICD-10-PCS guidelines. They are grouped into conventions followed by guidelines. Guidelines for the Medical and Surgical section are further grouped by character. The guidelines are numbered sequentially within each category.

CONVENTIONS

A1 ICD-10-PCS codes are composed of seven characters. Each character is an axis of classification that specifies information about the procedure performed. Within a defined code range, a character specifies the same type of information in that axis of classification.

Example: The fifth axis of classification specifies the approach in sections 0 through 4 and 7 through 9 of the system.

A2 One of 34 possible values can be assigned to each axis of classification in the seven-character code: they are the numbers 0 through 9 and the alphabet (except I and O because they are easily confused with the numbers 1 and 0). The number of unique values used in an axis of classification differs as needed.

Example: Where the fifth axis of classification specifies the approach, seven different approach values are currently used to specify the approach.

A3 The valid values for an axis of classification can be added to as needed.

A4 As with words in their context, the meaning of any single value is a combination of its axis of classification and any preceding values on which it may be dependent.

Example: The meaning of a body part value in the Medical and Surgical section is always dependent on the body system value. The body part value 0 in the Central Nervous body system specifies Brain and the body part value 0 in the Peripheral Nervous body system specifies Cervical Plexus.

A5 As the system is expanded to become increasingly detailed, over time more values will depend on preceding values for their meaning.

Example: In the Lower Joints body system, the device value 3 in the root operation Insertion specifies Infusion Device and the device value 3 in the root operation Fusion specifies Interbody Fusion Device.

A6 The purpose of the alphabetic index is to locate the appropriate table that contains all information necessary to construct a procedure code. The ICD-10-PCS Tables should always be consulted to find the most appropriate valid code.

A7 It is not required to consult the index first before proceeding to the tables to complete the code. A valid code may be chosen directly from the tables.

A8 All seven characters must be specified to be a valid code. If the documentation is incomplete for coding purposes, the physician should be queried for the necessary information.

A9   Within a ICD-10-PCS table, valid codes include all combinations of choices in characters 4 through 7 contained in the same row of the table.

A10   "And," when used in a code description, means "and/or."

Example: Lower Arm and Wrist Muscle means lower arm and/or wrist muscle.

A11   Many of the terms used to construct ICD-10-PCS codes are defined within the system. It is the coder's responsibility to determine what the documentation in the medical record equates to in the ICD-10-PCS definitions. The physician is not expected to use the terms used in ICD-10-PCS code descriptions, nor is the coder required to query the physician when the correlation between the documentation and the defined ICD-10-PCS terms is clear.

Example: When the physician documents "partial resection" the coder can independently correlate "partial resection" to the root operation Excision without querying the physician for clarification.

MEDICAL AND SURGICAL SECTION (SECTION 0)

Body System

B2.1a The procedure codes in the general anatomical regions general guidelines body systems should only be used when the procedure is performed on an anatomical region rather than a specific body part (e.g., root operations Control and Detachment, drainage of a body cavity) or on the rare occasion when no information is available to support assignment of a code to a specific body part.

Example: Control of postoperative hemorrhage is coded to the root operation Control found in the general anatomical regions body systems.

B2.1b Body systems designated as upper or lower contain body parts located above or below the diaphragm respectively.

Example: Vein body parts above the diaphragm are found in the Upper Veins body system; vein body parts below the diaphragm are found in the Lower Veins body system.

Root Operation

B3.1a In order to determine the appropriate root operation, the general guidelines full definition of the root operation as contained in the ICD-10-PCS Tables must be applied.

B3.1b Components of a procedure specified in the root operation definition and explanation are not coded separately. Procedural steps necessary to reach the operative site and close the operative site are also not coded separately.

Example: Resection of a joint as part of a joint replacement procedure is included in the root operation definition of Replacement and is not coded separately. Laparotomy performed to reach the site of an open liver biopsy is not coded separately.

Multiple Procedures

B3.2 During the same operative episode, multiple procedures are coded if:

- The same root operation is performed on different body parts as defined by distinct values of the body part character.

  Example: Diagnostic excision of liver and pancreas are coded separately.

- The same root operation is repeated at different body sites that are included in the same body part value.

  Example: Excision of the sartorius muscle and excision of the gracilis muscle are both included in the upper leg muscle body part value, and multiple procedures are coded.

- Multiple root operations with distinct objectives are performed on the same body part.

  Example: Destruction of sigmoid lesion and bypass of sigmoid colon are coded separately.

- The intended root operation is attempted using one approach, but is converted to a different approach.

  Example: Laparoscopic cholecystectomy converted to an open cholecystectomy is coded as percutaneous endoscopic Inspection and open Resection.

Discontinued Procedures

B3.3 If the intended procedure is discontinued, code the procedure to the root operation performed. If a procedure is discontinued before any other root operation is performed, code the root operation Inspection of the body part or anatomical region inspected.

Example: A planned aortic valve replacement procedure is discontinued after the initial thoracotomy and before any incision is made in the heart muscle, when the patient becomes hemodynamically unstable. This procedure is coded as an open Inspection of the mediastinum.

Biopsy Followed By More Definitive Treatment

B3.4 If a diagnostic Excision, Extraction, or Drainage procedure (biopsy) is followed by a more definitive procedure, such as Destruction, Excision or Resection at the same procedure site, both the biopsy and the more definitive treatment are coded.

Example: Biopsy of breast followed by partial mastectomy at the same procedure site, both the biopsy and the partial mastectomy procedure are coded.

Overlapping Body Layers

B3.5   If the root operations Excision, Repair or Inspection are performed on overlapping layers of the musculoskeletal system, the body part specifying the deepest layer is coded.

Example: Excisional debridement that includes skin and subcutaneous tissue and muscle is coded to the muscle body part.

Bypass Procedures

B3.6a   Bypass procedures are coded by identifying the body part bypassed "from" and the body part bypassed "to." The fourth character body part specifies the body part bypassed from, and the qualifier specifies the body part bypassed to.

Example: Bypass from stomach to jejunum, stomach is the body part and jejunum is the qualifier.

B3.6b   Coronary arteries are classified by number of distinct sites treated, rather than number of coronary arteries or anatomic name of a coronary artery (e.g., left anterior descending). Coronary artery bypass procedures are coded differently than other bypass procedures as described in the previous guideline. Rather than identifying the body part bypassed from, the body part identifies the number of coronary artery sites bypassed to, and the qualifier specifies the vessel bypassed from.

Example: Aortocoronary artery bypass of one site on the left anterior descending coronary artery and one site on the obtuse marginal coronary artery is classified in the body part axis of classification as two coronary artery sites and the qualifier specifies the aorta as the body part bypassed from.

B3.6c   If multiple coronary artery sites are bypassed, a separate procedure is coded for each coronary artery site that uses a different device and/or qualifier.

Example: Aortocoronary artery bypass and internal mammary coronary artery bypass are coded separately.

Control vs More Definitive Root Operations

B3.7   The root operation Control is defined as, "Stopping, or attempting to stop, postprocedural bleeding." If an attempt to stop postprocedural bleeding is initially unsuccessful, and to stop the bleeding requires performing any of the definitive root operations Bypass, Detachment, Excision, Extraction, Reposition, Replacement, or Resection, then that root operation is coded instead of Control.

Example: Resection of spleen to stop postprocedural bleeding is coded to Resection instead of Control.

Excision vs Resection

B3.8   PCS contains specific body parts for anatomical subdivisions of a body part, such as lobes of the lungs or liver and regions of the intestine. Resection of the specific body part is coded whenever all of the body part is cut out or off, rather than coding Excision of a less specific body part.

Example: Left upper lung lobectomy is coded to Resection of Upper Lung Lobe, Left rather than Excision of Lung, Left.

Excision for Graft

B3.9   If an autograft is obtained from a different body part in order to complete the objective of the procedure, a separate procedure is coded.

Example: Coronary bypass with excision of saphenous vein graft, excision of saphenous vein is coded separately.

Fusion Procedures of the Spine

B3.10a   The body part coded for a spinal vertebral joint(s) rendered immobile by a spinal fusion procedure is classified by the level of the spine (e.g. thoracic). There are distinct body part values for a single vertebral joint and for multiple vertebral joints at each spinal level.

Example: Body part values specify Lumbar Vertebral Joint, Lumbar Vertebral Joints, 2 or More and Lumbosacral Vertebral Joint.

B3.10b   If multiple vertebral joints are fused, a separate procedure is coded for each vertebral joint that uses a different device and/or qualifier.

Example: Fusion of lumbar vertebral joint, posterior approach, anterior column and fusion of lumbar vertebral joint, posterior approach, posterior column are coded separately.

B3.10c   Combinations of devices and materials are often used on a vertebral joint to render the joint immobile. When combinations of devices are used on the same vertebral joint, the device value coded for the procedure is as follows:

- If an interbody fusion device is used to render the joint immobile (alone or containing other material like bone graft), the procedure is coded with the device value Interbody Fusion Device
- If bone graft is the only device used to render the joint immobile, the procedure is coded with the device value Nonautologous Tissue Substitute or Autologous Tissue Substitute
- If a mixture of autologous and nonautologous bone graft (with or without biological or synthetic extenders or binders) is used to render the joint immobile, code the procedure with the device value Autologous Tissue Substitute

Examples: Fusion of a vertebral joint using a cage style interbody fusion device containing morselized bone graft is coded to the device Interbody Fusion Device.

Fusion of a vertebral joint using a bone dowel interbody fusion device made of cadaver bone and packed with a mixture of local morselized bone and demineralized bone matrix is coded to the device Interbody Fusion Device.

Fusion of a vertebral joint using both autologous bone graft and bone bank bone graft is coded to the device Autologous Tissue Substitute.

Inspection Procedures

B3.11a Inspection of a body part(s) performed in order to achieve the objective of a procedure is not coded separately.

Example: Fiberoptic bronchoscopy performed for irrigation of bronchus, only the irrigation procedure is coded.

B3.11b If multiple tubular body parts are inspected, the most distal body part inspected is coded. If multiple non-tubular body parts in a region are inspected, the body part that specifies the entire area inspected is coded.

Examples: Cystourethroscopy with inspection of bladder and ureters is coded to the ureter body part value.

Exploratory laparotomy with general inspection of abdominal contents is coded to the peritoneal cavity body part value.

B3.11c When both an Inspection procedure and another procedure are performed on the same body part during the same episode, if the Inspection procedure is performed using a different approach than the other procedure, the Inspection procedure is coded separately.

Example: Endoscopic Inspection of the duodenum is coded separately when open Excision of the duodenum is performed during the same procedural episode.

Occlusion vs. Restriction for Vessel Embolization Procedures

B3.12 If the objective of an embolization procedure is to completely close a vessel, the root operation Occlusion is coded. If the objective of an embolization procedure is to narrow the lumen of a vessel, the root operation Restriction is coded.

Examples: Tumor embolization is coded to the root operation Occlusion, because the objective of the procedure is to cut off the blood supply to the vessel.

Embolization of a cerebral aneurysm is coded to the root operation Restriction, because the objective of the procedure is not to close off the vessel entirely, but to narrow the lumen of the vessel at the site of the aneurysm where it is abnormally wide.

Release Procedures

B3.13 In the root operation Release, the body part value coded is the body part being freed and not the tissue being manipulated or cut to free the body part.

Example: Lysis of intestinal adhesions is coded to the specific intestine body part value.

Release vs. Division

B3.14   If the sole objective of the procedure is freeing a body part without cutting the body part, the root operation is Release. If the sole objective of the procedure is separating or transecting a body part, the root operation is Division.

Examples: Freeing a nerve root from surrounding scar tissue to relieve pain is coded to the root operation Release.
Severing a nerve root to relieve pain is coded to the root operation Division.

Reposition for Fracture Treatment

B3.15   Reduction of a displaced fracture is coded to the root operation Reposition and the application of a cast or splint in conjunction with the Reposition procedure is not coded separately. Treatment of a nondisplaced fracture is coded to the procedure performed.

Examples: Putting a pin in a nondisplaced fracture is coded to the root operation Insertion.

Casting of a nondisplaced fracture is coded to the root operation Immobilization in the Placement section.

Transplantation vs. Administration

B3.16   Putting in a mature and functioning living body part taken from another individual or animal is coded to the root operation Transplantation. Putting in autologous or nonautologous cells is coded to the Administration section.

Example: Putting in autologous or nonautologous bone marrow, pancreatic islet cells or stem cells is coded to the Administration section.

Body Part General Guidelines

B4.1a   If a procedure is performed on a portion of a body part that does not have a separate body part value, code the body part value corresponding to the whole body part.

Example: A procedure performed on the alveolar process of the mandible is coded to the mandible body part.

B4.1b   If the prefix "peri" is combined with a body part to identify the site of the procedure, the procedure is coded to the body part named.

Example: A procedure site identified as perirenal is coded to the kidney body part.

Branches of Body Parts

B4.2   Where a specific branch of a body part does not have its own body part value in ICD-10-PCS, the body part is coded to the closest proximal branch that has a specific body part value.

Example: A procedure performed on the mandibular branch of the trigeminal nerve is coded to the trigeminal nerve body part value.

Bilateral Body Part Values

B4.3   Bilateral body part values are available for a limited number of body parts. If the identical procedure is performed on contralateral body parts, and a bilateral body part value exists for that body part, a single procedure is coded using the bilateral body part value. If no bilateral body part value exists, each procedure is coded separately using the appropriate body part value.

Example: The identical procedure performed on both fallopian tubes is coded once using the body part value Fallopian Tube, Bilateral. The identical procedure performed on both knee joints is coded twice using the body part values Knee Joint, Right and Knee Joint, Left.

Coronary Arteries

B4.4   The coronary arteries are classified as a single body part that is further specified by number of sites treated and not by name or number of arteries. Separate body part values are used to specify the number of sites treated when the same procedure is performed on multiple sites in the coronary arteries.

Examples: Angioplasty of two distinct sites in the left anterior descending coronary artery with placement of two stents is coded as Dilation of Coronary Arteries, Two Sites, with Intraluminal Device.

Angioplasty of two distinct sites in the left anterior descending coronary artery, one with stent placed and one without, is coded separately as Dilation of Coronary Artery, One Site with Intraluminal Device, and Dilation of Coronary Artery, One Site with no device.

Tendons, Ligaments, Bursae and Fascia Near a Joint

B4.5   Procedures performed on tendons, ligaments, bursae and fascia supporting a joint are coded to the body part in the respective body system that is the focus of the procedure. Procedures performed on joint structures themselves are coded to the body part in the joint body systems.

Example: Repair of the anterior cruciate ligament of the knee is coded to the knee bursae and ligament body part in the bursae and ligaments body system. Knee arthroscopy with shaving of articular cartilage is coded to the knee joint body part in the Lower Joints body system.

Skin, Subcutaneous Tissue and Fascia Overlying a Joint

B4.6   If a procedure is performed on the skin, subcutaneous tissue or fascia overlying a joint, the procedure is coded to the following body part:

- Shoulder is coded to Upper Arm
- Elbow is coded to Lower Arm
- Wrist is coded to Lower Arm

- Hip is coded to Upper Leg
- Knee is coded to Lower Leg
- Ankle is coded to Foot

Fingers and Toes

B4.7   If a body system does not contain a separate body part value for fingers, procedures performed on the fingers are coded to the body part value for the hand. If a body system does not contain a separate body part value for toes, procedures performed on the toes are coded to the body part value for the foot.

Example: Excision of finger muscle is coded to one of the hand muscle body part values in the Muscles body system.

Approach Guidelines

B5.2   Procedures performed using the open approach with percutaneous endoscopic assistance are coded to the approach Open.

Open Approach with Endoscopic Assistance

Example: Laparoscopic-assisted sigmoidectomy is coded to the approach Open.

External Approach

B5.3a   Procedures performed within an orifice on structures that are visible without the aid of any instrumentation are coded to the approach External.

Example: Resection of tonsils is coded to the approach External.

B5.3b   Procedures performed indirectly by the application of external force through the intervening body layers are coded to the approach External.
Example: Closed reduction of fracture is coded to the approach External.

Percutaneous Procedure via Device

B5.4   Procedures performed percutaneously via a device placed for the procedure are coded to the approach Percutaneous.

Example: Fragmentation of kidney stone performed via percutaneous nephrostomy is coded to the approach Percutaneous.

Device General Guidelines

B6.1a   A device is coded only if a device remains after the procedure is completed. If no device remains, the device value No Device is coded.

B6.1b   Materials such as sutures, ligatures, radiological markers and temporary post-operative wound drains are considered integral to the performance of a procedure and are not coded as devices.

B6.1c   Procedures performed on a device only and not on a body part are specified in the root operations Change, Irrigation, Removal and Revision, and are coded to the procedure performed.

Example: Irrigation of percutaneous nephrostomy tube is coded to the root operation Irrigation of indwelling device in the Administration section.

Drainage Device

B6.2.   A separate procedure to put in a drainage device is coded to the root operation Drainage with the device value Drainage Device.

OBSTETRICS SECTION GUIDELINES (SECTION 1)

Products of Conception

C.1   Procedures performed on the products of conception are coded to the Obstetrics section.

Procedures performed on the pregnant female other than the products of conception are coded to the appropriate root operation in the Medical and Surgical section.

Example: Amniocentesis is coded to the products of conception body part in the Obstetrics section. Repair of obstetric urethral laceration is coded to the urethra body part in the Medical and Surgical section.

Procedures Following Delivery or Abortion

C.2   Procedures performed following a delivery or abortion for curettage of the endometrium or evacuation of retained products of conception are all coded in the Obstetrics section, to the root operation Extraction and the body part Products of Conception, Retained. Diagnostic or therapeutic dilation and curettage performed during times other than the postpartum or post-abortion period are all coded in the Medical and Surgical section, to the root operation Extraction and the body part Endometrium.

ICD-10-PCS DEVICE AND SUBSTANCE CLASSIFICATION

THIS APPENDIX DISCUSSES the distinguishing features of device, substance and equipment as classified in ICD-10-PCS, to provide further guidance for correct identification and coding. The appendix includes discussion of the ICD-10-PCS definitions and classification of device, substance and equipment, and is accompanied by specific coding instruction and examples.

ICD-10-PCS DEVICE CLASSIFICATION

In most ICD-10-PCS codes, the 6th character of the code is used to classify device. The 6th character device value "defines the material or appliance used to accomplish the objective of the procedure that remains in or on the procedure site at the end of the procedure." If the device is the means by which the procedural objective is accomplished, then a specific device value is coded in the 6th character. If no device is used to accomplish the objective of the procedure, the device value NO DEVICE is coded in the 6th character.

For example, an aortocoronary bypass that uses saphenous vein graft to accomplish the bypass is coded to the device value AUTOLOGOUS VENOUS TISSUE in the 6th character of the ICD-10-PCS code. A coronary bypass that uses the patient's internal mammary artery directly to accomplish the bypass uses the device value NO DEVICE in the 6th character of the ICD-10-PCS code

DEVICE AND PROCEDURAL OBJECTIVE

Whether or not the material used in a procedure should be coded using a specific ICD-10-PCS device value can be determined primarily by asking the question

- Is this material central to achieving the objective of the procedure, or does it only support the performance of the procedure?

For example, radiological markers are put in the procedure site to guide the performance of a primary procedure such as excision of a tumor, whereas radioactive brachytherapy seeds are put in the procedure site as an end in themselves, to treat a malignant tumor. The radiological marker is not classified as a device in ICD-10-PCS, but the brachytherapy seeds are classified to the device value RADIOACTIVE ELEMENT in the root operation INSERTION.

The same device coded as a specific device value for one procedure may not be coded at all for another procedure where it is not central to the procedural objective. For example, a procedure performed specifically to place a drain in a body part for diagnostic or therapeutic purposes is coded to the root operation DRAINAGE with the specific device value DRAINAGE DEVICE in the 6th character of the code. However, a wound drain placed at an incision site at the conclusion of the procedure to promote healing is not central to the procedural objective and therefore not coded separately as a device in ICD-10-PCS. For this reason, materials such as wound dressings and operative site drains that support the performance of the procedure are not coded separately.

Sutures and suture alternatives (e.g., fibrin glue, Dermabond, specialized vessel closures) are not coded as devices in ICD-10-PCS, because in most cases using material to bring the edges of a procedure site together is not central to the procedural objective, but is used to support the performance of the procedure (to close the site). For procedures where the sole objective is to close a wound created by trauma or other incident, the procedure is coded to the root operation REPAIR with the device value NO DEVICE in the 6th character of the ICD-10-PCS code.

DEVICE AND LOCATION

Whether material or an appliance is coded as a device cannot be determined by the size, shape or complexity of the object or material being used. A device may be too small to be seen with the naked eye (microcoils used to occlude a vessel) or two feet long (external fixator for a long bone). A device may be of a predetermined shape (prosthetic heart valve) or no particular shape (morselized bone graft). A device may be a highly complex machine (cardiac synchronization pacemaker/defibrillator) or a simple piece of hardware (internal fixation bone screw).

However, material that is classified as a ICD-10-PCS device is distinguished from material classified as a ICD-10-PCS substance by the fact that it has a specific location. A device is intended to maintain a fixed location at the procedure site where it was put, whereas a substance is intended to disperse or be absorbed in the body. Indeed, a device that does not stay where it was put may need to be "revised" in a subsequent procedure, to move the device back to its intended location.

DEVICE AND REMOVABILITY

Material that is classified as a ICD-10-PCS device is also distinguishable by the fact that it is removable. Although it may not be *practical* to remove some types of devices once they become established at the site, it is *physically possible* to remove a device for some time after the procedure. A skin graft, once it "takes," may be nearly indistinguishable from the surrounding skin and so is no longer clearly identifiable as a device. Nevertheless, procedures that involve material coded as a device can for the most part be "reversed" by removing the device from the procedure site.

DEVICE DISTRIBUTION IN ICD-10-PCS

The general distribution and use of the 6th character when specified as a device is summarized in the table below. The sections and root operations that specify device in the 6th character are listed. Also included are examples of 6th character values and corresponding procedure examples.

PCS Section	Root Operation	Device Value Example	Procedure Example
Medical and Surgical	Alteration	Autologous Tissue Substitute	Nasal tip elevation using fat autograft
Medical and Surgical	Bypass	Synthetic Substitute	Femoral-popliteal bypass using synthetic graft
Medical and Surgical	Change	Drainage Device	Foley catheter exchange
Medical and Surgical	Creation	Nonautologous Tissue Substitute	Sex change operation using tissue bank graft material
Medical and Surgical	Dilation	Intraluminal Device	Percutaneous coronary angioplasty using stent

Medical and Surgical	Drainage	Drainage Device	Drainage of pleural effusion using chest tube
Medical and Surgical	Fusion	Interbody Fusion Device	Spinal interbody fusion
Medical and Surgical	Insertion	Infusion Pump	Insertion of infusion pump for pain control
Medical and Surgical	Occlusion	Extraluminal Device	Fallopian tube ligation using clips
Medical and Surgical	Removal	Spacer	Removal of joint spacer
Medical and Surgical	Replacement	Autologous Tissue Substitute	Skin graft using patient's own skin
Medical and Surgical	Reposition	Internal Fixation Device	Fracture reduction with plate and screw fixation
Medical and Surgical	Restriction	Extraluminal Device	Laparoscopic gastric banding, adjustable band
Medical and Surgical	Revision	Neurostimulator Lead	Reposition of spinal neurostimulator lead
Medical and Surgical	Supplement	Zooplastic Tissue	Pulmonary artery patch graft using bovine pericardium
Obstetrics	Insertion, Removal	Monitoring Electrode	Insertion of fetal monitoring electrode
Placement	Change	Cast	Forearm cast change
Placement	Compression	Pressure Dressing	Application of pressure dressing to lower leg
Placement	Dressing	Bandage	Application of bandage to chest wall
Placement	Immobilization	Splint	Splint placement to wrist
Placement	Packing	Packing Material	Nasal packing
Placement	Removal	Brace	Removal of back brace
Placement	Traction	Traction Apparatus	Skin traction of lower leg using traction device

ICD-10-PCS SUBSTANCE CLASSIFICATION

The 6th character substance value "defines the blood component or other liquid put in or on the body to accomplish the objective of the procedure." The 6th character is defined as substance in the ADMINISTRATION section. Administration is the only section where a substance is classified as a separate code, and not included as information in a more definitive procedure.

SUBSTANCE AND PROCEDURAL OBJECTIVE

Many different substances are typically put in or on the body in the course of an inpatient hospital stay, both during surgical procedures and at the bedside. Only those which meet UHDDS and facility coding guidelines are coded separately. Most material classified as a substance in the ADMINISTRATION section is in liquid form and intended to be immediately absorbed by the body or, in the case of blood and blood products, disseminated in the circulatory system. An exception is the substance value ADHESION BARRIER. It is a non-liquid substance classified in the Administration section, and coded separately for tracking purposes.

SUBSTANCE AND REMOVABILITY

Most substances cannot be removed once they are administered, because the whole point of administering them is for them to be dispersed and/or absorbed by the body. Imaging contrast is sometimes extracted from the bloodstream at the conclusion of a procedure to minimize the possibility of adverse effects.

SUBSTANCE DISTRIBUTION IN ADMINISTRATION SECTION

The general distribution and use of the 6th character specified as a substance in the ADMINISTRATION section is summarized in the table below. All root operations that specify substance in the 6th character are listed. Also included are examples of 6th character values and corresponding procedure examples.

Root Operation	Substance Value Example	Procedure Example
Introduction	Nutritional substance	Infusion of total parenteral nutrition
Irrigation	Irrigating Substance	Irrigation of eye
Transfusion	Frozen Plasma	Transfusion of frozen plasma

CLASSIFICATION OF SUBSTANCE IN ANCILLARY SECTIONS

Three ancillary sections record their own specific substance values as part of the ICD-10-PCS code, where a substance is used to support the objective of the procedure. They are the IMAGING, NUCLEAR MEDICINE and RADIATION ONCOLOGY sections, and they specify CONTRAST, RADIONUCLIDE and RADIOISOTOPE respectively. However, these substance values are unambiguously included as part of a more definitive procedure code, to be recorded when the substance is used to support the objective of the procedure. Substances in these three ancillary sections are therefore not likely to be confused with separately coded substances in the ADMINISTRATION section.

SUBSTANCE DISTRIBUTION IN ANCILLARY SECTIONS

The three ancillary sections that specify a type of substance used in the procedure are summarized in the table below. The sections and the type of substance classified are listed along with the ICD-10-PCS character where this information is recorded. Also included are examples of the values used and corresponding procedure examples.

PCS Section	Substance Classified	Substance Value Example	Procedure Example
Imaging	Contrast (5th character)	Low Osmolar Contrast	Left heart ventriculography using low osmolar contrast
Nuclear Medicine	Radionuclide (5th character)	Fluorine 18	PET scan of brain using Fluorine 18
Radiation oncology	Isotope (6th character)	Iodine 125	HDR brachytherapy of thyroid using Iodine 125

EQUIPMENT AND ICD-10-PCS CODING

For the most part, equipment used to assist in the performance of the procedure is not coded in ICD-10-PCS.

The only exception to this rule occurs in the REHABILITATION AND DIAGNOSTIC AUDIOLOGY section, where the 6th character is specified as *equipment*. The 6th character values in the REHABILITATION AND DIAGNOSTIC AUDIOLOGY section are used to capture information about the machine, physical aid, or other equipment used to assist in performing the procedure.

EQUIPMENT AND PROCEDURAL OBJECTIVE

For all other sections in ICD-10-PCS, equipment is distinguished from a codeable device by the fact that equipment is a method used to support the performance of a procedure. For example, the machine used to maintain cardiovascular circulation during an open heart bypass procedure is equipment that performs the circulatory functions for the heart so that the heart bypass can be performed. This support procedure is coded to the root operation PERFORMANCE in the EXTRACORPOREAL ASSISTANCE AND PERFORMANCE section, and the type of equipment used is not captured in the code. The primary procedure is coded to the root operation BYPASS in the MEDICAL AND SURGICAL section, and any graft material used is coded to the appropriate 6th character device value.

EQUIPMENT AND LOCATION

Equipment is also distinguished from a codeable device in ICD-10-PCS by the fact that equipment resides primarily outside the body during the procedure. Cardiopulmonary circulatory support is coded to the EXTRACORPOREAL ASSISTANCE AND PERFORMANCE section and the type of equipment used is not recorded in the ICD-10-PCS code. With cardiovascular support equipment, the machinery resides primarily outside the body. The outtake and return cannulae are the only portions of the machine directly connected to the patient.

On the other hand, insertion of intra-aortic balloon pump is coded as a separate INSERTION procedure in ICD-10-PCS, in addition to the ICD-10-PCS code in the EXTRACORPOREAL ASSISTANCE AND PERFOR-MANCE section specifying assistance with cardiac output. The intra-aortic balloon pump resides principally in the patient's body. The balloon mechanism that supports cardiac output is in the aorta itself.

Mechanical ventilation is also coded to the EXTRACORPOREAL ASSISTANCE AND PERFORMANCE section and the equipment used is not recorded in the ICD-10-PCS code. As with cardiovascular support equipment, the mechanical ventilation machine resides primarily outside the body. The endotracheal tube is the only portion of the machine directly connected to the patient. Insertion of the endotracheal tube as part of a mechanical ventilation procedure is not coded as a separate device insertion procedure, because it is merely the interface between the patient and the equipment used to perform the procedure, rather than an end in itself.

On the other hand, insertion of an endotracheal tube in order to maintain an airway in patients who are unconscious or unable to breathe on their own is the central objective of the procedure. Therefore, insertion of an endotracheal tube as an end in itself is coded to the root operation INSERTION and the device ENDOTRACHEAL AIRWAY.

EQUIPMENT AND REMOVABILITY

Equipment used solely to support the performance of a procedure and therefore not coded in ICD-10-PCS can be further distinguished by the fact that the equipment is used only for the duration of the procedure. Once the procedure is completed, any portions of the equipment attached to the patient are disconnected. For example, a patient no longer requiring mechanical ventilation is "extubated," or disconnected from the equipment that provides ventilation support.

SUMMARY

Three distinguishing features have been identified to enable correct identification and coding of device, substance and equipment: procedural objective, location, and removability. The procedural objective alone is sufficient in most cases to determine whether material or an appliance used in a procedure should be coded in ICD-10-PCS. Once it is determined that the information should be coded in ICD-10-PCS, location and removability are useful in determining whether the item is classified as a device or substance. The following table summarizes the distinguishing features of device, substance, and equipment in relation to each other, along with examples.

PCS 6th Character	Procedural Objective	Location	Removability	Procedure Example
Device	Material or appliance put in or on the body is central to accomplishing the procedural objective	Resides at the site of the procedure, not intended to change location	Capable of being removed from the procedure site	Neurostimulator lead insertion
Substance	Liquid or blood component is central to accomplishing the procedural objective	No fixed position, intended to be absorbed or dispersed	Not removable, once dispersed or absorbed	Antibiotic injection
Equipment	Machinery or other aid used to perform a procedure	Resides primarily outside the body	Temporary, used for the duration of the procedure only	Mechanical ventilation

INDEX